ARTIFICIAL REPRODUCTION AND REPRODUCTIVE RIGHTS

Titles in the series:

All titles are provisional

ARTIFICIAL REPRODUCTION AND REPRODUCTIVE RIGHTS

ATHENA LIU
University of Hong Kong

Dartmouth
Aldershot • Brookfield • USA • Hong Kong • Singapore • Sydney
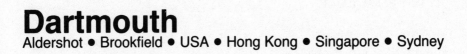

Published by
Dartmouth Publishing Company Limited
Gower House
Croft Road
Aldershot
Hants GU11 3HR
England

Dartmouth Publishing Company Limited
Distributed in the United States by
Ashgate Publishing Company
Old Post Road
Brookfield
Vermont 05036
USA

British Library Cataloguing in Publication Data
Liu, Athena
  Artificial reproduction and reproductive rights
  (Medico-legal series).
  1. Man. Reproduction.   Scientific innovation.   Social aspects
  I. Title   II. Series
  362.1042

Library of Congress Cataloging-in-Publication Data
Liu, Athena.
  Artificial reproduction and reproductive rights / Athena Liu.
     p.   cm. – (Medico-legal series)
  Includes bibliographical references and index.
  1. Human reproductive technology–Moral and ethical aspects.
  2. Human reproductive technology–Law and legislation.   I. Title.
  II. Series.
  RG133.5.L58   1991   90–47831
  176–dc20   CIP

  ISBN 1–85521–022–3

Printed in Great Britain by
Billing & Sons Ltd, Worcester

To my parents

Contents

Preface

The family is the basic and fundamental unit of human societies, and reproduction is imperative for the continuation of the human race, societies and cultures. The desire to have children has sometimes been said to be biological and innate, and having children is sometimes regarded as essential to a happy human existence and the fulfilment of human potential and self-development. Although the theory of an innate need to reproduce has long been doubted, and voluntary childlessness is not unknown to human societies, these assumptions regarding reproduction lend support to the view that there is a human right to reproduce and to have children, something which is inalienable and inseparable from human existence. Interference with human reproduction, therefore, has often been viewed with extreme sensitivity. The discriminatory nature of the Nazi laws prohibiting the freedom of marriage and authorizing compulsory sterilization prompted the provision in the Universal Declaration on Human Rights that men and women of marriageable age have 'the right to marry and found a family' – a provision which is predicated on the assumption that marriage and founding of a family are fundamental to human existence and can be categorized as fundamental human rights.

Modern conceptualization of human reproduction has moved far from simply seeing it as an innate desire or urge to reproduce. Over the last century, increased medical knowledge has rendered it possible to control reproduction by the use of contraception and sterilization. These birth-controlling methods make it possible to dislodge the connecting link between sexual intercourse and reproduction. More recently, scientific and technological developments of a different kind allow for the possibility of separating sexual intercourse and reproduction altogether. These techniques (artificial insemination, in vitro fertilization and the use of donated gametes) were not developed to divorce sex further from reproduction. They were developed to cater to a group of people for whom such a connection is meaningless or unfruitful; that is, the infertile. With these new techniques, reproduction is no longer confined to those who are involved in sexual intercourse, as in natural reproduction, but extends to situations where there is no such process and to parties who are not part of the process.

The 'reproductive revolution' does not just stop there. It brings along with it a whole host of ethical, social and legal issues, vexing problems which many people would prefer not to see. Direct confrontation with these issues is emotionally and intellectually taxing, particularly when they look seemingly insurmountable. When the controversy first started, the moral acceptability of artificial insemination dominated the debate. Gradually, artificial insemination using semen of a donor became an accepted method of treating certain types of infertility. The success of the first test-tube birth widened the scope of the discussion in infertility treatment to a topic which is still fervently debated, namely, experimentation on embryos. The polemic escalated when surrogacy – 'renting or borrowing the womb of another woman temporarily' for the purpose of having a child – was introduced into the field. A few of the many questions which accompany these situations can be identified: what about artificial insemination of the wife using the husband's semen after his death? What about artificial insemination using donor semen by a poor, welfare-dependent single woman? Surrogacy for altruistic reasons may be passively condoned by society, but what about surrogacy for profit? And what if the surrogate refuses to hand over the baby as agreed, or the child is born handicapped and neither the surrogate nor the commissioning parties wants it?

One societal approach to these problems is to pretend that they do not exist, and thus turn a blind eye to them. Another way is to legislate against their use, proscribing with criminal sanctions. On the whole, the UK Parliament has been slow in reacting to these developments. It has taken a long time to deliberate and reflect on these issues, until finally – five years after *The Warnock Report* – it introduced the Human Fertilisation and Embryology Bill 1989 which received the Royal Assent in November 1990. This book takes the view that the Act is an important step in the right direction, since neither avoidance nor prescription is desirable.

Since the issues involved in the reproductive revolution are potentially infinite, what is presented here does not claim to be a comprehensive review of them all. Instead, some of the fundamental moral, social and legal issues in the field have been selected. Recent discussion on the use of artificial reproductive methods to assist those who would otherwise be infertile to have children of their own has brought to the forefront the argument of whether the infertile have the right to procreate. Do they have the right to found a family by resorting to these new techniques? This book examines the 'right to procreate' and the 'right to found a family' in the context of the debate on artificial reproductive techniques; it explores the validity of the claims of the infertile in a day and age when modern techniques can enhance their chances of fertility but when the potential legal, ethical and social implications of these techniques are still to be explored.

This book is based on my doctoral thesis entitled 'Artificial Reproduction: the right to reproduce and the right to found a family', completed in the summer of 1987. Converting the thesis into a book took much longer than I had anticipated, with other commitments consuming available time for writing and researching. The lapse of time has meant that recent developments have had to be incorporated, including the Human Fertilisation and Embryology Act. Developments are covered up to November 1990.

Finally, a word of appreciation must be conveyed to those who have helped in my endeavours to write this book. My thanks to my Ph.D. supervisor, Sheila McLean, who is also the general editor of the series in which this book appears. My gratitude is also due to Sonia Bridgman, the editor for Dartmouth Publishing Company, who has assisted in polishing this book; and to my colleague Nihal Jayawickrama who has so generously spared his time to read the draft of the manuscript and has made many valuable suggestions for its improvement. Any remaining errors are, of course, my own responsibility.

Athena Liu
University of Hong Kong, December 1990.

1 Introduction

INFERTILITY AND ITS EXTENT

The problem of human infertility is as old as humanity. For instance, it was recorded in *Genesis* XVI that Sarah, Abraham's wife, could not have children and she asked her maid to bear him a child.

There are certain intrinsic difficulties in trying to construct an accurate assessment of the number of people who are affected by infertility. Some people do not want to have children; others seek no professional help or assistance if they find they do not conceive. There may be a number of reasons for not seeking help. Also, few data are available on the extent of infertility, the provision of services and their location and the numbers treated.[1] Having said that, it is widely estimated that approximately 10 per cent[2] of British married couples are infertile for one reason or another[3] and that the husband's infertility is responsible in about one-third of these cases.[4] This indicates an incidence of 16 000 marriages a year which will be infertile because of the husband.[5] In other words, the total number of infertile marriages per annum in the UK is about 48 000. Others maintain that infertility is a problem affecting one in six of the reproductive population at some point in their lives. Some suggest that at least one in six couples need specialist help at some time.[6]

CONVENTIONAL MEANS FOR ALLEVIATING INFERTILITY

An obvious means whereby infertile couples can have children is by adoption. Up to 100 000 British couples at any one time would like to adopt babies.[7] However, the number of babies available for adoption has been declining since the 1970s.[8] As *The Warnock Report* noted,[9] there are at least four reasons for this: (1) the widespread use of contraceptive devices, (2) the increase in the number of abortions, (3) changing attitudes to, and state support for, single parents, and (4) the freer availability of sterilization. As a result, there are fewer babies available for adoption.[10] In 1983, there were only 9029 adoptions in

1

England and Wales.[11] Over half of these were 'step-parent adoptions' (that is, where one of the adoptive parents was already the child's biological parent).[12] Fewer than 2000 of the remaining adoptees were under one-year old, and the most sought-after group of healthy white babies were adopted at a rate of about 1200 a year.[13] The demand, therefore, is in no way reflected by the supply.[14] Consequently, only a relatively small number of couples can succeed in adopting a baby.

THE POSSIBLE EFFECTS OF INFERTILITY

Whether the desire for a child emanates from an innate biological drive, or relates to social pressures, or a combination of these factors, is not the issue here.[15] The reality is that a large number of infertile couples desperately want either children of their own (that is, they wish to procreate) or other children, in order that they may establish a family.[16] This is borne out by the fact that a large number of infertile couples seek medical advice and assistance on how to achieve pregnancy.[17] Some couples are even willing to go through often very complicated fertility diagnostic procedures,[18] in some cases to the extent of exhausting the last personal, emotional and medical possibility, in an attempt to have a child.

The diagnostic procedure for infertility involves the use of a basal temperature chart, blood and urine studies for various hormonal levels, semen analysis, biopsies of tissue, X-ray examination of the reproductive tract or even direct visualization, by surgical means, of internal organs. Depending on the diagnosis, treatment may consist in the provision of hormones or steroids, which may be hazardous or have unpleasant side effects. Surgically, an individual may require resection or repair of organs or a delicate operation in an attempt to open passageways.

The final verdict of infertility is always traumatic. The initial shock generally gives way to a protracted period of human suffering, with an eventual resolution of feelings and, hopefully, recovery. Nijs and Rouffa[19] reported a sequence of four stages which embrace a feeling of confusion for one week, puzzlement, rebellion and doubting for two or three weeks, sexual dysfunction for two or three months and a depressive reaction which may last six months. According to them, this sequence is reminiscent of the changes which follow bereavement. The initial sense of shock is accompanied by feelings of confusion and numbness, often with an associated sense of isolation and loneliness. They reported that the individual may experience anger at the sense of losing control of his or her body. Lowered self-esteem may lead to feelings of despair, and guilt feelings may be evoked. Grief is felt not only over the loss of the body's fertility function but also over the implicit loss of a natural child (potential, anonymous and idealized).

Furthermore, infertility may have serious social and psychological consequences in both men and women. In a survey of patients in an *in vitro* fertilization programme, some of the important reasons given for wanting children are that one has a strong desire to have a child, life is incomplete without a child, or the feeling of uselessness without a child.[20] An infertile woman may therefore feel that her life is incomplete, unfulfilled and that she is not quite a 'woman' because she is unable to have a child or to undertake the role of parenting. If a man is infertile, he is somehow seen to be inadequate and lacking manhood. This, perhaps, explains partly why AID (that is, artificial insemination using semen from a donor) is almost invariably kept secret.[21] A wife who has received AID writes,[22]

> . . . I personally would prefer to adopt a child but my husband was absolutely against it. He was scared by the thought that people should know he was no good . . . .

Infertility may also put great strain on marriages. One infertile woman described her feelings in this way:[23]

> I gave myself to the end of this year to become pregnant (having tried to have a baby for the past five years), and I decided that if I wasn't, then I had best leave my husband and let him look for a younger, more productive lady to have a baby with. This will be a very sad thing, as Martin and I have everything going for us, but children.

Infertility, therefore, is a genuine and sometimes destructive human problem which affects a sizeable proportion of the population. Its circumvention has considerable importance both for the happiness of individuals and for the future of the species. Since the conventional means for the circumvention of infertility (for example, adoption) are inadequate to meet all these needs, and alternative artificial reproductive methods (artificial insemination,[24] *in vitro* fertilization[25] and surrogacy) have been developed which can circumvent various causes of infertility, the contention is often that these methods should be available to enable people to found a family (whether through reproduction or not – for example a wife, with a sterile husband, undertaking artificial insemination using semen of a donor will be founding a family through reproduction, whereas the husband may be said to be founding a family *without* reproduction)[26] and that they should also be part of state-funded infertility treatments.

Yet, decisions taken in this respect have both moral and legal implications which must be considered in tandem with social consequences. It is not sufficient, therefore, merely to state that there is a problem causing human suffering and demanding attention. If already limited resources are to be channelled into this area, a consistent ideology is needed to explain the commitment to infertility circumvention and to delineate the extent to which services can, or should, be made available. If such a rationale can be found and adequately explained, then there are implications for society, for medicine and for the law.

Before embarking on an appraisal of the strength of this contention, Chapter 2 will explain the nature, usefulness and current status of the artificial reproductive methods which will be considered. The importance of these methods will be apparent in Chapter 3 which examines the nature of rights, if any, of the infertile.

The use of artificial reproductive methods for the founding of a family (whether through reproduction or not) has been the subject of concern both in the UK and in many other affluent societies such as the USA and Australia. Although debates today are mainly centred on the acceptability of, and possible approaches to, surrogacy, rather than AI and IVF, an examination and appraisal of the debates regarding the latter, and not simply the former, can and will furnish a wider picture concerning the claim of the infertile to have access to artificial reproductive methods. In considering this, one is clearly dealing with moral and social issues as well as legal ones. Although the law is not the exact mirror of morality, the reaction and role of the law regarding artificial reproductive methods must, and should, be anchored on conclusions reached after rational discussion of the issues involved.[27] Nonetheless, debates regarding the acceptability of artificial reproductive methods have often been conducted in a vacuum in which no specific conceptual position is adopted or referred to. This is so even in relation to AI and IVF which have largely been accepted by the British society at large as viable alternative methods of enabling the founding of a family (whether through reproduction or not). The relative absence of a theoretical perspective is especially striking, and significant. It may therefore prove to be fruitful to consider analytically the value of such discourse in relation to those whose condition militates against the satisfaction of a need which is strongly felt to be both legitimate and desirable.

To that end, endeavours will be made to examine what rights, if any, people have in the areas of reproduction and founding of a family. To assist in this project, analysis will be made of Anglo-American cases concerning reproductive rights. Appeals are often made to Article 12 of the European Convention on Human Rights which recognizes the 'right to marry and to found a family',[28] and therefore the extent of its protection will be examined.

In Chapter 3, reproduction and founding of a family will be viewed as two separate concepts and their significance in the context of the infertile and the use of artificial reproductive techniques will be explained. If individuals have certain rights in the areas of reproduction and founding of a family, some social and legal implications can be drawn from this regarding the use of artificial reproductive methods. Moreover, the nature of any identifiable rights may significantly affect the expectations which may legitimately attach to the behaviour of a given state.

Having examined what rights people have in the areas of reproduction and founding of a family, the question is, is the use of artificial reproductive methods in order to exercise these rights acceptable? In other words, are there compelling moral, social or legal reasons which may hinder or defeat the exercise of these rights? Chapters 4 and 6 deal with the moral and social acceptability of artificial techniques (AI, IVF and the use of donated gametes) and surrogacy, respectively, in founding a family (whether through reproduction or not).

Chapters 4 and 6 essentially involve analysis of the validity, compulsion and superability of certain arguments – whether personal, social or moral in nature – against the use of artificial reproductive methods. This is consistent with the theme, established in Chapter 3, that the burden of proof in arguments seeking to deny access to artificial reproductive methods for the founding of a family (whether through reproduction or not) is on those who maintain such a view. It will be argued, in both Chapters 4 and 6, that artificial reproductive methods, as means of founding a family (whether through reproduction or not) should be accommodated. A proper set of regulatory schemes will furnish a bedrock for these methods, and a proper legal foundation for their use, which is also important, can be shaped.

Chapters 5 and 7 deal with certain vital legal issues involved in founding a family through artificial reproductive methods. One such legal issue is the definition of parenthood. The law and society are obviously interested in this question, since all children have legally defined parents unless they are unknown (for example, in cases of babies abandoned at birth, or where fathers are unknown). Up until *The Warnock Report* and its recommendations on status, parenthood was seen to be a mind-boggling morass which few dared to track. The Family Law Reform Act 1987 and the Human Fertilisation and Embryology Act attempt to tackle the question of parenthood. However, many questions are yet to be resolved.

Surrogacy as a means of founding a family generates additional legal issues, including questions of enforceability and the means of securing a legally recognized relationship between the commissioning parties and a surrogate-born child. These will be examined in Chapters 6 and 7.

Finally, consideration will be given to a further implication of accepting artificial reproductive methods: do identification and exposition of reproductive rights necessarily imply a certain type of access? Do they demand state provision of these methods?

The use of artificial reproductive methods for the founding of a family can raise many social and legal issues. This book, therefore, is only an inceptive attempt, amongst the voluminous literature in the area, to examine the questions consequential on medical advance. It is hoped that it will generate, and contribute to, debate both in respect of the issues discussed and on a wider range of important issues in the field of artificial reproduction.

NOTES

1   See *The Report of the Committee of Inquiry into Human Fertilisation and Embryology*, London, HMSO, Cmnd. 9314, 1984, para. 2.1 (hereinafter cited as *The Warnock Report*).

2   Ibid. The basis on which this figure is arrived at is not mentioned. It was said that 75 per cent of couples engaging in normal sexual intercourse without using contraceptive devices achieve pregnancy within 12 months. Where this is not the case, a couple may be potentially infertile. See Pepperill, R.J., Hudson, B. and Wood, C., *The Infertile Couple*, Edinburgh, Churchill Livingstone, 1980, p. 1.

3   For the various causes of infertility, see Chapter 2.

4   Snowden, R. and Mitchell, G.D., *The Artificial Family*, London, Allen & Unwin, 1981, p. 14.

5   Snowden, R. and Mitchell, G.D., op. cit., p. 14.

6   See Mathieson, David, 'Infertility services in the NHS: what's going on?' (1986), a report prepared for Frank Dobson MP.

7   See 'Is buying babies bad?', *The Economist*, 12 January, 1985, p. 12.

8   'Is buying babies bad?', loc. cit.

9   *The Warnock Report*, para. 2.1.

10 However, there are some 20 000 'special needs' children in the care of British local authorities. For the work of adoption agencies in finding homes for these children, see Ingram, Miranda 'Adopting the unadoptable', *New Society*, 9 August, 1985, pp. 206–7.

11 'Is buying babies bad?', loc. cit.

12 Ibid.

13 Ibid.

14 Ibid. The demand and supply ratio in the UK is 80:1.

15 For a discussion regarding the tenability of the procreational instinct theory, see Ruut, Veenhoven, 'Is there an innate need for children?', *European Journal of Social Psychology* (1975) **4**, pp. 495–501.

16 *Vide infra*, Chapter 3, pp. 25–43, for the distinction between procreation and founding of a family.

17 See Menning, B.E., 'The infertile couple: a plea for advocacy', *Child Welfare* (1975) **54**, p. 454.
18 Menning, B.E., loc. cit.
19 Nijs, P. and Rouffa, L., 'AID couples: psychological and psychopathological evaluation', *Andrologia* (1975) **7**, p. 187.
20 Singer, P. and Wells, D., *The Reproduction Revolution*, Oxford, Oxford University Press, 1984, p. 237.
21 *Vide infra*, Chapter 4, pp. 60–3.
22 Snowden, R. and Mitchell, G.D., op. cit., p. 40. See also Snowden, R. and Mitchell, G.D., *Artificial Reproduction: a Social Investigation*, London, Allen & Unwin, 1984.
23 See Singer, P. and Wells, D., op. cit., p. 54.
24 Hereinafter referred to as AI.
25 Hereinafter referred to as IVF.
26 *Vide infra*, Chapter 3, pp. 25–43, for a fuller exposition of the distinction between the concepts of reproduction and founding of a family.
27 This is particularly vital in the context of surrogacy, where emotion and sentiment can run high.
28 See generally, Jacobs, F.G., *The European Convention on Human Rights*, Oxford, Clarendon Press, 1975, p. 162.

2 Artificial Reproductive Methods

INTRODUCTION

Artificial reproduction is probably well known to most people. The extended press coverage of Louise Brown, the first child born as a result of the technological breakthrough, has stimulated popular debate on the scientific frontier of human reproduction. Although the birth of Louise Brown in 1978 was the watershed date for *in vitro* fertilization (IVF) – a technique which has captured the imagination of people ever since – artificial reproduction is a generic term which embraces a multifaceted combination of means of having children. These include techniques ranging from the relatively simple artificial insemination using semen of the husband (AIH), to artificial insemination using semen of an anonymous donor (AID), to the high tech of IVF which involves the fertilization of gametes *extra corporeal* followed by the transfer or replacement of the resulting embryo into the womb, sometimes of a surrogate woman. This chapter will seek to provide a brief exposition of both the nature and the estimated efficacy of artificial reproductive methods in the circumvention of infertility (whether through reproduction or not). Since the book concerns artificial reproduction, surrogacy as implemented by natural means will not be discussed. Thus, no consideration will be given to pregnancies achieved by means of sexual intercourse even on the understanding that the subsequent child will be handed over to the social mother.

In this chapter, three main artificial reproductive methods as options for the infertile who seek to found a family (whether through reproduction or not) will be considered.

ARTIFICIAL INSEMINATION (AI)

AI is a technique whereby semen of a man is mechanically introduced into a woman's vagina with the intention that conception will take place. The first recorded human artificial insemination was in 1790

8

when a British doctor, John Hunter, succeeded in inseminating the wife of a linen draper in London with the seed of her husband who was suffering from a disability which made normal intercourse impossible. It was reported that normal pregnancy and delivery ensued.[1]

The first recorded successful human insemination by donor (AID) was not performed until 1884 in the USA. This was revealed when, in 1909, Addison Davis Hard published a letter in an American journal – *Medical World* – in which he claimed that the first human donor insemination had been performed at Jefferson Medical College in 1884. The operation was performed when it was found that the patient's husband was azoospermic.[2] The surgeon discussed the case in the medical school with a group of students, one of whom was Hard. They suggested that semen should be collected from the 'best looking member of the Class' and used to inseminate the patient. According to Hard, the operation was performed under anaesthetic and neither the wife nor the husband was informed. The wife became pregnant and a son was born. The secret was kept until the son was 25, when Hard published information concerning the experiment.

In the UK, the issue of artificial insemination was discussed seriously in the 1930s.[3] In 1945, the general public, the press[4] and Parliament became involved. The Archbishop of Canterbury set up a commission to enquire into the development of AI. The commission's report, published in 1948, strongly criticized AID and recommended that the practice should be made a criminal offence.[5] In 1960, the *Feversham Committee Report* concluded that AID was undesirable.[6] Nonetheless, AID continued to be practised on a small scale. By 1970, public opinion had changed considerably regarding AID, and a Panel of Inquiry under the chairmanship of Sir John Peel reported more favourably on AID.[7] In 1979, the practice had become so widespread that the Royal College of Obstetricians and Gynaecologists (RCOG) provided the following written information to prospective recipients:[8]

> Artificial insemination has been practised in this country for many years. Each year several hundred children are born following this procedure, bringing a great deal of happiness to parents. . . . The treatment is straight-forward and painless. It will be carried out by a doctor or nurse who will insert a single instrument into the vagina to place the sperm in the mucus at the neck of the womb.

The actual number of human artificial inseminations performed from nation to nation is unknown. This is due partly to the secrecy surrounding artificial insemination, and partly to the fact that the introduction of regulation and control is a recent phenomenon in many countries.[9] Recent estimates are that about 1700 children a year are born as a result of AID in the UK,[10] and there are a number of medical centres in the UK performing AI either as a private service or as part of the NHS. Developments in the last few decades clearly show that AI has gradually become an acceptable method of circumventing certain causes of infertility.

Types of Artificial Insemination

There are three kinds of artificial insemination which may be used to enable the founding of a family[11] (whether through reproduction or not).

Artificial Insemination Using Husband's Semen

This form of artificial insemination uses semen from a husband to inseminate his wife (AIH) and is sometimes referred to as *homologous insemination*. This is not frequently resorted to because the husband's semen is rarely of any value. However, it is appropriate in the following situations:[12]

(i) Where there are factors (such as physical difficulties) on the part of either a husband or a wife or both preventing successful intercourse, but where the fertility of both parties is otherwise adequate. Male physical difficulties include retrograde ejaculation,[13] physical impotence, penile deformity and obesity. Female physical difficulties may include obesity, vaginal scarring or tumours, abnormal uterine position, vaginismus[14] and cervical hostility.[15]

(ii) Where a husband is subfertile because of defective spermatozoa, the chances of conception may be improved if the fertile part of the semen can be separated from the less fertile part. Since semen can be preserved, several specimens of a husband's semen can be collected to form one single insemination. AI, therefore, may be more effective than natural intercourse. AIH can also be used where a husband's subfertility is caused by poor motility of sperm cells.

(iii) If a man is about to undergo vasectomy, he may wish to obtain a store of his semen to be retained and utilized, if necessary, in the future.

The advantage of AIH is that a husband and wife can found a family through reproduction. Consequently, a husband will not feel left out of the reproductive process. Furthermore, there is no difficulty or ambiguity with a resulting child's legal status,[16] and the question of parenthood is not raised.[17] AIH is, thus, the least controversial of the available artificial techniques, morally, socially and legally.[18]

Artificial Insemination by Donor

Artificial insemination by donor is sometimes called *heterologous insemination*. This involves the insemination of a woman (usually a married woman) with the semen of a donor, and may be the answer to certain causes of infertility. There are three situations where AID can be used:

(i) AID is mainly used where a husband's semen is defective for one reason or another, causing sterility or gross subfertility. This may be due to the following conditions: his semen may contain no living sperm cells (azoospermia); it may have no sperm cells at all (aspermia); it may contain too few spermatozoa (oligospermia), or very few motile sperm cells (oligozoospermia).[19] The first two conditions result in absolute sterility.

(ii) AID may be used where a husband suffers from a hereditary disease such as Huntington's Chorea, haemophilia, hereditary blindness or certain types of muscular dystrophy, which are likely to be transmitted to his children. AID can sometimes be used in cases of rhesus incompatibility, or where the wife has a history of spontaneous abortion which may be due to abnormality in her husband's sperm.

   The advantage of AID in these situations is obvious. It gives an infertile couple an opportunity to have a child of whom the wife is the biological mother. Furthermore, AID does not necessarily entail public admission of male sterility, and a wife can experience pregnancy, which may be very important to some women.

(iii) The third possible use of AID is where a single woman wants a child but is unwilling to conceive by conventional means for one reason or another.

At present, semen in AID is mainly collected from medical students and husbands of obstetric patients.[20] General criteria for selection of semen donors are as follows: the donor should be of reasonable intelligence and should understand the nature of the donation, and he should have a good medical background, with no record of mental disease or other transmittable hereditary diseases. In addition, a donor with matching physical characteristics to that of the husband is often preferred. The donor's identity is kept anonymous. Thus, neither the donor nor the couple know each other.[21] The success rate of AID depends on the selection of the participants, but it may be as high as 75 per cent.[22] On average, it takes three or four cycles for conception to occur and it can sometimes take much longer.[23]

Artificial Insemination Using Combined Semen of a Husband and Donor

This technique is known as CAI or *confused artificial insemination*, and is sometimes used where a husband is not completely sterile but has only a few motile sperm cells (oligozoospermia). A child conceived as a result of the use of this method of conception may well be the biological child of the husband. There is no way to determine whether this is so without paternity testing.[24] However, opinion in medical circles is against CAI on the ground that it diminishes the effectiveness of AID.[25] Moreover, it confuses the status of resulting children.

IN VITRO FERTILIZATION (IVF), EMBRYO REPLACEMENT AND EMBRYO TRANSFER

Whereas artificial insemination essentially dominated artificial reproductive technology until fairly recently, additional techniques are now available which may be useful in cases of infertility where AI is of little or no assistance.

Whilst AI functioned mainly when the infertility was that of the male partner, female difficulties in conception may also now be overcome in some cases. Perhaps the commonest, and best known, of these techniques is that of *in vitro* fertilization (IVF). The publicity surrounding the development and use of this technique has rendered the phrase 'test-tube baby' a part of everyday language. In fact, this is something of a misnomer, since '*in vitro*', is Latin for 'in glass', and therefore IVF simply means fertilization of a female ovum by male sperm in a shallow saucer.[26]

The technique of IVF was developed in order to facilitate conception by bypassing damaged or blocked Fallopian tubes whose functions were inadequate to produce pregnancies.[27] Unsuccessful tubal surgery is the major reason for turning to IVF which in humans is a recent development. Most of the early technical advances were made in England by Edwards and Steptoe.[28] These included collection of oocytes by laparoscopy,[29] fertilization of oocytes matured *in vitro*, and *in vitro* development of embryos to the blastocyst stage.[30] In 1976, they reported a tubal ectopic pregnancy[31] resulting from IVF.[32] The first successful replacement of an embryo to a uterus was made by them in 1978 in the treatment of Mrs Lesley Brown, resulting in the birth of the first IVF baby.[33]

It has been said that IVF may be useful for about 5 per cent of women who have damaged or diseased Fallopian tubes.[34] It will be useful, for example, where a woman's fertility cannot be alleviated by tubal surgery because of the severity of the blockage or disease, or where the tube has been removed altogether. Where a woman is not ovulating, IVF of a donated ovum may be achieved. IVF may also be used in cases where a husband's semen contains an insufficient number of spermatozoa (oligospermia). In such cases, fertilization may take place under laboratory conditions rather than after sexual intercourse. Additionally, IVF may be useful to couples who suffer from unexplained sterility.[35]

In other words, IVF can be useful to some infertile people for the founding of a family (whether through reproduction or not). Thus, where a couple's infertility is due, for instance, to the female partner's blocked Fallopian tubes, IVF allows the couple both to reproduce and to found a family. The technique is completed by the reimplantation of the fertilized ovum – otherwise known as *embryo replacement* (hereinafter referred to as ER). Thus, the woman who provides the ovum may have it fertilized outside of her womb and reimplanted. Where reimplantation is successful, she is both the biological and the bearing mother.

The same technique can also be applied in situations where the woman is sterile, but is able to carry a child. In this case, fertilization is undertaken of a donated ovum, and the resulting embryo is then implanted in the womb of the bearing, but not biological, mother. This technique is referred to as *embryo transfer* (hereinafter referred to as ET).

Additionally, donated semen can be used in IVF. For instance, where a male partner is sterile, and the female partner has blocked Fallopian tubes, fertilization of the female's ovum can be achieved *in vitro* using donated semen.

Although the permutations of IVF are varied, and the social and legal implications may differ, IVF remains simply a fertilization technique in its purest form, and need not be associated with surrogacy.[36] Thus, in the situations described above, surrogacy is not involved, and the arguments which may be used against surrogacy cannot be taken to apply automatically or fully to these uses of IVF.[37]

Success Rate of IVF[38]

It is difficult to give a uniform assessment of the 'success rate' of IVF because scientists use the term in different ways. However, one way of assessing the issue is to consider the number of pregnancies per laparoscopy. In England, the figures given by Edwards and Steptoe in 1983 were 967 laparoscopies and 192 pregnancies, that is, a pregnancy rate of between 19 and 20 per cent.[39]

Another way of looking at the success rate of IVF is to ask how many embryos created actually result in pregnancies. One trial in Melbourne resulted in a pregnancy rate of 12–18 per cent when only one embryo was put back into the uterus.[40] This, however, does not indicate the survival rate of all embryos created, which depends on the practice of particular IVF centres. For instance, the practice of Carl Wood's team in Melbourne is to collect as many oocytes as possible in one single laparoscopy, fertilize them all and select the best for implantation.[41] Thus, some embryos may be found to be unsuitable for implantation whilst others are 'spare' embryos and are frozen. Since the survival rate for frozen embryos is very low, they are counted amongst those that do not survive. With this practice, one achieves a higher birth rate per laparoscopy but a lower rate of birth per embryos created. According to the figures supplied by Dr Alan Trounson, between 1980 and 1982, Wood's team obtained 876 oocytes and succeeded in fertilizing 633 of them for 272 patients. Out of these 633, there were 45 live births – that is, for every 14 embryos created, one finally became a baby.[42] In England, the practice is similar, except that where embryos are not implanted, they are thrown away or used for research and experiments.[43] Some may be frozen. These practices have met with some moral objections.[44] As a result, in Norfolk, Virginia, the practice is to fertilize only as many oocytes as a woman is willing to have transferred to her womb.[45]

Available data do not suggest an increased frequency of congenital abnormalities among IVF conceptuses.[46] In experienced IVF clinics, the frequency of spontaneous abortions also does not seem to be in excess of that anticipated in natural conception (12–18 per cent).[47] Finally, several tubal pregnancies have been reported following IVF, but these are not unexpected since most of the women in question had remnants of severely damaged Fallopian tubes, which might predispose them towards ectopic pregnancies.[48]

SURROGACY

A third artificial method to which the infertile may have access in order to found a family (whether through reproduction or not) is surrogacy. Surrogacy, as has been said,[49] is not a distinct artificial reproductive technique. Rather it is a particular situation in which these techniques are applied. Essentially, surrogacy involves a woman (the surrogate) agreeing to bear a child, and subsequently to surrender that child to be brought up by a person or persons other than herself. The terms commissioning mother and father (or parties) are generally used to denote the persons who intend to bring up a surrogate-born child.[50]

Surrogacy may be useful where a woman is unable to bear a child. This may be because she suffers severe pelvic disease or has had a hysterectomy, or because she has a medical condition (e.g. heart or kidney disease) and pregnancy may seriously threaten her life or health.[51]

Surrogacy is not a novel, but rather an ancient, method for the circumvention of infertility. For instance, as noted in the Introduction, it was recorded in the Bible that Abraham's wife, Sarah, could not bear him a child. Sarah gave Abraham her slave girl so that she could bear him a child.[52] Another example of ancient surrogacy was the story of Jacob and his barren wife Rachel.[53] In these cases, the surrogates conceived by natural means and thus they were also the biological mothers.

One of the novel aspects of surrogacy today is the capacity to implement it by use of artificial techniques. These techniques replace conception by natural means, and a surrogate-born child may have a number of possible genetic links. He or she may be genetically connected with two of the following people: the surrogate, the commissioning parties and the donors of gametes. One may classify surrogacy according to whether a surrogate has any biological link with the child.

Where a surrogate has a biological link with the child, this can be achieved by artificial techniques in the following ways. The most common form of surrogacy is where a couple arrange for a surrogate to undertake artificial insemination using the semen of the commissioning male partner. This will hereinafter be called *partial surrogacy*.[54] Alternatively, a surrogate may have a biological link with the child she bears by virtue of the fact that fertilization was achieved by means of the technique of IVF followed by embryo replacement.[55] This form of surrogacy and will hereinafter be referred to as *IVF & ER surrogacy*.

A surrogate-born child may have no genetic link with the surrogate at all. In other words, the surrogate is merely offering her gestational function to an embryo. The embryo may be genetically linked to the commissioning parties. This is possible because of the availability of IVF followed by embryo transfer. Such a case will hereinafter be referred to as *full surrogacy*.

A more unlikely possibility, where the surrogate has no genetic link with the child, is where the commissioning parties also have no genetic link with the child – for instance, where an embryo is donated by anonymous gamete donors. This will be referred to as *donated embryo surrogacy*.

Surrogacy can also be classified according to whether or not money is involved. It is important to bear this aspect in mind, since the nature of the arguments both for and against surrogacy may change significantly according to the circumstances under which it is entered into. Moreover, the response of society to the parties involved, and to the acceptability of a surrogacy arrangement, may also be coloured or influenced by the presence or absence of money payment. Thus the media often calls surrogacy 'baby-selling'.[56] However, money is not necessarily an inevitable part of surrogacy which may be purely an altruistic act. For instance, a sister may bear a child for her infertile sister, and the whole transaction may involve no payment of money or other rewards.[57] This will be called *surrogacy in principle*.

Where money payment is involved, depending on the sort of payment and to whom it is made, one can envisage at least three different possibilities. The first possible situation arises where a woman agrees to be a surrogate, providing that the commissioning parties will compensate her for all expenses she is likely to incur – for instance, medical expenses for the conception and birth of the child, and any loss of earnings by the surrogate during the period of confinement. This will be called *surrogacy with reasonable compensation*.

The second possibility is where a surrogate may receive payment besides that which represents a reasonable compensation. This will be called *surrogacy for a fee*.

The distinction between surrogacy with reasonable compensation and surrogacy for a fee may not, however, always be easily drawn. Surrogacy arrangements in the USA, for example, may involve payment to the surrogate of about US$10 000–12 000, but it will often be unclear whether such payment is a genuine costing of out-of-pocket expenditure, or whether it represents compensation plus a fee, and if the latter, which proportion relates to which aspect of the transaction. Approximately the same amount (that is, about £6500) was paid in the *Baby Cotton case*[58] and the *Adoption Application: Surrogacy case*.[59] The judge in the latter case, in fact, said that the £5000 paid was insufficient to compensate the surrogate's loss of earnings and expenses.[60]

The distinction between surrogacy with reasonable compensation and surrogacy for a fee must depend on the individual circumstances of each case, and no fixed line can be drawn which divides the two categories. Thus, a large amount paid to a surrogate who has to give up a highly paid job may be reasonable compensation to that particular surrogate. Yet, when that same amount is paid to a surrogate with a low income, it may be a case of surrogacy for a fee.

As will be seen later,[61] a rough distinction is important for subsequent discussions on the permissibility of surrogacy with money payment, but a precise distinction between the two categories is not vital.

The third possibility regarding money payment in surrogacy is where payment may be made to a party other than the surrogate. An agency may operate on a commercial basis, arranging surrogacy and charging both surrogates and commissioning parties for linking the two parties together and for the provision of counselling services. These will be called *commercial surrogacies*.[62]

CONCLUSION

The current status of all these reproductive methods is not uniform. The provision of AI seems to be relatively uncomplicated.[63] Whether AIH or AID, the technique is relatively simple and in terms of its use, AI is now a well-established technique. Issues of interest have tended to centre on certain social and legal problems which are consequential to the technique itself – for example, the status of AID children, the issue of fatherhood, registration and recording of AID births[64] – rather than on the acceptability or legality of the technique itself.[65]

IVF, in comparison with AI, is a much newer artificial reproductive technique. It has generated a number of wider issues which have moral, social and legal implications.[66] Nonetheless, as an artificial reproductive technique which aims at circumventing certain causes of infertility in order to enable some infertile people to found a family, it is now widely accepted. For instance, the British Medical Association's working group on *In Vitro Fertilisation and Embryo Replacement and Transfer* (1982) took the view that IVF was an acceptable means to circumvent certain forms of infertility.[67] *The Warnock Report* took the same view, and recommended that IVF 'should continue to be available within the NHS'.[68]

Consistent with the acceptance of the use of donated semen in AI, the BMA considers the use of a male partner's sperm and a donated ovum for IVF & ET to a female partner not unethical.[69] The same view was also reached by *The Warnock Report*, which endorsed the use of donated embryos by infertile couples where a female partner is capable of carrying a child to term.[70]

In 1984, there were some hundreds of babies born throughout the world as a result of IVF,[71] and some 36 medical teams offering IVF in the UK, Australia, the USA and most of Western Europe.[72] The Government *Consultation Paper* published in 1986 stated that about 1000 births in total in the UK were thought to have involved IVF.[73]

It can be seen, therefore, that – whatever objections there may be to this practice – it is now widely used and relatively uncontentious. Of course, this explains only its use, and says nothing about its social and moral acceptability.[74] However, the apparently general acceptance of IVF does say something about its value as a technique in circumventing infertility.

More recently, GIFT – Gamete Intra-Fallopian Transfer – has also been practised:[75]

[T]his new method has been devised for the treatment of couples where the woman has unexplained infertility or her partner has a low sperm count. The treatment is analogous to IVF in that the woman is stimulated to produce a number of eggs which are removed at laparoscopy and the most mature selected for replacement. In the meantime, the partner's semen sample is treated in the same way as for IVF to select the most active sperm. However, rather than allowing fertilisation to take place *in vitro* eggs and sperm are returned to the woman's fallopian tubes so that it can occur *in vivo*. As this method dispenses with the need for pre-embryo culture and associated laboratory facilities it would appear attractive to a larger number of centres with limited resources. However, the preparation of semen samples and identification and handling of eggs requires expertise. Clinicians should take advice before embarking on such procedures.

In 1988 there were 44 centres in the UK offering GIFT and in 27 of these GIFT was offered in conjunction with an IVF programme.[76]

Surrogacy, however, is much more controversial. Since it was first reported that an American lawyer[77] had set up a commercial agency, surrogacy has been a hotly debated issue.[78] Because of its potential moral, social and legal implications, the debate about surrogacy continues,[79] and the UK Parliament has been ambivalent toward the issue. In the UK, Section 2 of the Surrogacy Arrangements Act 1985 has criminalized the activities of commercial surrogacies. The Act has also made it a criminal offence to advertise in respect of or for surrogacy.[80] Surrogacy itself is not illegal or unlawful.[81] Nonetheless, the general attitude towards surrogacy seems to be one of disapproval and rejection, and doctors have been advised by the BMA not to participate in such arrangements.[82] Indeed, *The Warnock Report* by a majority of 16:14 rejected all forms of surrogacy.[83]

The preceding brief description of the three main types of artificial methods currently available has been undertaken to provide some information as to the situations in which they are relevant. It also serves to illustrate that their use may vary according to the nature of the infertility problem. A distinction has also been highlighted between those methods which are generally used to circumvent

n *Vitro* Fertilisation and Embryo Replacement
rnal (1983) **286**, p. 1594.

6.6. and 7.4.
.5.
'IVF: the major issues', *Journal of Medical Ethics*

oluntary Licensing Authority for Human In Vitro
1987, p. 11.
Voluntary Licensing Authority for Human In Vitro
1988, p. 13.
, D.L., *The Surrogate Mothers*, New York, Everest

idered by various reports. See *The Warnock Report*;
984; *Surrogate Motherhood, Report of the Board of Science*
. Reports in other jurisdictions include, *Report on the*
oduced by IVF, the Committee to Consider the Social,
Arising from IVF, chaired by Professor Louis Waller,
(hereinafter cited as *The Waller Report*); *Report on Human*
nd Related Matters (2 Vols), Ministry of the Attorney
(hereinafter cited as *The Ontario Report*). For two more
e Final Report on Surrogate Motherhood, the New South
mmission (LRC 60), March 1989 and *The Surrogate Report*,
the British Medical Association, 1989.
rated by the *Baby M case*, see 'Judges press for guidelines',
87, p. 8; 'The future of baby M', *The Daily Telegraph*, 3 April,

7.
May, 1987, p. 3 and *The Surrogate Report*, the Working Party
cal Association, 1989.
t, Chapter 8.
r 3, pp. 23–47.
e Singer, P. and Wells, D., op. cit., pp. 1–69; *Artificial*
OG, 1979. See also Cusine, D., *New Reproductive Techniques*,
mouth, 1988.

infertility by involving both of the partners in the actual reproduction, and those which do not. This distinction and its significance for the rights to which the infertile may lay claim will be considered in context later.[84] It is not, however, considered necessary to describe the practicalities of these artificial methods in more depth, since they have been extensively reviewed elsewhere.[85] Their significance for the purpose of this book lies essentially in the extent to which they facilitate reproduction and founding of a family, or merely permit the founding of a family. Whilst these two concepts may tend to be thought of as inseparable, it may be that distinctions can be drawn which, whilst not suggesting that they *never* coincide, may nonetheless serve to highlight what it is about the rights (if any) of an individual, and particularly, the infertile, that is truly significant, especially in view of the possibility of artificial reproduction. Analysis of the value of conceptualizing procreation and founding a family separately, and of the significance of using the language of rights, is therefore undertaken in Chapter 3 in order to provide a sound conceptual basis from which moral deductions can be drawn, and which may serve to stimulate and inform relevant social and legal change.

NOTES

1 Finegold, Wilfred J., *Artificial Insemination*, Springfield, Illinois, Charles C. Thomas, 1964, pp. 5–9.
2 That is, the husband's semen contained no living sperm cells, and thus he was sterile.
3 See Snowden, R. and Mitchell, G.D., *The Artificial Family*, London, Allen & Unwin, 1981, p. 15.
4 See Snowden, R. and Mitchell, G.D., op. cit., p. 15.
5 See the *Report of the Commission, Human Artificial Insemination*, published in 1948, reprinted in 1952 by S.P.C.K.
6 Departmental Committee on Human Artificial Insemination, London, HMSO, Cmnd. 1105, 1960, para. 239 (hereinafter cited as *The Feversham Report*).
7 Peel Committee, 'Report of the Panel on Human Artificial Insemination', *British Medical Journal* (1973) **2**, Suppl., Appendix V, p. 3, para. 12.
8 RCOG, *Artificial Insemination*, explanatory information booklet for patients, London, 1979.
9 Thus, in December 1972, at the CIBA Foundation Symposium on Law and Ethics of AID and Embryo Transfer held in London, it was said that no nation kept a register recording details of AID. See *Law and Ethics of AID and Embryo Transfer*, London, Associated Scientific Publishers, 1973, p. 4.
10 See *Legislation on Human Infertility Services and Embryo Research – A Consultation Paper*, London, HMSO, Cmnd. 46, 1986 (hereinafter cited as the *Consultation Paper*.
11 Ibid., Note 9.
12 See generally, *The Warnock Report*, Chapters 4–9.

13   Patients suffering from this condition have the sensation of ejaculation but semen is deflected into the bladder instead of being discharged externally. Sperm can be salvaged for AIH.

14   This entails painful spasms of the vagina associated with an aversion to intercourse.

15   This is where sperm are killed or rendered inactive by cervical mucus.

16   Compare this with an AID child, *vide infra*, Chapter 5, pp. 73–81.

17   *Vide infra*, Chapter 5, pp. 73–81.

18   *Vide infra*, Chapters 4 and 5.

19   In a normal man, there may be 100 million or more spermatozoa per cubic centimetre of semen; 60 million may be regarded as below normal but not low enough for AID to be considered. However, it is not possible to say that a man with less than a certain number of sperm cells is completely sterile. The number of sperm cells per cubic centimetre varies from one week to another. Therefore, a husband's semen is usually examined on several occasions before a practitioner decides whether AID is necessary. This is a precaution taken to avoid a situation where after the birth of an AID child, the husband is found to be capable of fathering a child.

20   Joyce, D.N., 'Recruitment, selection and matching of donors', in Brudenell, M. et al. (eds), *Artificial Insemination, Proceedings of the Fourth Study Group of the Royal College of Obstetricians and Gynaecologists*, RCOG, 1976, pp. 60–9 (hereinafter cited as *Artificial Insemination*, RCOG, 1976).

21   See Snowden, R. and Mitchell, G.D., op. cit., pp. 62–72.

22   See Kerr, M.G. and Rogers, C., 'Donor insemination', *Journal of Medical Ethics*, (1975) **1**, pp. 30, 31. See also *Artificial Insemination*, RCOG, 1976.

23   See *Artificial Insemination*, RCOG, 1976.

24   See Maidment, Susan, 'DNA fingerprinting', *N.L.J.* (1986) **136** (1), p. 326.

25   See *Human Procreation, Ethical Aspects of the New Techniques, Report of a Working Party Council for Science and Society*, Oxford, Oxford University Press, 1984, p. 40 (hereinafter cited as *Human Procreation*, CSS, 1984). Neither *The Warnock Report* nor the *Consultation Paper* mentioned this particular type of artificial insemination.

26   See *Human Procreation*, CSS, 1984, pp. 13–27.

27   The functions of Fallopian tubes include the collection of oocytes, transportation of sperm from the uterus to the outer end of the Fallopian tube, nutrition and transportation of an early embryo down the Fallopian tube to the uterine cavity. Inadequacies in any of these functions would make pregnancy difficult or impossible. The major kind of tubal pathology which causes infertility is adhesions – inflammation of the lining of the uterus to which the Fallopian tubes connect directly on either side, by way of a structure known as the horn of the uterus. Such inflammation can be caused by intrauterine devices (IUDs), pelvic inflammatory disease, or gonorrhoea.

28   See Edwards, R.G. and Steptoe, P., *A Matter of Life*, London, Hutchinson, 1980; Hann, Judith, *The Perfect Baby*, London, Weidenfeld & Nicolson, 1982, Chapter 7.

29   Laparoscopy is an operation performed under local anaesthesia whereby a telescope is passed into the abdominal cavities enabling the inspection of internal organs and the collection of ova from the ovaries.

30   Hann, Judith, op. cit.

31   Foetus growing in the Fallopian tube instead of the womb.

32   Hann, Judith, op, cit.

33   Edwards, R.G. and Steptoe, P., op. cit.

34   See *The Warnock Report*, para. 5.1.

35   See *The Warnock Report*, para. 5.1.

36   For a discussion on surrogacy, *vide infra*, Chapters 5 and 6.

45

46

47

48   S

49   *Vid*

50   See

51   See *The*

52   *Genesis* xv

53   *Genesis* xiii

54   See Singer,

55   For instance, wh

56   *Vide infra*, Chapter

57   Although the British

58   [1985] FLR 846.

59   [1987] 2 All ER 826.

60   Ibid.

61   *Vide infra*, Chapter 6.

62   Section 2 of the Surrogacy A

63   See *Artificial Insemination*, RC

64   *Vide infra*, Chapter 5, pp. 81–

65   See generally, Snowden, R. an
Mitchell, G.D., *Artificial Reproa*
Unwin, 1983.

66   *Vide infra*, Chapter 5.

67   See 'Interim Report on Human
and Transfer', British Medical Jou

68   See para. 5.10.

69   Ibid., Note 68.

70   See *The Warnock Report*, paras.

71   See *The Warnock Report*, para.

72   See Singer, P. and Wells, D.
(1983) **9**, p. 192.

73   See Note 10, para. 8.

74   *Vide infra*, Chapter 4.

75   *The Second Report of the*
Fertilisation and Embryology,

76   *The Fourth Report of the*
Fertilisation and Embryology

77   See Keane, Noel and Bre
House, 1981.

78   The issue has been cons
Human Procreation, CSS,
and Education, BMA, 198
Disposition of Embryos P
Ethical and Legal Issues
Victoria, Australia, 1984
Artificial Reproduction
General, Toronto, 198
recent reports, see *Tr*
Wales Law Reform C
the Working Party of
the debates gene

79   For *The Times*, 2 April, 19
1987, p. 15.

80   Section 3.

81   *Vide infra*, Chapter
See *The Guardian*,

82   See the British Med
of *The Warnock Repo*

83   *Vide infra*, Chapt

84   For example, s

85   *Insemination*, RC
Aldershot, Dart

3 Artificial Reproductive Methods: The Right to Reproduce and the Right to Found a Family

INTRODUCTION

Debates about the use of artificial reproductive methods have often suggested that the infertile have the 'right to reproduce'. What does that mean? Does anybody have a 'right to reproduce'? This chapter examines whether an individual indeed has any *right* to reproduce and to found a family and, if so, whether such a right will support the claim of the infertile to have access to artificial reproductive methods.

The use of rights-talk may sound strange or eccentric. To some, procreation and having children is perhaps something which one takes for granted. People may deliberate over the question of family planning – how many children to have and when to have them – but procreation is rarely presented as a question of the exercise of a right. It is no different from an individual who has the freedom to stroll down a street without interference unless he is causing a nuisance to the neighbourhood or conducting himself in a manner which constitutes a breach of the peace; he would rarely conceptualize this activity as an exercise of one's right to walk down a street.

Rights-talk however, is a very useful tool in asserting one's entitlement and legitimate expectation. As Feinberg states:

> A right is something a man can stand on, something that can be demanded or insisted upon without embarrassment or shame. . . . A world with claim-rights is one in which all persons, as actual or potential claimants, are dignified subjects of respect, both in their own eyes and in the eyes of others.[1]

In the context of procreation and having children, the significance of the moral coinage of rights cannot be underscored. During the past few decades, the concept of rights has set the scene for debates in women's struggles for reproductive control and freedom,[2] in issues relating to population control[3] and on the question of compulsory sterilization.[4] Its value can also be seen in the context of novel issues which have arisen concomitant to advances in medical technology and knowledge, the consequences of which are, on the one hand, to expand the parameters of reproductive choice and freedom (and thus their importance) and, on the other, create conflicting interests which have hitherto not been encountered. Thus individuals may have interests in using medical technology to control certain aspects of reproduction (such as the sex of children), which may conflict with the interests of the community as a whole. One of the ways of analysing and balancing these conflicting interests is in terms of rights. To that extent, conflicts of interest regarding the use of artificial reproductive methods may be so analysed.

Nonetheless, specific rights are not the starting premise of this chapter. Rather, endeavours will be made to demonstrate that fundamental values are involved, justifying the claim that certain reproductive rights do exist by reference to Anglo-American judicial jurisprudence and pronouncements (whether these rights are positively recognized or not), and they should be vindicated. This chapter, therefore, is concerned with examining the claim of the infertile to use artificial reproductive methods to reproduce and have children, an issue which has undergone extensive debate and discussion in affluent societies.

Rights have been subject to considerable analysis and classification by jurisprudentialists and jurists.[5] Therefore, it is sufficient, for the purpose of this chapter, to identify the rights, if any, an individual has in the areas of reproduction and founding of a family, and to explain briefly the nature and classification of these rights.

The term 'claim-rights' is sometimes used to denote a right-holder having control over others' duties. For example, if A has a right to repayment of a sum of money from B, the duty of B is to pay A that sum. The parameter of control that A, the right-holder, has in relation to B's duty is the choice of enforcing that duty, waiving or even extinguishing it. In simple terms, the right-holder is at liberty to choose whether or not to enforce or exercise a claim-right. A slightly different notion is represented by the term 'liberty-rights'. This denotes a right-holder having control over his or her own acts through freedom from an imposed duty or absence of duty to do, or not to do, certain things. For example, A is at liberty to look at, or not to look at, a neighbour's (B's) garden. In this context, there is no strictly correlative duty to A's liberty protecting its exercise, but there are other general rights the correlative duties of which may suffice to protect A's liberty in this respect. Thus if B were to assault A in an attempt to prevent A from looking at B's garden, A can assert a right not to be assaulted. Since the major characteristics of 'liberty-rights' are the absence of obligation on the part of the right-holder to do, or not to do, a certain thing, and the absence of strictly correlative duties on others not to interfere (B can erect an obstacle obstructing A's view of B's garden), 'liberty-rights' may not provide sufficient protection in certain circumstances. It is precisely for this reason that the concept of 'claim-rights' becomes significant. It is also worth noting the two possible aspects of this concept. A positive claim-right entails a right-holder having control over others' duties to do something, whereas a negative claim-right involves controlling others' duties not to do something. For instance, if X has a positive claim-right to education, others have the obligation to provide it. If X has a negative claim-right to education, the obligation of others would simply be one of not interfering with X's educational pursuits. These two aspects will be examined further in later chapters in the context of the use of various means of bypassing infertility.

THE RIGHT TO REPRODUCE

An initial difficulty with this subject is: what does the right to reproduce mean? Literature on the subject has tended to overlook the importance of formulating a working definition which will ultimately affect one's view as to whether or not there is such a right and, if so, what are its nature and scope. As Suzanne Uniacke said:[6]

> . . . hardly anyone would agree that the right to have children means that infertile people have a right to be supplied with children to adopt, or that someone has a right to participation of another, non-consenting person as a co-parent, or that a couple has a right intentionally to reproduce without incurring any subsequent responsibility for their offspring.

Although Suzanne Uniacke talks about 'the right to have children', the multi-faceted dimension of the phrase is immediately apparent. Similarly, the term 'the right to reproduce' is also capable of being understood in various ways, each of which denotes a slightly different concept and involves different consideration, rendering separate analysis and evaluation necessary.

First, the term can mean the right to have one's biological children (whether by natural or artificial means). This is the literal and obvious meaning of the term. Second, apart from biological reproduction *per se*, the term can include the concomitant responsibility of the procreator to parent the offspring. In this sense, 'the right to reproduce' means 'the right to reproduce and the right to parenting'. A third possible meaning of the term is the narrower concept denoting the right to parenting, where an individual has no biological connection with the child. In this sense, the term appears to be a misnomer for the 'right to parenting'. As will be seen later, a clear distinction has to be made between the three different dimensions to reproduction and parenting. Therefore, in the analysis of rights of the infertile, appropriate terms will be used to separate the different concepts.

The right to reproduce and the right to parenting is the broadest of the three concepts. Consequently, considerations which may be relevant in defining the nature and scope of this right may be extensive.[7] But the right to reproduce and the right to parenting, if considered separately, are each narrow concepts. Indeed, each of these rights may be said to be a separate and distinct entity. For example, a woman may reproduce but be deemed in certain circumstances not to have the right to be a parent.[8] Conversely, a right to parenting may be used to vindicate one's claim to be a child's adoptive parent,[9] or to resist state interference with one's role as parent,[10] and an appeal to the right to reproduce (which is generally taken to include the converse – that is, not reproducing)[11] may be used as a means to validate a choice not to be a parent.

In this chapter and throughout later chapters, the term 'right to reproduce' is used to denote the bringing of one's biological children into the world. To that extent, one is distinguishing the concepts of reproduction and founding of a family, the latter being concerned with the right to parenting. Nonetheless, this in no way implies that the two concepts, reproduction and founding of a family, are unconnected. Indeed, the claim of most infertile people is not simply the right to reproduce or the right to parenting, but rather, where possible, both – the right to have children.

Michael Freeman summarized the history of the debate on the 'right to reproduce' in these terms:

> The right to reproduce is first heard of in the latter part of the nineteenth century. It is then that feminists demand the right to 'voluntary motherhood'. The 'right to reproduce' emerges as a demand for birth control. . . . The right not to reproduce that was being identified in these debates was that of self-determination or freedom of choice. . . . At roughly the same time as feminists were demanding freedom from biological roulette, early genetic knowledge began to leave its mark on the debate . . . The [eugenics movement] argued that compulsory reproductive control was essential if societies were not to be swamped by the unfit.[12]

The influence of the eugenics movement left its mark in the often cited case of *Buck* v. *Bell*.[13] The Supreme Court there upheld a Virginia statute providing for the sterilization of mentally defective inmates of state hospitals upon the order of an impartial board after reasonable notice to all parties interested and an opportunity for a hearing. Procedural due process was upheld by the court on the ground that there was available notice, hearing and appeal. Limitation of the law to inmates of institutions was found acceptable. Thus it was said that 'the law does all that is needed when it does all that it can, indicates a policy, applies it to all within the lines, and seeks to bring within the line all similarly situated so far and so fast as its means allow.'[14] On the question of substantive due process, the view taken was that the statute could stand if it met the standard of rationality. Justice Holmes's statement manifested the thinking at the time:

> The 'right to reproduce' was not perceived to be a right and it was more as a privilege. We have seen more than once that the public welfare may call upon the best citizens for their lives. It could be strange if it could not call upon those who already sap the strength of the State for these lesser sacrifices, often not felt to be such by those concerned, in order to avoid our being swamped with incompetence. It is better for all the world if instead of waiting to execute degenerated offspring for crime or to let them starve for their imbecility, society can prevent those who are manifestly unfit from continuing their kind. The principle that sustains compulsory vaccination is broad enough to cover cutting the Fallopian tubes. Three generations of imbeciles are enough.[15]

Buck has been widely criticized, and its precedential value is very limited today. The court was ready to impose limits on the right to procreate on certain people on the flimsy pretext of the public good, although there was no evidence that Buck offspring were inclined towards crime and no evidence that the starvation was imminent.[16] But, as will be seen later, it is with this legacy that the US Supreme Court then began to consider the question of reproductive freedom. In the meantime, developments in European human rights laws confirm the fundamental importance of reproduction and the creation of family life. Unfortunately, European human rights laws have little to say about the right to procreate, and the protection it offers to an individual (fertile or otherwise) is very limited.

ARTICLES 8 AND 12 OF THE EUROPEAN CONVENTION ON HUMAN RIGHTS

The importance of family units to society has been recognized in a number of international agreements. For instance, Article 16(3) of the Universal Declaration on Human Rights (1948) states that the 'family is the natural and fundamental group unit of society and is entitled to protection by society and the State . . .'.[17] Article 12 of the European

Convention for the Protection of Human Rights and Fundamental Freedoms says:[18]

> Men and women of marriageable age have the right to marry and to found a family, according to the national laws governing the exercise of this right.

Article 8 of the Convention protects the 'private and family life' of an individual from unwarranted interference of public authorities. It says that '(1) everyone has the right to respect for his private and family life . . .'.[19]

Article 12 is succinctly drafted but has not been extensively analysed and its precise scope is far from clear. It talks about marriage and founding of a family.

Article 12 is subject to limitations 'according to the national laws governing the exercise of this right'. This does not mean that national laws governing the exercise of the right to marry and to found a family cannot amount to a breach of Article 12; otherwise, the very purpose of the Convention, which was to guarantee certain minimum rights irrespective of national laws, would be defeated. Thus, in relation to the right to marry, it was said that,[20]

> . . . although the right to marry is thus to a large extent subjected by A12 itself to the domestic legislation, . . . this reference to the domestic law cannot authorise States completely to deprive a person or category of persons of the right to marry.

Limitations regarding Article 12, therefore, must relate to legitimate purposes, such as the prevention of polygamy or incest. Lord Kilbrandon, for example, suggests that,[21]

> it might well be . . . that the European Court would not condemn 'national laws governing the exercise of' the right to found a family if these laws were designed to prohibit the wilful transmitting of genetic defects. Such laws would stand on exactly the same footing as those which, for genetic reasons, forbid marriage and punish sexual intercourse between persons of particular degrees of consanguinity.

In simple terms, the protection of Article 12 could extend to situations even where there was a breach of national laws.

Article 12 is formulated in such a way that it appears to link marriage with the founding of a family. Very little has been said, however, about these two aspects and their relationship with each other.[22] The question arises, therefore, as to whether the two are to be treated as one right or whether they are two rights separate and distinct from one another. There is no case directly on the point which defines the exact scope of Article 12. It has been argued that the right to marry and the right to found a family are two separate rights.[23] While these may indeed be intended as two separate rights, the wording of the Article appears to suggest that only married couples can claim the right to found a family. If Article 12 had stated that 'everyone has the right to marry and to found a family', it might have been easier to infer that unmarried people also had the right to found a family. It may also be significant that the Article ends with a reference to 'this right', rather than 'these rights', thus apparently envisaging a close connection between the two.[24]

In the *Van Oosterwijck case*,[25] the applicant brought an action against the Belgian authority for violations of Articles 8 and 12. The complainant had a sex change operation but was not allowed to have his birth certificate changed to reflect the reality of the situation. The question was whether the failure to rectify the statement as to sex in the birth certificate constituted in itself, or by implication, an interference with the right to respect for private life. A further question was whether the effect of the legal status imposed on the applicant deprived him of the right to marry as guaranteed by Article 12. On Article 12, the Commission took the view that the Belgian authority's failure to rectify his birth certificate had deprived him of the right to marry and found a family.[26] The opinion of the Commission was not considered by the court, which found that there was a failure to exhaust domestic remedies. The Commission said that,[27]

[A]dmittedly the government argues that the operations the applicant has undergone have deprived him of the capacity to procreate; he has thus rendered himself unable to exercise the right to found a family which A12 attaches indissolubly to the right to marry . . . although marriage and the family are in fact associated in the Convention and in domestic legal systems, there is nothing to support the conclusion that the capacity to procreate is an essential condition of marriage or even that procreation is an essential purpose of marriage.

In another case, the Commission considered whether there was a right to adopt,[28] and it was said that 'the provision [Article 12] does not guarantee the right to have children born out of wedlock. Article 12, in fact, foresees the right to marry and to found a family as one simple right.'[29] This again seems to suggest unity of the two aspects in Article 12. It further said that,

However, even assuming the right to found a family may be considered irrespective of marriage, A13 recognizes in fact the right of man and woman at the age of consent to found a family i.e. to have children. The existence of a couple is fundamental.

In the present case, the adoption of an adolescent by an unmarried person cannot lead to the existence of a family life in the meaning of the Convention.

In another case, the Commission said that,[30]

> . . . adoption of a child and its integration into a family with a couple might, at least in some circumstances, be said to constitute the foundation of a family by that couple. It is quite conceivable that a 'family' might be 'found' in such a way. Nevertheless, whilst it is implicit in Article 12 that it guarantees a right to procreate children, it does not as such guarantee a right to adopt or otherwise integrate into a family a child which is not the natural child of the couple concerned. The Commission considers that it is left to national law to determine whether, or subject to what conditions, the exercise of the right in such a way should be permitted.

Article 12 offers a very limited scope of protection of an individual's right to reproduce. Indeed it perceives it as a right of a married couple. There is no right to adopt or to found a family by alternative means. The use of artificial reproductive methods to create a family was never in the minds of the draftsmen. However, it appears that the State cannot interfere with family life without a valid justification. Thus it was said that the fact that,

> the applicant cannot claim 'the right to found a family' does not mean, however, that the relationship between an adoptive parent and an adoptive child is not of the same nature as the family relations protected by Article 8 of the Convention . . . A State cannot separate two persons united by an adoption contract, or forbid them to meet, without engaging its responsibility under Article 8 of the Convention. But one should not deduce from this a positive obligation on the State to grant a particular status – that of adoption – to the applicant and the person in his care.[31]

Thus once a family unit comes into existence, state interference will bring into operation Article 8 and it must be justified. 'Family' in Article 8 therefore has a much wider meaning than in Article 12, but it is confined to existing family life, not family life to be constituted.[32]

Since there is no exhaustive definition on the other aspect of Article 8 – 'private life' – it is difficult to gauge its potential. In one case, the Commission was of the view that 'not every regulation of the termination of unwanted pregnancies constitutes an interference with the right to respect for the private life of the mother. Article 8(1) cannot be interpreted as meaning that pregnancy and its termination are, as a principle, solely a matter of the private life of the mother.[33]

The indeterminate nature of this statement demonstrates that the

Commission was reluctant to offer any clear view on the point of reproductive freedom on which the American courts have been particularly vocal.[34]

Judicial Recognition of the Right to Reproduce

In the USA, the right to reproduce, after *Buck* v. *Bell*, has only recently been given judicial support. It was first manifested in the landmark decision of *Skinner* v. *Oklahoma*[35] where it was suggested that procreation was a fundamental individual right. In that case, an Oklahoma statute provided for the sterilization of persons who had been convicted for larceny three times. But the statute specifically exempted persons convicted of embezzlement, although the crime was often the same in nature and attracted the same punishment. The Supreme Court struck down the statute on the ground that it violated the equal protection clause of the Fourteenth Amendment. In other words, the statute was held to be unconstitutional because differential treatment of different classes of people was based on criteria wholly unrelated to the objectives of that statute. The court, nonetheless, recognized the significant nature of sterilization operations which generally deprived people of their reproductive capacities. Chief Justice Stone, utilizing the broad concept of liberty, talked of compulsory sterilization as 'an invasion of personal liberty'.[36] More importantly, Justice Douglas spoke of the statute as one which 'touches a sensitive and important area of human rights. *Oklahoma* deprives certain individuals of a right which is basic to the perpetuation of a race – *the right to have offspring*'.[37] To that extent, it was a matter of constitutional significance requiring strict scrutiny (rather than mere rationality).

> We are dealing here with legislation which involves one of the basic civil rights of man. Marriage and procreation are fundamental to the very existence and survival of the race. The power to sterilize, if exercised, may have subtle, far-reaching and devastating effect. In evil or reckless hands it can cause races or types which are inimical to the dominant group to wither and disappear. There is no redemption for the individual whom the law touches. Any experiment which the State conducts is to his irreparable injury. He is forever deprived of a basic liberty. We mention these matters not to re-examine the scope of the police power of the State. We advert to them merely in emphasis of our view that strict scrutiny of the classification which a State makes in a sterilization law is essential, less unwittingly or otherwise, invidious discriminations are made against groups or types of individuals in violation of the constitutional guaranty of just and equal laws.[38]

The clear implication of this statement is that there is a right not to have one's procreative capacities interfered with. The judge thus perceived the fundamental value pertaining to one's procreative capacity and the potential grave injustice to the individual of state interference with that capacity. A statute which compulsorily deprived an individual of the opportunity of exercising this right would need to be stringently justified. This judgement marked a distinct move in American judicial attitude, since, in a number of earlier cases, the right to reproduce had received little or no attention or credibility. As a result, *Skinner* has often been considered the milestone in claims that it was appropriate to discuss procreation in terms of human rights.

This attitude has continued to pervade subsequent American decisions and has formed a significant part of debates relating to many aspects of reproductive choice. Procreation is offered protection as a penumbra right to the wider constitutional rights of liberty and privacy. Thus in *Griswold* v. *Connecticut*,[39] a state statute which made the use of contraceptives a criminal offence, was held to be unconstitutional on the ground that it violated the right of marital privacy. Justice White (concurring) said:[40]

> . . . the liberty entitled to protection under the Fourteenth Amendment includes the right 'to marry, establish a home and bring up children'. . . . there is a 'realm of family life which the state cannot enter' without substantial justification.

Although *Griswold* was decided on the ground of marital privacy, the right to make one's own choice as to whether to procreate (or whether to use contraceptive devices) is not restricted to married couples. It is the right of an individual, the deprivation of which requires the existence of a compelling state interest.

Thus it was said that '*Skinner* . . . did not guarantee the individual a procreative opportunity; it merely safeguarded his procreative potential from state infringement'.[41] In other words, the right to reproduce was significant even where it attached to a single person who had no opportunity to exercise it. This view was restated in the judgement of *Eisenstadt* v. *Baird*,[42] in which the Supreme Court held a Massachusetts statute banning the distribution of contraceptives to unmarried persons to be unconstitutional. The court held that the statute violated the equal protection clause of the Fourteenth Amendment by providing dissimilar treatment for married and unmarried persons who were in similar situations. Justice Brennan, delivering the opinion of the court, said:[43]

> If the right of privacy means anything, it is the right of the individual, married or single, to be free from unwarranted governmental intrusion into matters so fundamentally affecting a person as the decision whether to bear or beget a child. . . .

The decision of *Roe* v. *Wade*[44] extended the individual's right to privacy in procreation a step further. In that case, the majority of the court took the view that the right of privacy encompassed a woman's right to decide whether or not to terminate her pregnancy during the first trimester. Justice Blackmun, delivering the opinion of the court, said:[45]

> . . . the right [of personal privacy] has some extension to activities relating to marriage, procreation, contraception, family relationships and child rearing and education. . . . [W]here certain 'fundamental rights' are involved, the Court has held that regulation limiting these rights may be justified only by a 'compelling state interest' . . . and that legislative enactments must be narrowly drawn to express only the legitimate state interests at stake.

The series of cases from *Skinner*[46] to *Roe*[47] therefore demonstrates two essential points. First, that the essence of the right to reproduce in the US is based on the constitutionally protected concepts of liberty and privacy. The application of these concepts to procreation protects an individual's freedom to choose, free from unwarranted governmental interference.[48] The right to reproduce, therefore, is a negative claim-right.[49] Moreover, the right to reproduce applies to individuals, irrespective of marital status. In other words, if liberty to choose in relation to procreation is valued, such freedom has the same value regardless of one's marital status.[50]

In the US, the appeal to constitutional freedoms, couched in terms of human rights, has therefore significantly clarified the extent and nature of the right to reproduce. The freedom to make reproductive choices is the basis against which derogation is tested, and courts have been obliged to justify in strong terms any denial of this right.

Recognition of the importance of reproductive choices is also evident in Canada. Prior to the 1988 ruling of the Supreme Court of Canada (S.C.C.) in the *Morgentaler case*, the abortion law in Canada was governed by Section 251 of the Criminal Code.[51] That provision limited a pregnant woman's access to abortion by requiring her to obtain a certificate from a therapeutic abortion committee of an accredited or approved hospital.[52]

One of the constitutional questions which arose was whether Section 251 infringed or denied the rights and freedoms guaranteed by Section 7 of the Canadian Charter of Rights and Freedoms which states that:[53]

> Everyone has the right to life, liberty and security of the person and the right not to be deprived thereof except in accordance with the principles of fundamental justice.

The S.C.C., by a majority of 5:2, held that Section 251 of the Criminal Code constituted state interference with bodily integrity. Forcing a woman, by threat of criminal sanction, to carry a foetus to term unless she met certain criteria unrelated to her own priorities and aspirations, was a profound interference with a woman's body and an infringement of the security of the person. The mandatory procedure by Section 251 also led to a second breach of the right to security of the person which occurred independently in consequence of the delay in obtaining therapeutic abortions resulting in a higher probability of complications and greater risk. The harm to the psychological integrity of women seeking abortions was also clearly established. Thus, it was said that the right to security of the person protected both the physical and psychological integrity of the individual. Section 251 was more deeply flawed: apart from subjecting a woman to considerable emotional stress and unnecessary physical risk, it asserted that the woman's capacity to reproduce was subject, not to her own control, but to that of the State. This was a direct interference with the woman's physical 'person'.

In regard to 'liberty', the court observed that Section 7 guaranteed to every individual a degree of personal autonomy over important decisions intimately affecting his or her private life. Liberty in a free and democratic society does not require the State to approve such decisions but it does require the State to respect them. Section 251 took a personal and private decision away from the woman and gave it to a committee.

In assessing whether the infringement of the right to life, liberty and security of the person was in conformity with the principles of fundamental justice, the court found that the administrative and procedural requirements in Section 251 were unfair; they impaired more than necessary the rights in Section 7, and the effects of the limitation on the rights in Section 7 were out of proportion to the objective sought to be achieved and might actually defeat the objective of protecting the life and health of the woman.[54]

British Judicial Attitude

British legal tradition differs markedly from that of America. For one, British judges are less receptive to the employment of rights terminology. There is also in Britain no written constitution – enshrining the rights of the people – setting the standards against which legislation is to be scrutinized. Parliament is supreme and it can make any law restricting individual liberty. Although there are no British cases which analyse in detail the concept of the right to reproduce,[55] whatever evidence is available suggests that English law and attitudes of judges seem to incline towards according considerable freedom to individuals in relation to procreation. What is not prohibited is permissible and this represents the residual freedom of an individual under the law.

There is no British law directly prohibiting or interfering with the free choice of individuals, whether married or not, in relation to procreation. However, some restriction is applied in situations where one of several competing values must be given priority. For example, the Abortion Act of 1967 does not recognize[56] a woman's absolute right to terminate a pregnancy at any stage.[57] Indeed, that Act was not framed in terms of rights at all, but was based rather on a more pragmatic concern to ensure that, where terminations *were* carried out, they were done so safely and competently so as to reduce the toll in terms of human life.[58] Other restrictions which stipulate the age at which women may lawfully consent to sexual intercourse, and the prohibition of incestuous relationships, strike at the sexual act rather than at the right to reproduce.

Whether the general assertion that an individual is free to make her choices in relation to procreation is further qualified by the recent House of Lords' decision in *Re B (a Minor) (Wardship: Sterilisation)*,[59] which will be considered below.[60] Leaving that case aside for the moment, in general an individual may choose to have one child, many children or no children at all. The decision not to procreate is no longer confined to the deliberate choice of celibacy or abstinence. The spacing and timing of procreation can, in most cases, be controlled according to one's preference and by the use of various contraceptive devices, voluntary sterilization and abortion (within the ambit of the law).[61] Therefore, what is central to rights in reproduction is an individual's freedom to decide whether, when and how often one should reproduce. The freedom to choose regarding reproduction is accentuated by Justice Peter Pain, in *Thake* v. *Maurice*, where he said (emphasis added):[62]

> The policy of the state, as I see it, is to provide the widest *freedom of choice*. It makes available to the public the means of planning their families or planning to have no family. If plans go awry, it provides for the possibility of abortion. But there is no pressure on couples either to have children or not to have children or to have only a limited number of children. Even the one-parent family, whether that exists through choice or misfortune, is given substantial assistance.

A further example demonstrating this attention to freedom of choice being derivative from, and descriptive of, the right of an individual to make autonomous choices can be seen in the recent growth in, and recognition of, wrongful conception claims.[63] This type of claim accepts that there is a wrong to parents where, as a result of a defendant's (usually a physician's) negligence, they are not given an opportunity to consider all possible options regarding procreation or non-procreation. Compensation is thus given for the wrong done to the parents.[64]

In sum, although the British courts have never attempted to elaborate on the concept of the right to reproduce as exhaustively as the US judiciary have done, the underlying assumption is that individuals should be given the widest possible choice regarding procreation, and that invasion of what may be called one's right to self-determination or autonomy requires careful consideration and considerable justification.[65]

A decision that may be cited as reinforcing this view is the case of *Re D (a Minor) (Wardship: Sterilisation)*.[66] In that case, an 11-year-old minor suffered from a rare condition known as Sotos syndrome.[67] Her IQ was about 80. She had the capacity to marry and could possibly have a reasonable family life. A proposal to sterilize her to avoid an unwanted pregnancy was successfully challenged. Justice Heilbron in the Queen's Bench Division said that the operation involved the deprivation of a *basic human right* (that is, the right of a woman to reproduce).[68] The judge also mentioned the girl's prospect of marriage and having children. Because the judge's reference to the right to reproduce was interchanged with the concept of the right to marry and found a family,[69] it is difficult to identify whether the decision was a vindication of the girl's right to reproduce or her right to found a family, or both. In other words, the court made no serious distinction between the concepts of reproduction and founding of a family which, as will be seen later,[70] can be very important in the context of the infertile.

Re D was distinguished in the recent House of Lords' decision in *Re B (a Minor) (Wardship: Sterilisation)*,[71] where the court exercised its wardship jurisdiction and ordered a 17-year-old mentally retarded girl, with a mental age of five, to be sterilized. The Law Lords unanimously came to the decision after considering the evidence in the case which demonstrated that there was an unacceptable risk of pregnancy which could only be obviated by sterilization in order to prevent childbirth in circumstances of uncomprehending fear and pain and risk of physical injury.

In the first instance, Justice Bush said that, in sterilizing Jeanette, 'one is in effect depriving her of nothing because she will never desire the basic human right to reproduce'.[72] In the Court of Appeal, Justice Dillon said that the minor would remain incapable of giving informed consent to sterilization, abortion or marriage, and she would not be capable of looking after a baby. If she became pregnant, the pregnancy would have to be terminated. In effect, she has no right to reproduce (and/or to found a family).[73] Again, in the House of Lords it was said:[74]

But [the right to reproduce] was only such when reproduction was the result of informed *choice* of which the ward in the present case was incapable. . . . To talk of the 'basic right' to reproduce of an individual who was not capable of knowing the causal connection between intercourse and childbirth, the nature of pregnancy, what was involved in delivery, unable to form any maternal instincts or to care for a child, appeared to his Lordship wholly to part company with reality.

It may be argued that this decision and others[75] are getting dangerously close to suggesting that a particular group of people do not have the right to reproduce[76] and, consequently, that it is a step towards narrowing the application of the concept. However, as the Law Lords stressed, the decision involved no general principle of public policy and was concerned solely with what was in the best interests of the ward. The right of the mentally handicapped to reproduce involves complicated issues;[77] consideration of the merits of this decision is outside the ambit of this book, which is concerned with the rights of individuals, particularly the infertile, to use artificial reproductive methods to found a family (whether through reproduction or not). In any event, the decision does not affect the conclusion drawn so far regarding the right to reproduce. Indeed, judges and society alike clearly recognize the fundamental import-ance of the freedom to procreate, and it is precisely for this reason that there was considerable anxiety concerning the implications of *Re B*.[78] The whole episode of *Re B*[79] can well buttress the conclusion arrived at earlier that the right to reproduce means that one's reproductive capacity should not be unwarrantedly interfered with unless compelling interests dictate otherwise.

Moreover, even if the decision in *Re B*[80] were to be taken as having wider implications in respect of the right to reproduce, it must be borne in mind that, in reality, some of the most fundamental of human rights may be subject to exceptions. Thus, the right to life may be denied, for example, after due process of law.[81] Equally, the court has declared that a decision to sterilize a mentally handicapped girl can be taken *only* after consideration by the appropriate court.[82] The fact that the right to reproduce may not be extended to *all* individuals in *every* situation is not fatal to the claim that the right exists, nor to the assertion of its fundamental significance.

THE RIGHT TO REPRODUCE AND ARTIFICIAL REPRODUCTIVE METHODS

So far, the right to reproduce in the Anglo-American legal context has been analysed. It may be said that the right to reproduce, as a negative claim-right, denotes freedom of choice relating only to *whether* and *when* to procreate. All the cases mentioned so far deal with the right of a person to retain his/her procreative capacities, opposition to government interference with an individual's reproductive capacities, or the use of contraceptive devices and abortion for the purposes of controlling reproduction. Consequently, it could be argued that what has been said thus far has no implication or bearing on the use of artificial reproductive methods, since those matters relate essentially to *how* to procreate.[83]

Nonetheless, if the right to procreate raises a strong presumption against interference unless it is proved to be warranted, this presumption applies equally in respect of a person's freedom to choose to use artificial reproductive methods. In other words, the right to reproduce does not have to be justified, or argued for, whenever a new situation arises. The burden of proof is for those who argue against freedom and choice. Two points follow on from this premise. One concerns the use of artificial reproductive methods in general, not specifically relating just to the infertile. The other concerns the use of artificial reproductive methods, in particular by the infertile.

The possibility of using artificial reproductive methods to procreate can increase the range of choices available to those whose fertility is not in question. For instance, a couple may prefer artificial, as opposed to natural, reproduction for reasons other than their infertility. If freedom to choose is the essential aspect of the right to reproduce, interference with people's options can only be justified by a compelling state interest.

Indeed, the facts of *Baby M*[84] may be close to one end of the spectrum of choice. There, the wife was told that she might have multiple sclerosis, which rendered pregnancy a serious health risk. According to the Supreme Court, '[h]er anxiety appears to have exceeded the actual risk, which current medical authorities assess as minimal. Nonetheless, that anxiety was evidently quite real, Mrs Stern fearing that pregnancy might precipitate blindness,[85] paraplegia, or other forms of debilitation.'

This libertarian philosophy underlies what the Supreme Court judge had in mind in the *Baby M* case. The various aspects of the case will be considered later. At this stage, it would suffice to say that the case involved a partial surrogacy arrangement. The surrogate mother, however, changed her mind and refused to hand over the child to the commissioning (and biological) father. The Superior Court judge, Harvey Sorkow, considered the Supreme Court cases on procreation and privacy and said that, although those decisions did not address non-coital procreation,[86] it must be reasoned that if one has a right to procreate coitally, then one has a *right to reproduce non-coitally*. If it is the reproduction that is protected, then the *means of reproduction* are also to be protected. . . . This court holds that *the protected means extends to the use of surrogates*.

The thesis propounded in this statement by Judge Harvey is in no way affected by the Supreme Court's decision.[87] Indeed the Supreme Court's decision recognized Mr Stern's right to use a surrogate mother for the purposes of having a child.[88] One principle to be drawn from the case of *Baby M*, therefore, is that from the perspective of an individual, he or she should have the choice to resort to artificial reproductive methods for procreation. From the point of view of a surrogate, the concepts of liberty and privacy, as exemplified by *Roe* v. *Wade*,[89] would be wide enough to encompass a woman's choice to be a surrogate even though that may entail merely the use of her gestation function.[90] To put the matter in another way, if an individual has the right to reproduce, then the services of those who may facilitate the exercise of that right must be inextricably linked with that right. Thus, even in situations where the surrogate makes no genetic contribution to the embryo, it could be argued that to prohibit surrogacy interferes with the right of the other individual(s) to reproduce. Where the surrogate is genetically linked to the child, then the freedom of both the surrogate and that of the other individual to reproduce would be equally restricted were surrogacy to be outlawed.[91] In other words, the right to reproduce would include the right to choose *how* to procreate. Consequently, only if other, and compelling, values compete would restrictions on artificial reproductive methods be consistent with validation of the right to reproduce as described here.

For present purposes, however, it is essential to establish in greater depth what relevance, if any, the existence of this right to reproduce has to the infertile.

The fact that those whose procreative capacities are unimpaired can validly demand their protection (with the limited exclusions noted above)[92] may not necessarily seem directly relevant to the position of those who have no such capacity or those whose capacity is impaired for one reason or another.[93] The significance of the judgement in the *Baby M case* is that it seemed to extend the right to reproduce beyond the mere capacity to procreate. It contemplated the right as including access to artificial assistance. The question remains, however, as to the extent to which capacity is a prerequisite for the exercise of the right.

THE RIGHT OF THE INFERTILE TO REPRODUCE

The initial hypothesis of this chapter was that once the nature and scope of the right to reproduce was explored and unravelled, the concept may provide a satisfactory justification for the claim of the infertile to use artificial reproductive methods. This is satisfactory only up to one level of enquiry. If the view taken in the *Baby M case*[94] is adopted, then the right to reproduce may be taken to imply an incorporation not simply of the right to decide whether or not to procreate, but also of the right to choose *how* to procreate. As with all other human rights, a compelling justification would be needed if the exercise of the right is to be interfered with.

This formulation of the right to reproduce, however, is inadequate in respect of the infertile in two aspects. First, it fails to accommodate the claim of some infertile people. Second, the right to reproduce, as a negative claim-right, will clearly not advance any claim of the infertile to state funding of artificial reproductive techniques, without which the right may be meaningless. This latter claim can only be understood by reference to the notion of a positive claim-right to reproduce. Questions of state responsibility will be considered in more depth later.[95] For the moment, the situation of the infertile will be considered.

In the case of a sterile individual, any claim that there is a right to use artificial reproductive methods to have a child so that he or she can found a family would obviously not be covered by the concept of the right to reproduce. The individual's claim to have access to AID is not in reproduction, but rather in founding a family or parenting. However, the inability to reproduce may relate to circumstances other than the lack of capacity of a given individual. This is of particular importance since reference to 'infertility' is often made in the context of the infertile couple even though one of the parties may have unimpaired procreative capacity. Such a person within that relationship lacks the natural opportunity to vindicate his or her right to reproduce. Nonetheless, the right to reproduce, as explicated here, provides protection for the individual's freedom to choose not only whether or not to exercise that capacity, but also *how* to exercise it.

Indeed, if the right to reproduce did not include the right of access to artificial reproductive methods, the right to reproduce of individuals who are in the situation described above would be rendered nugatory. This is so because the choice confronting them is either not to procreate,[96] or to engage in sexual relations outside the relationship with a fertile partner. This latter option, whilst it would allow the exercise of the right to reproduce, may be regarded as immoral or unacceptable in itself. Indeed, much of the earlier debate concerning artificial reproduction has centred on similar questions as to the morality of the techniques.[97]

If the right to reproduce is of value, then it would be strange indeed were its vindication to depend on an individual being forced to indulge in activities which could be regarded as immoral. In other words, unless artificial reproductive methods are themselves sufficiently immoral so as to amount to a compelling justification to limit their accessibility in order to vindicate the right to reproduce, it would seem that where a husband is sterile, his wife's right to reproduce includes the right to choose to employ AID. Similarly, in a case where a wife is sterile and wombless, the husband has a right to choose partial surrogacy in order to procreate.

Yet to describe these couples' interests in artificial reproductive methods purely in terms of an individual right to reproduce – though technically correct and impeccable – may not reflect a major or equally important dimension or interest at stake. The claim to use artificial reproductive methods in those cases may not be related entirely to the wife's or the husband's claim to exercise an individual's right to reproduce. It may additionally, and as importantly, reflect the interest of these couples in founding a family. Indeed, the interest of a couple in founding a family (rather than in procreation) may be fundamental in some cases. For instance, in the case of a couple both of whom are sterile, their claim to use donated embryo surrogacy can hardly be a claim to reproduce by the couple. Rather, it is a claim reflecting their interest in founding a family.

Implicit in this analysis is that individuals who do not have the capacity to reproduce (because of sterility) cannot be in a position meaningfully to claim a right to reproduce.[98] Having said that an individual's right to reproduce may be too narrow a concept to encapsulate one crucial element of the interest of some infertile couples in founding a family, it does not necessarily follow that an individual's right to reproduce is totally inapplicable and inappropriate when one is dealing with an infertile couple. Thus, both the right to reproduce and the interest in founding a family co-exist in a case where a couple is childless because the female partner has blocked Fallopian tubes. Here, both partners can seek to vindicate both their individual rights to reproduce and their interest (as a couple) in founding a family. In other words, functional incapacity which is not irremediable is not a bar to the application of the right to reproduce. Obviously, an individual, as well as a couple, may have an interest in founding a family. To what extent this interest can be accommodated in the context of the use of artificial reproductive methods will be considered later.

The above discussion demonstrates that reproduction and founding of a family can be seen as distinct concepts, albeit that they are often inextricably connected. For instance, although an individual who has the right to reproduce may also claim an interest in founding a family, not all those who can claim the latter may be in a position meaningfully to claim the right to reproduce, which depends on capacity. The distinctiveness of the two concepts is reinforced by the fact that families can be founded by means other than through biological procreation (for instance, by adoption and step-parenting),[99] the necessary corollary being that reproduction may not always be followed by founding of a family.[100]

Two points which emerge from this discussion can be recapitulated here. First, the right to reproduce extends to an individual who has the capacity to reproduce, but is unable to exercise that capacity because of the infertility of his or her partner. In practical terms, the use of the language of rights in such a case may seem to point to the desirability of allowing access to artificial reproductive methods in order that the person having the right may vindicate it. Second, it has also been noted that the claim of the infertile to have access to artificial reproductive methods is not always based solely on the right to reproduce. In some cases, it may be based also on the interest in founding a family, which will be the sole claim of a couple both of whom are sterile. It is important, therefore, when discussing the rights of the infertile in respect of the use of artificial reproductive methods, to consider in more depth both the strength of this interest and its place and consequences in the catalogue of rights.

CONCLUSION

To say that someone has a right to something is to say that the right-holder has a strong claim to its fulfilment, a claim that may be defeated only if there is another equally strong competing claim, or if the exercise of that right will seriously jeopardize the existence of society, fundamental social institutions or moral values. The right to reproduce, when exercised, can have obvious implications for others and for society in general. To the extent that reproduction involves the procreation of a child, the child's rights, if any, are implicated and can become crucial to the debate about the parameters of the right to reproduce. Society cannot be oblivious to the ramifications which the use of artificial reproductive techniques may have on science, morals and the law. To the extent that a third party's genetic material or body is used for the production of a child, that individual's rights will also have to be examined. The use of artificial reproductive methods to have children therefore draws together a very complex system of claims and interests which have hitherto lain dormant. In many respects, the exact dimensions of the numerous issues involved in artificial reproduction have still to reveal themselves. The claim to the right to reproduce, however, has raised some obvious fundamental arguments which must be assessed and weighed, along with the strength of the claim of each individual involved.

NOTES

1 Coleman, Phyllis, 'Surrogate motherhood: analysis of the problems and suggestions for solution', *Tennessee Law Review* (1982) **50**, p. 71; Rushevsky, Cynthia, 'Legal recognition of surrogacy gestation', *Women's Rights Law Reporter* (1982) **7**, p. 107; Fineburg, Joel, 'The nature and values of rights', in Fineburg, Joel (ed.), *Rights, Justice and the Bounds of Liberty*, Guildford, Princeton, 1980.

2 See Gordon, Linda, *Woman's Body, Woman's Right*, Harmondsworth, Penguin Books, 1977.

3 See Bayles, M.D., 'Limits to a right to reproduce', in O'Neil, Onora and Ruddick, William (eds), *Having Children: Philosophical and Legal Reflections on Parenthood*, Oxford, Oxford University Press, 1979, p. 13. Hardin, Garrett, 'The tragedy of the commons', in Bayles, M.D. (ed.), *Ethics and Population*, Cambridge, Mass., Schenkman, 1976.

4 A new conflict between medicine, mother and the unborn child can be seen in the debate on foetal surgery. See Lenow, Jeffrey, 'The fetus as a patient: emerging rights as a person?', *American Journal of Law and Medicine*, **9**; Weinberg, S.R., 'A maternal duty to protect fetal health?', *Indiana Law Journal* (1983) **58**, p. 531; Robertson, John A., 'The right to procreate and *in vitro* fetal therapy', *The Journal of Legal Medicine* (1982) **3**, p. 333.

5 See, for example, Hart, H.L.A., 'Bentham on legal rights', in Simpson, A.W.B. (ed.), *Oxford Essays in Jurisprudence*, 2nd Series, Oxford, Clarendon Press, 1973; p. 170; MacCormick, D.N., 'Rights in legislation', in Hacker, P.M.S. and Raz, J., *Law, Morality and Society*, Oxford, Clarendon Press, 1977, p. 139. MacCormick, Neil, *H.L.A. Hart*, London, Edward Arnold, 1981, Chapter 7, p. 88.

6 'IVF and the right to reproduce', *Bioethics* (1987) **1**, p. 241.

7 See O'Neil, Onora, 'Begetting, bearing and rearing', in *Having Children*, op. cit., p. 25.

8 See *Re D (a minor)* [1987], All ER 20, a case which will be discussed later.

9 Thus surrogacy is sometimes seen as antenatal adoption. See for example, *Report on Human Artificial Reproduction and Related Matters* (2 Vols), Ministry of the Attorney General, Toronto, 1985.

10 Ibid.

11 McLean, S.A.M., 'The right to reproduce', in Campbell, T.D., *et al.* (eds), *Human Rights: From Rhetoric to Reality*, Oxford, Basil Blackwell, 1986, p. 80.

12 'Is there a right to reproduce?' (unpublished paper).

13 274 US 200 (1927).

14 Ibid., 208.

15 Ibid., 207.

16 See Bergdorf and Bergdorf, 'The wicked witch is almost dead: *Buck* v. *Bell* and the sterilisation of handicapped persons', 50 *Temp. L.Q.* 995 (1977). See generally Meyers, D.W., *The Human Body and the Law*, Chicago, Aldine, 1970, Chapter 2.

17 See also similar provisions in Article 10(1) of the International Covenant on Economic, Social and Cultural Rights, and Article 23(1) of the International Covenant on Civil and Political Rights.

18 Similarly, Article 16(1) of the Universal Declaration on Human Rights (1948) says, 'Men and women of full age . . . have the right to marry and found a family . . .'. A similar article appears in Article 23(2) of the International Covenant on Civil and Political Rights.

19 Article 8(2): There shall be no interference by a public authority with the exercise of this right except such as is in accordance with the law and is necessary in a democratic society in the interests of national security, public safety or the economic well-being of the country, for the prevention of disorder or crime, for

the protection of health or morals, or for the protection of the rights and freedoms of others.

20 See Jacobs, F.G., *The European Convention on Human Rights*, Oxford, Clarendon Press, 1975, p. 162.

21 See 'The comparative law of genetic counselling', in Hilton, B., *et al.* (eds) *Ethical Issues in Human Genetics*, New York, Plenum, 1973, p. 254.

22 It was held that the right to marry did not guarantee a right to divorce: *Johnston* v. *Ireland* [1987]9 EHRR 203. However, a temporary prohibition on remarriage was held to be a violation of Article 12; see *F* v. *Switzerland* [1988] 10 EHRR 411.

23 See Jacobs, ibid.

24 Ibid. See also *Rees case*, 17 October, 1986, Series A, No. 106 and *Cossey case*, 27 September, 1990, Series A, No. 184.

25 Op. Com., 1 March, 1979, Public Court B, Vol. 36, p. 27.

26 On Article 8, the Commission took the view that Article 8 essentially imposes an obligation on a member state to abstain from acting. It does not expressly guarantee the right to be protected by the law against interference with private life. There are however cases where failure to act may be caught by Article 8. The state properly takes action to regulate a situation, confer legal effects on certain facts or certain documents may, by failing to take account of subsequent changes in such facts or documents, interfere with the respect for private life without any positive new act of interference. Here asking the complainant to have a birth certificate clearly incompatible with his appearance would in fact require him to expose information relating to his private life.

27 The *Van Oosterwijck Case, vide supra*, at p. 28.

28 The case was brought by a Dutch national living in Belgium. The applicant, an unmarried person, wanted to adopt an abandoned child who had been living with the applicant for a number of years. The Belgian law required that the applicant, being a foreign national, fulfil the conditions imposed by his personal status which was Dutch law. Under the Dutch Civil Code, however, an unmarried person was not entitled to adopt. See Dec. Adm. Com. Ap. 6482/74, 10 July, 1975, *D and R* 7, p. 55 (77).

29 Ibid.

30 The case concerned a married couple who were citizens of the United Kingdom and Colonies. They adopted Z in accordance with Indian law whilst they were there. They complained that the refusal of the United Kingdom authorities to allow Z to join them constituted an interference with their private and family life under Article 8, and the right to found a family under Article 12. See Dec. Adm. Com. Ap. 7229/75, 12 December, 1977, *D and R* 12, p. 32 (34–5).

31 See 6482/74, 10 July, 1975, *D and R* 7, p. 55 (77).

32 '[Article 8] does not oblige a state to grant a foreign citizen entry to its territory for the purpose of establishing a new family relationship there.' See Dec. Adm. Com. Ap. 7229/75, 12 December 1977, *D and R* 12, p. 32 (34–5). Article 8 has been concerned with other matters, particularly the parent and child relationship. For the denial of access to children taken into care, see e.g. *R* v. *UK* [1987] 10 EHRR 74; *O* v. *UK* [1987] 10 EHRR 82; *W* v. *UK* [1987] 10 EHRR 29. These cases deal with the mutual enjoyment by parent and child of each other's company, which constitutes a fundamental element of family life. This sometimes takes Article 8 into the area of immigration control and its consequential upheaval on family and private life. See e.g. *Application No. 11970/86* v. *UK* [1987] 10 EHRR 48; *Application No. 12513/86* v. *UK* [1987] 10 EHRR 49.

33 See the case of *Bruggemann and Scheuten*, Op. Com., 12 July, 1977, *D and R* p. 100 (166–7).

34 There is only one case on sterilization that has been considered by the Commission, albeit not under Article 12 or Article 8. The applicant alleged that

his wife was sterilized without her consent shortly after she had a child and that the operation had completely changed his married life. The Commission declared the application inadmissible on a number of grounds: the applicant did not state the Articles on which he relied; it appeared that the wife had given her consent, and the applicant did not dispute this fact but was solely contesting that his consent was not obtained; there was no indication that the wife was associated with the application; and the case did not disclose any appearance of a violation of the applicant's individual rights and freedoms. However, the Commission did express the view that an operation of that nature without the consent of the husband might in some circumstances involve a breach of the Convention, in particular Articles 2 and 3, which concern deprivation of life and inhuman and degrading treatment, respectively.

35 316 US 535 (1942).
36 Ibid., p. 544.
37 Ibid., p. 536.
38 Ibid., p. 541.
39 281 US 479 (1965).
40 Ibid., p. 502.
41 *Poe et al.* v. *Gerstein et al.* 517 F. 2d, 787, 795 (1975).
42 405 US 438 (1972).
43 Ibid., p. 453.
44 410 US 113 (1973).
45 Ibid., pp. 152–5.
46 *Vide supra.*
47 *Vide supra.*
48 But there is no right to federal funding of abortion. See *Harris* v. *McRae*, 488 U.S. 297 (1980); and see generally, Petersen, K.A., 'Public funding of abortion services: comparative developments in the United States and Australia', *International Comparative Law Quarterly* (1984) **33**, p. 158.
49 For an argument that the right to reproduce may be a positive claim-right that demands public funding to assist one to reproduce, *vide infra*, Chapter 8.
50 A woman's right to abortion as established in *Roe* is irrespective of marital status. See *Planned Parenthood Association* v. *Danforth*, 428 US 52 (1976).
51 Section 251(1) says:
    Every one who, with intent to procure the miscarriage of a female person, whether or not she is pregnant, uses any means for the purpose of carrying out his intention is guilty of an indictable offence and liable to imprisonment for life.
    Section 251(4) says:
    Subsections (1) and (2) do not apply to (a) a qualified medical practitioner, other than a member of a therapeutic abortion committee for any hospital, who in good faith uses in an accredited or approved hospital any means for the purpose of carrying out his intention to procure the miscarriage of a female person, or (b) . . . if, before the use of those means, the therapeutic abortion committee for that accredited or approved hospital, by a majority of the members of the committee and at a meeting of the committee at which the case of the female person has been reviewed, (c) has by certificate in writing stated that in its opinion the continuation of the pregnancy of the female person would or would be likely to endanger her life or health, and (d) has caused a copy of such certificate to be given to the qualified medical practitioner.
52 The appellants were doctors who set up a clinic to perform abortions upon women who had not obtained a certificate from a therapeutic abortion

committee. They were charged with conspiring with each other with intent to procure abortions contrary to Section 251 of the Criminal Code.

53   Section 1 of the Charter says:
The Canadian Charter of Rights and Freedoms guarantees the rights and freedoms set out in it subject only to such reasonable limits prescribed by law as can be demonstrably justified in a free and democratic society.

54   As a result of the S.C.C.'s decision, the Minister of Justice has introduced new abortion legislation compatible with the *Morgentaler* decision. The Bill introduced establishes that the question of abortion is a medical decision to be made between a woman and her doctor, based on health grounds. It balances the rights of the woman with society's interest in the protection of the foetus. The new section proposed by the Bill says:
Every person who induces an abortion on a female person is guilty of an indictable offence and liable to imprisonment for a term not exceeding two years, unless the abortion is induced by or under the direction of a medical practitioner who is of the opinion that, if the abortion were not induced, the health or life of the female person would be likely to be threatened.
For the purposes of this section, 'health' includes, for greater certainty, physical, mental and psychological health.

55   The concept of the right to reproduce has been briefly considered in two English cases: *Re B (a Minor) (Wardship: Sterilisation)* [1976] 1 All ER 326; *Re B (a Minor) (Wardship: Sterilisation)* [1987] 2 All ER 206; [1987] 2 All ER 209 (C.A.); [1987] 2 All ER 211 (H.L.); *Vide infra* for a fuller discussion of the case. See also *T* v. *T* [1988] 1 All ER 613 and *F* v. *West Berkshire Health Authority* [1989] 2 All ER 545.

56   See *Paton* v. *British Pregnancy Advisory Service Trustees* [1978] 2 All ER 887.

57   See also the Abortion Act as amended by the Human Fertilisation and Embryology Act 1990.

58   H.C., Vol. 732, Col. 1067–77.

59   *Re B (a Minor) (Wardship: Sterilisation)*, Note 55 above.

60   *Vide infra*, pp. 36–43.

61   For further discussion, see Skegg, P.D.G., *Law, Ethics and Medicine*, Oxford, Clarendon Press, 1984, Chapter 1.

62   [1984] 2 All ER 513, 526. Other aspects of the case were considered in the Court of Appeal, see [1986] 2 All ER 497.

63   See, for example, *Sciuriaga* v. *Powell* (1980, unreported), CA transcript 597; *Emeh* v. *Kensington, Chelsea & Fulham Area Health Authority* [1984] 3 All ER 1044; *Udale* v. *Bloomsbury Area Health Authority* [1983] 2 All ER 522; *Thake* v. *Maurice* [1986] 2 All ER 497.

64   See generally, Hillard, Lexa, ' "Wrongful birth": Some growing pains', *M.L.R.* (1985) **48**, p. 224; Taylor, Ann Spowart, 'Compensation for unwanted children', *Family Law* (1985) **5**, p. 147; Brahmas, Diana, 'Damages for unplanned babies – a trend to be discouraged?', *N.L.J.* (1983) **133**(1), p. 643.

65   See Lord Hailsham in *Re B (a Minor) (Wardship: Sterilisation)*, where he stressed that this case is not to be taken as a precedent in all cases relating to the mentally handicapped; [1987] 2 All ER 211, 212.

66   [1976] 1 All ER 326.

67   This involved, amongst other symptoms, epileptic seizures, clumsiness, dull intelligence, precocious growth and personality problems.

68   [1976] 1 All ER 326, 332.

69   See Article 12 of the Convention on Human Rights which says: 'Men and women of marriageable age have the right to marry and to found a family, according to the national laws governing the exercise of this right.'

70   *Vide infra*, pp. 38–43.

71   Cited above.

72   Ibid., at p. 208 (i.e. [1987] 2 All ER 206, 208).

73 Ibid., p. 210.
74 Lord Hailsham, L-C., *The Times*, 1 May 1987, p.37. Ibid., p. 213.
75 See also *F* v. *West Berkshire Health Authority*; *T* v. *T* cited above.
76 *Vide supra*.
77 See the Canadian approach in the case of *Re Eve* (1986) 31 DLR (4th) 1, where the court concluded that sterilization should never be performed for non-therapeutic purposes under the *parens patriae* jurisdiction. See Bowker, W.F., 'Sterilisation of the mentally retarded adult: the Eve case', *McGill Law Journal*, (1981) **26**, p. 931.
78 Cited above.
79 *Vide supra*.
80 *Vide supra*.
81 Article 2(1) of the European Convention on Human Rights says,
    Everyone's right to life shall be protected by law. No one shall be deprived of his life intentionally save in the execution of a sentence of a court following his conviction of a crime for which his penalty is provided by law.
    See generally Jacobs, F.G., *The European Convention on Human Rights*, Oxford, Clarendon Press, 1975. But note *Soering* v. *United Kingdom*, 11 EHRR, 439 (1989); Protocol No. 6 to the European Convention for the Protection of Human Rights and Fundamental Freedoms and Protocol No. 2 to the International Convenant on Civil and Political Rights.
82 *Vide supra, Re B*.
83 Coleman, Phyllis, 'Surrogate motherhood: analysis of the problems and suggestions for solutions', *Tennessee Law Review* (1982) **50**, p. 71.
84 217 N.J. super. 313; 525 A. 2d 1128 (1987).
85 537 A.2d 1227 (1988) at 1235.
86 217 N.J. 313; 525 A.2d 1128 at 1164 (1987), emphasis added.
87 109 N.J. 396; 537 A.2d 1227 (1988).
88 *Vide infra*, pp. 110–11.
89 410 US 113 (1973).
90 See *Carey* v. *Population Services International*:'individual autonomy in matters of child-bearing' and 'the teaching of *Griswold* is that the Constitution protects individuals' decisions in matters of child-bearing from unjustified intrusion of the state'. Ibid., 687.
91 See Chapter 6 for further discussions on the acceptability of surrogacy.
92 *Vide supra*, pp. 25–7.
93 *Vide supra*, Chapter 2.
94 *Vide supra*.
95 *Vide infra*, Chapter 8.
96 As the state is not obliged to provide a sexual partner, nor presumably to provide a fertile sexual partner, see *Poe et al.* v. *Gerstein et al., vide supra*, p. 795.
97 *Vide infra*, Chapter 4.
98 Unless the concept of the right to reproduce includes the right to be rendered fertile. This is clearly incompatible with the notion of a negative claim-right. *Vide infra*, Chapter 8 for a discussion on the positive claim right to found a family.
99 For example, the Commission on Human Rights noted that (Dec. Adm. Com. Ap. 7229/75, 12 December 1977. D & R 12 p. 32 (34–5), see later):
    . . . adoption of a child and its integration into a family with a couple might, at least in some circumstances, be said to constitute the foundation of a family by that couple. It is quite conceivable that a 'family' might be 'found' in such a way.
100 See, for example, where children are given up for adoption.

4 Moral and Social Acceptability of Artificial Reproductive Techniques

INTRODUCTION

In Chapter 2, reference was made to three possible artificial reproductive methods (AI, IVF and surrogacy) to which the infertile may have resort in order to found a family (whether through reproduction or not). The nature and use of these methods have been the subject of concern and have generated varying degrees of debate. Concern is understandable, because these are not purely medical techniques, as applied to reproduction and founding of a family, which exist in a vacuum without moral, social and legal implications.[1] In this chapter, one of the questions addressed is whether artificial reproductive techniques (AI, IVF and the use of donated gametes) which enable the infertile to found a family (whether through reproduction or not) are, as some have argued, inherently objectionable. To a certain extent, the debate is dated as the question of acceptability has largely been superseded by their use in various centres in the UK and in various countries. But in a work of this nature, the acceptability of these techniques cannot be assumed simply by reference to their practical use since it does not necessarily in itself suggest that their acceptability is a non-issue. If these techniques are indeed morally and socially objectionable, there seems to be no reason why society cannot legitimately prohibit their use. Conversely, if there is nothing inherently objectionable about them and their use, there is no reason why the rights of the infertile to have children should not be vindicated, although the exercise of these rights may have to be subjected to regulations which reflect legitimate social interests. Thus one of the issues considered in this chapter is the acceptability and feasibility of these techniques in the light of the various moral and social complications they may create, and the approach of the law and society towards their use, bearing in mind the rights of the infertile to have children and to found a family.[2]

Analysis of some of the fundamental objections against AI and IVF indicates that they are proffered on the basis of common and deep-rooted beliefs, which may be marshalled and appraised under the same headings. It is to these common features that the first section of this chapter will be directed. Following this, the arguments applicable uniquely to IVF will be considered. The acceptability of the use of donated gametes will be considered in the last section of this chapter.

OBJECTIONS TO ARTIFICIAL REPRODUCTIVE TECHNIQUES: ARTIFICIAL INSEMINATION AND *IN VITRO* FERTILIZATION

Unnatural Procreation[3]

It has been argued that artificial reproductive techniques (that is, AI and IVF) are unacceptable because they are 'unnatural'. There are two ways of comprehending this argument. First, artificial reproductive techniques may be considered by some to be 'unnatural' in the sense that the 'sacred process' of life is the prerogative of God and should not be interfered with. This argument would suggest that the infertile should accept their condition rather than attempt to procreate against God's 'will' by using artificial reproductive techniques.[4] This line of argument is certainly vague. Would taking drugs to destroy a life-threatening bacterium be an interference with the 'sacred process' of life, and an usurpation of God's prerogative? Further, the belief that procreation should be dictated by God's prerogative is clearly a belief not adhered to rigidly by those who are prepared to use artificial techniques to procreate, and there is no serious suggestion that these people's view should be converted.

A second interpretation of the 'unnatural' argument is based on the belief that these techniques contravene the 'natural law'. One theory of natural law is that the laws of nature can be discovered by reference to the ends of natural things.[5] That is, all things and all human beings have certain goals in whose pursuit they flourish; in addition, human acts have certain ends (or purposes) which define the appropriate way in which they should be performed.

The argument that AI and IVF are 'unnatural' goes like this: since the only natural and legitimate end of sex is procreation, modes of procreation, such as AI and IVF which sever such a link, are contrary to the natural law.[6] Notwithstanding the unpopularity of this procreational model of sex and the lack of credibility of its original basis,[7] it is unclear what useful purpose this argument serves regarding the acceptability of artificial reproductive techniques. As Singer and Wells have said,[8] even if procreation is the essential legitimation for sexual intercourse, it would not necessarily be wrong to achieve procreation in some other way when infertility prevents the achievement of this essential goal through sexual intercourse. This leads to the next objection to AI and IVF.

Natural Procreation

To some people, AI and IVF are wrong because 'true' procreation is achieved solely by a man–woman relationship. This argument turns the procreational model of sex on its head. In other words, instead of arguing that sex is for procreation, the contention here is that procreation should only be achieved naturally, that is, as a result of sexual intercourse. Thus, it has been argued that:[9]

> The true character of procreation is secured by its belonging to the man–woman relationship . . . The procreative and relational aspects of marriage strengthen one another, and that each is threatened by the loss of the other. This is a knot tied by God, which men should not untie. It is clear that any attempt to covert begetting into making constitutes a loosening of that knot . . .

According to this view, AI and IVF are not 'true' procreation. Yet, defining one mode of procreation as 'true' or 'false' is rather extraneous to the main issue. Why is artificial procreation unacceptable? The author seems to suggest that AI and IVF which separate the relational and procreational aspects of marriage, threaten the former.[10] However, there is no concrete or substantive evidence to support this assertion. Indeed, it may equally be argued that couples who resort to AI and IVF in order to have children demonstrate their love and commitment to each other, possibly even to a greater extent than some fertile couples.

To sum up, the 'unnatural' argument, and the argument that natural procreation should be the only mode of procreation, are based on fundamental personal beliefs and values. Consequently, individuals who ascribe to those views may legitimately eschew artificial reproductive techniques. These arguments, however, are not sufficient to establish by themselves that others, who do not share the same beliefs, should be prohibited from having the choice to use them in the exercise of their right to reproduce and to found a family. Consistent with Mill's[11] classic explanation of the justification for interference with others, these beliefs would be enforceable on others only if they represent harm to the general good.

OBJECTIONS TO IVF

In the preceding section, fundamental objections common to both artificial reproductive techniques have been discussed. The conclusion is that they are not morally and socially unacceptable. However, some unique features of IVF may require some modification to this conclusion. Whereas certain objections may be common to both AI and IVF, the nature of the latter may provide a further source of debate for those who would advocate its use. The crucial distinguishing characteristic of IVF is that it involves more than simply the facilitation of a process which takes place naturally. Rather, it entails the extracorporeal creation of a human embryo. Thus, extracorporeal fertilization and its subsequent implantation or use raises other subtle arguments.

The existence of embryos outside the womb causes concern for some people who argue that embryos should be protected and be equated with the status of human beings. But even those who take the position that an embryo, from the moment of conception, ought to be treated with the respect accorded to a human being, may accept that as long as it is given the chance to fulfil its potential, IVF is not unacceptable.[12] Consequently, debates on IVF usually centre on its practical use and the many scientific possibilities it opens up, such as experiments on human embryos, freezing embryos and genetic studies[13] rather than on the acceptability of IVF *per se*. For instance, responding to moral concern regarding wastage of embryos during the selection and reimplantation process, the IVF centre in Norfolk, Virginia, has adopted the practice of fertilizing eggs only if a woman wishes them to be transferred to her womb.[14] In the UK, the Unborn Children (Protection) Bill 1985[15] which generated much passionate debate on the moral status of embryos was essentially an attempt to ensure that embryos were created *in vitro* only for the purpose of enabling a woman to have a child.[16] In other words, IVF as a technique is not automatically regarded as unacceptable. Rather, anxieties are directed primarily to the way in which it is carried out or ancillary scientific activities.[17]

However, some may contend that, although IVF is not an unacceptable technique in itself, it becomes unacceptable in view of the possible consequences to which it may lead. This is called the slippery slope argument.[18] For instance, it may be argued that, if IVF is allowed, it may be a step on the road to the Brave New World – a society in which genetic engineering enables human beings to be produced with certain characteristics in a state-controlled laboratory for the benefit of the state. IVF, therefore, is unacceptable because its potential danger outweighs its possible benefits. Opponents to IVF, therefore, argue that 'if medicine turns to doctoring desires instead of medical conditions . . . is there any reason for doctors to be reluctant to accede to parents' desires to have a girl rather than a boy, blonde hair rather than brown, a genius rather than a Clout . . . ?'.[19]

Although the slippery slope argument (a type of consequentialist argument) can often sound persuasive, it may also be inherently illogical. The thrust of the argument, in relation to IVF, runs like this: IVF is used to satisfy the desire of the infertile to have their own children and, if this is accepted, the principle of consistency will require the acceptance of other technical extensions, such as genetic engineering, to create, for example, a genius, if this is what parents desire. This will eventually lead us to the Brave New World. Accepting IVF does not necessarily force acceptance of other technological extensions. The two situations mentioned above may be equated in the sense that both are concerned with satisfying people's desires, and thus, if these desires are accorded the same weight consistency will require acceptance of the latter situation if the former is permitted. Yet the two situations are not identical, since one relates to a situation where people desire to have their own children and the other is where parents desire to have particular kinds of children. These desires and the reasons for them may not be equally ranked or regarded equally acceptable, and hence the two cases need not be treated as identical. Accepting the former does not necessarily oblige one, on grounds of consistency, to accept the latter. Moreover, the desire to have children is validated by acceptance of the right to reproduce and to found a family.[20] No such equivalent rights adhere to the wish for a particular kind of child. In any event, technological advances alone will not lead to Aldous Huxley's Brave New World. This is because Huxley's society is one where not only has the state mastered genetic engineering and artificial human reproduction, but it is a society with a rigid caste system, intense brainwashing and human enslavement. Transformation of our present society to that of the Brave New World could not be achieved by successes in genetic engineering alone.

Nonetheless, fear of potential abuse of genetic engineering techniques is not entirely unjustifiable. Even if the above scenario is unlikely, other more plausible consequences, which could be equally unacceptable, may follow from IVF techniques. On the question of ancillary scientific developments or activities, fears have been voiced that embryos not used for implantations may be used for scientific experiments and that this is ethically unacceptable. Proponents of experimentation argue that embryonic research is necessary for human welfare, firstly for the development and refinement of the IVF procedure itself (for example, improving the means of storage and the transfer mechanism leading to greater success and reducing the rate of wastage). Research could also lead to a greater understanding of early embryonic development, survival, implantation and its subsequent evolution – knowledge which is neeeded to reduce not only the incidence of infertility but also the rate of spontaneous abortion. A review of these arguments led to *The Warnock Report's* recommendation of a statutory licensing authority.[21] In the absence of legislative backing for this recommendation, a voluntary licensing authority was set up in 1985 to monitor the activities of those who wish to carry out research involving human embryos and/or the treatment of IVF.[22] The Human Fertilisation and Embryology Act now provides a legal regulatory framework for embryonic research be limited to 14 days and that such research could be carried out for the following specific purposes: the promotion of treatment for infertility; increased knowledge of the causes of congenital diseases; increased understanding of miscarriage; the development of more effective contraception; the detection of genetic or chromosomal abnormality, and increasing knowledge about embryos before implantation.[23] The Act prohibits the creation of hybrids, cloning or genetic engineering and set up the Human Fertilisation and Embryology Authority to control research.[24] The Act, it is hoped, will temper some of the fiercest opposition to work on embryology.

The weight of public opinion, therefore, is in favour of the right of the infertile to reproduce and to found a family. Indeed this has been tacitly recognized by virtue of the fact that no prohibition of these techniques has been seen as appropriate despite strong condemnation from some sections of the community. The balance of morality, therefore, may be said to favour the vindication of human rights over practical, but avoidable, problems which can arise in the attempts to facilitate access to these rights.

However, it must be noted that the arguments described above have been deliberately confined to the relatively straightforward situation where a couple are artificially assisted to reproduce and to found a family by the use of their own genetic gametes. Whilst the same arguments may be levelled against the use of donated ova and sperm, their characteristics may change. Equally, additional arguments may arise in this situation.

OBJECTIONS TO THE USE OF DONATED GAMETES

If AI and IVF are not unacceptable *in se* as means of reproduction and of founding a family, is the use of donated gametes which will enable the founding of a family (whether through reproduction or not) equally acceptable?

The Married Couple

It has been argued that the use of donated gametes (whether sperm or ova) is unacceptable because it amounts to a third party intervention in a marriage relationship which is a covenant-relationship between a man and a woman to the exclusion of all others.[25] If this argument stands, it will rule out the use by married couples of donated gametes. Another argument against the use of donated gametes is the possible harm to a child when he or she comes to know about the circumstances of his or her conception. The effects of both of these arguments on the rights of individuals to found a family (whether through reproduction or not) will be examined in turn. Since they are normally raised in respect of the use of donated semen in AI (AID), the following discussion will refer to AID. However, what is said is equally applicable to the use of donated gametes in artificial reproductive techniques in general.

Third Party Intervention

The essence of this contention against AID is that, since donated semen of a person not party to a marriage is used for procreation, it amounts to a third party intervention in a marriage. It is comparable to an extra-marital relationship, and is therefore objectionable.[26] AID has sometimes been equated to adultery. However, such a comparison can hardly be justified.[27] The nature, motive and elements are totally different.[28] An adulterous relationship involves sexual intercourse between two people, often with emotional involvement; AID does not. Again, the motives of the two acts are not parallel. AID is used in the hope that conception will occur so that a couple can have a family.[29] This is not generally the case in an adulterous relationship which usually aims at the pleasure it will give, whereas AID is a means to an end.[30] The legal position seems settled. In Scots law, AID is not adultery even if it is undertaken without a husband's consent.[31] This is almost certainly the English position, although no English court has yet considered the point.[32]

Other arguments also need to be examined. It has been suggested that the introduction of a third party into a marital relationship is undesirable because of the possible harmful consequences it may have, in that a husband will be reminded of his infertility by the existence of an AID child. This is clearly something that a couple will have to assess for themselves.[33] Moreover, the fact that some couples may be affected adversely by AID is not sufficient to exclude its use by others. In fact, this may merely serve to indicate the need for counselling for those contemplating using AID.[34]

In terms of a married couple, then, there may be some strength in the argument that AID is an intrusion into the marital relationship, since – at a practical level – there is the need for a donor. It is not clear, however, that an intrusion which is designed to develop the relationship and which is effective in vindicating basic rights, need be viewed as a bad thing. In other words, it is not morally imperative that intervention in a marriage is in itself wrong, particularly where the aim and likely outcome of the intervention is to cement a relationship rather than to disrupt it. In some cases, the use of donated gametes will provide the only method by which married couples may exploit their rights to reproduce and to found a family.

The Unmarried and Eligibility

The question of eligibility in the context of artificial reproductive methods (that is, people who should be allowed access to artificial reproductive technologies), like the question of 'licensing parents',[35] touches on the interplay between private morality and the complex matrices of public policy, the importance of marriage and the family as the fundamental unit of society, and society's perception of what is in the best interests of children. Much of the antipathy towards the use of artificial reproductive technologies is based on the apprehension that 'unsuitable' persons may be allowed to use them to become parents.

Although 'unsuitable' parents may be either married or single, the discussion tends to centre on groups who are not married or people who deviate from the traditional heterosexual relationship paradigm. This, to a a large extent, reflects society's perception of non-traditional family groups. Concern is expressed about the likelihood that these techniques may facilitate individuals who are otherwise regarded as 'unsuitable' for procreation and parenting to have children and become parents. Many of those who express such apprehension accept that no legal or social control can prevent or curb natural reproduction amongst fertile people who are 'unsuitable' for procreation and parenting, but feel that this should not prevent society from vetting 'unsuitable' parents and precluding them from participating in artificial reproduction.[36] This argument, if successful, would create the theoretical and conceptual anomaly of reproductive control over those who are infertile whilst ignoring parents who conceive naturally.[37]

Having said that, it must be noted that one of the strongest arguments against the use of artificial reproductive techniques is based on consideration of the interests of children.[38] This, to a large extent, helps to put the issue of eligibility into its proper focus.

Thus, it has been said that it might be possible to adopt an approach that the right to procreate should be restricted by using the same guiding principle that the courts use in resolving custody disputes – the best interests of the child. The pertinent line of enquiry here would take the form of asking 'Is it in the best interests of the child to be born in given circumstances?'[39] Yet, this is a nonsensical line of enquiry as it is impossible to assess the one alternative with another (non-existence is beyond the realm of human cognition).[40] According to this view, the best interests of the child is not a meaningful consideration when set off against the right to have children.

If we now move away from the philosophical and intuitive enquiry to the practical assessment of balancing conflicting claims: on the one hand, reproductive autonomy which advocates an individual-orientated approach and, on the other hand, the competing value of the welfare of children. One sees immediately that the use of artificial reproductive technologies is not simply and exclusively a question of satisfying the desire of the infertile; eligibility cannot be seen essentially as a private matter. Thus, whilst society has so far endorsed the use of artificial reproductive techniques for the alleviation of infertility, and social perception towards marriage and the family has changed – courts have recently been noticeably disinclined to devalue the one-parent family,[41] and society seems less inclined to regard it as necessarily a bad thing. There has not been a blanket acceptance of the use of these techniques by all infertile couples without qualification. After all, artificial reproduction is not the same as natural reproduction. It is the deliberate employment of human and technological endeavours to bring a child into being. Thus, it has been suggested that artificial reproductive techniques have placed the doctor in a unique position where he/she is an additional party to the pregnancy. A successful treatment brings into existence a child who would otherwise not have existed, and the medical profession may rightly see themselves as using a medical procedure which may have wider implications than simply curing an ordinary affliction. Similarly, society, which endorses the use of artificial reproductive techniques is also implicated in the child's existence. According to this view, it is appropriate for society to impose a degree of regulation in the case of artificial reproduction at the stage of eligibility; regulation which is neither desirable nor practical in natural reproduction.

What is the standard for testing suitability or fitness to have children? This is tied up with our perception of 'suitable' parents which is an ambiguous and amorphous social and psychological concept. Nonetheless, it has been said that there are several possible tests for judging a person's suitability to have access to artificial reproductive methods:[42]

> These include whether the potential parents could adopt a child under the particular jurisdiction or, less stringently, whether the child would be likely to be in need of protection . . . Perhaps the less stringent test which would be envisaged would be to assess parenting capacity for the purposes of access to birth technology according to whether a child born as a result of use of that technology would have any claim in a 'wrongful life' tort action, that is, a claim for damages for having been conceived and born.

The last option – using a wrongful life claim as the standard – does not appear to be a very valuable alternative for the reason stated above. Indeed, it is difficult to see how one can lend weight to the argument that being born in 'undesirable' family circumstances or environment is 'wrongful life'. The first option on adoption is not generally favoured as the operative circumstances – supply and demand – are not mirrored in artificial reproduction; the stringent standards used in adoption merely reflect the fact that there are more applicants to adopt than available children for adoption. The second, a middle course, is consistent with the value we put on reproductive freedom; existing constraints on the right to parenting and standards adoption for child protection. Here, eligibility intervention will admit most people for assistance except those against whom the state probably will have a clear case for depriving them of the right to parenting. Such an approach can be further defended by the argument that it is self-defeating to resort to birth technology with the aim of creating a child for parenting if the person in question has no such right.[43] In other words, assistance would be rendered only if there is no evidence that there is no impediment to the right to parenting after the assisted reproduction. Secondly, if the state is involved in funding infertility treatment,[44] it should use its resources in a sensible manner. Assisting reproduction in cases where the individual has no right to parenting runs counter to this, and it will lend credence to the idea that reproduction should be seen as an activity having its value irrespective of parenting.

In the context of eligibility, one of the major concerns is whether the unmarried and the single should have access to artificial reproductive techniques. *The Warnock Report*, which considered this issue, preferred married couples or couples in stable union. Thus it said that,[45]

> . . . as a general rule it is better for children to be born into a two-parent family, with both father and mother, although we recognise that it is impossible to predict with any certainty how lasting such a relationship will be.

The Victoria Infertility (Medical Procedures) Act 1984 provides that couples living in stable union are eligible for treatment.[46] But the Act expressly excluded a single woman from treatment.

Questions have therefore been raised as to whether the refusal to treat single (or homosexual) couples who do not conform with the traditional heterosexual paradigm is legitimate or whether it is no more than a reflection of popular prejudices against these people; is the decision based on any established empirical evidence that people who fall into those categories are less capable of parenting or that they make bad parents?

Susan Golombok and John Rust found that although children in fatherless (that is, single-parent) families were more likely to have emotional and behavioural problems, this was not the direct consequence of the absence of a father, as it is commonly assumed, but rather a direct consequence of experience of family discord, poverty or isolation or a combination of all these.[47] On the point of psychosexual development of fatherless children, the authors concluded that,[48]

[t]he vast number of empirical studies of the role of fathers in the psychosexual development of their children are contradictory and inconclusive in their findings. Most children in one-parent families, like children in two-parent heterosexual families, show typical psycho-sexual development, but it remains uncertain whether there is a slight effect on some behaviour and attitudes.

But as the authors continued,

This may, of course, be positive rather than problematic. After all, if as some researchers claim, boys in one-parent families are slightly less aggressive than their counterparts in two-parent families, is this such a bad thing? Many of the studies which are quoted today were carried out over 10 years ago. The divisions between male and female roles are now less clear-cut, and behaviour or attitudes which may have appeared odd a decade ago are quite acceptable now.

On the point of homosexual (lesbian) families, the authors found that there was no evidence of increased likelihood of psychiatric disorder or of gender identity disorder in children raised in lesbian families. Although there was no direct evidence of the effect on AID or IVF children born and raised in one-parent heterosexual or homosexual families, the authors felt that special concern for children raised in these circumstances was not warranted.[49] As Susan Golombok and John Rust asked rhetorically, 'Given the extent to which children are abused within the traditional system, surely the double standards which have so far permeated the debate about eligibility for AID and IVF should be recognized?'

Double standards, therefore, are what seem to be unacceptable. If genuine concern is expressed regarding suitability for parenting on the basis of the best interests of the child, then best interests and suitability of parenting should be the criteria, and a categorical rejection of particular social groups or groups of people is not called for in the absence of evidence that single, lesbian or homosexual parenting is positively detrimental to children in all cases.

The conclusion here is that excluding particular people or groups of people simply on the basis of membership of a particular group is tantamount to discrimination which cannot be justified on any legitimate ground and is, therefore, unacceptable. Indeed, if an individual has a right to procreate and have a family, a categorical exclusion of a certain group of people from access to artificial reproductive techniques is an infringement of a right which may not be justifiable on the basis that it is necessary for the protection of any legitimate interests of children. In a similar vein, the Ontario Law Reform Commission took the view that 'any *a priori* exclusions based simply on membership in a particular group (such as married persons) would automatically eliminate from consideration single persons or unmarried couples who, by any standard, would make suitable parents'. Thus, it seems that there is no convincing argument to exclude certain groups of people – on the grounds of their marital status – from using artificial reproductive techniques.

At the moment, the practice varies on selection of patients. For example, one IVF unit offers treatment to couples who have been living together for at least three years;[50] another makes no policy decision on the patients' relationship, or the lack of it, although cases are reviewed on a case by case basis.[51]

The recent Harriott case shows the complexities of the issues involved.[52] H was unable to have a child and her adoption application was rejected because of her criminal record for offences related to prostitution and the running of a brothel. She sought the help of the IVF unit of St Mary's hospital. At first she was put on the waiting list. The consultant, when she became aware of the reasons for the refusal of H's adoption application, decided that treatment should not be given to her and she was removed from the waiting list. In an action for judicial review, the court rejected the relief sought and said that even if it were to accept H's proposition that the consultant's decision was amenable to judicial review, 'it could not be suggested that no reasonable consultant could have come to a decision to refuse treatment to the applicant'.

One does not expect the court to get itself entangled with policy issues such as whether Harriott was a suitable potential parent. By implication, the decision of the consultant was to endorse the adoption criteria. As said before, had H not been infertile, her decision to have a child, and probably her right to parenting, might never be challenged. Yet, the judgement tacitly assumes that a reasonable decision by a consultant on who should be given IVF treatment cannot be challenged. A 'reasonable' decision may arguably embrace the exclusion of someone who is a rehabilitated juvenile offender, a homosexual or lesbian, although none of these statuses *per se* appear to warrant the deprivation of the right to reproduce and/or parenting. The whole process of decision making, as can be seen in the Harriott case, is potentially fraught with personal biases and prejudices. Can a person who is denied IVF treatment, which is the only means to have a child, claim to have a legitimate grievance? If some kind of selection is to be made on who is eligible and who is not, should there not be some kind of objective substantive criteria which would guide the decision-making process, making it less subjective and less likely to fall prey to irrelevant factors, thereby avoiding the challenge that the right to have children is arbitrarily denied or haphazardly negated? When the decision whether to provide assistance to someone fervently desiring a child is left to a single consultant, it is not surprising that the person denied treatment will feel a sense of grief. The lack of a consistent nationwide approach to the question of eligibility will only aggravate that feeling.[53]

Harm to an AID Child

Apart from the question of interests of children and eligibility for infertility treatment, one of the strongest objections to the use of AID is that an AID child may experience confusions of personal identity due to the circumstances of his or her conception. At the moment, the practice in AID appears to be that some practitioners advise couples not to disclose to the child his or her circumstances of conception, whilst others apparently leave the decision to the recipients:[54]

> . . . unless you decide to tell the child there is no reason for him (or her) even to know that he (or she) was conceived by AID. Whether or not you do so is entirely up to you.

A study[55] has found that most AID couples intended never to reveal the circumstances of their conception to AID children. These children therefore may never know of their AID conception nor be informed of the donors' identities. Some, therefore, argue against AID on the ground that it is wrong to deceive a child regarding the circumstances of his or her conception.[56] Despite the secrecy regarding AID in general, some AID children do discover the circumstances of their conception, either in the divorce proceedings of their 'parents', or indirectly from family conversation. The undesirable consequences of accidental disclosure have strengthened the case for openness with AID children regarding the circumstances of their conception.

Some may contend that possible harm to a child when he or she is told about his or her circumstances of conception is an important consideration against AID itself, and not merely a consequential issue. Those in favour of AID may seek to counter this argument by pointing out that the discovery by a child that his or her 'father' is in fact not genetically linked to him or her, does not necessarily entail greater distress than the discovery that one has been adopted. However, there are distinctions between the two situations which make this counter-argument of only limited value. Although adoption is a situation where the child may suffer when he or she is told about his or her true origin, it is nonetheless often the best option for a child who has already been born. To that extent, adoption is not comparable to the deliberate creation of a child, who may suffer as a result of his or her particular circumstances of conception.

Notwithstanding this, and conceding to the worst possible harmful scenario, it is difficult to contend with any strong conviction that an AID child would have been better off not being born in the first place (which he or she would not have been but for the use of AID), and that, conversely, people have no right to use AID to found a family (whether through reproduction or not).[57] In fact, courts have been notably loath to accept that non-existence could ever be preferable to existence even with handicap.[58]

Given that the strongest argument against AID (whether for individuals or couples) seems to relate to the resulting child, it is worth at this stage considering whether any unfavourable impact on the child could be minimized. In particular, considerable concern centres on the question as to whether or not a child has a right to have access to certain information about the donor. If the distress which forms the basis of this argument against AID is real, there seem to be two options. On the one hand, the child could simply be deceived – a practice which is relatively common, but can be frowned upon for several reasons.[59] On the other hand, the child could be told of the circumstances of his or her conception.

There appear to be a number of reasons why AID children are not told the truth. Some fear that the truth will adversely affect the relationship already established between the child and the family. Some couples consider that there is no reason to tell because they regard the AID child as 'their' child. Others fear that AID status will stigmatize the child. In one study,[60] it was concluded that the main reason for secrecy was in fact an attempt to protect the feelings of husbands, and to avoid publication of the fact of male infertility.

Because of the secrecy which has surrounded AID, thorough follow-up studies of the impact on AID children when they are told of the circumstances of their conception have not been possible. But from limited data, Snowden and Mitchell[61] found that the fear that telling an AID child the circumstances of his or her conception would damage the 'father'–child relationship might not be entirely justified. Those children who had been told appeared to be glad that their AID conceptions were not kept secret, and none found it a particularly traumatic experience. Some were surprised that their parents had found it necessary to keep AID secret. In some cases, the relationship between parents and child was enhanced rather than spoiled. Hence, it appears to be possible to tell a child about these circumstances without harming the 'father'–child relationship.[62]

Moreover, secrecy may be harmful to family relationships and to the child. The positive and/or negative deception necessary to conceal the circumstances of a child's conception may blemish or destroy the relationship of trust which ideally exists within the family. If a child suspects his or her origin, secrecy may also be harmful to his or her mental health.

Here, an analogy may be made with adoption. It is generally accepted in adoption practice that, in order to develop a proper sense of identity, an adopted person should know that he or she was adopted, and should be given this information in a way which takes account of his or her age and understanding.[63] In recognition of this principle, the Children Act 1975 gave an adopted person in England or Wales a right to ascertain his or her biological parentage at the age of 18.[64] In Scotland, an adopted person, on reaching 17, can go to Register House in Edinburgh and ask to see the original birth entry.[65] In England and Wales, a person adopted prior to 1975 is required to be counselled before information is given which would lead them to his or her original birth record. The purpose of counselling is to assist the adopted person to understand some of the possible effects of his or her enquiries. It was also thought that there should be some protection for the mother who gave the child up for adoption.

One may therefore argue that, by analogy with adoption, AID children should not be deceived about the circumstances of their conception, and that they should have the right to know the identities of donors. If so, provisions similiar to those in adoption could be made enabling them to find out if they so wish.

Nonetheless, opinions are relatively divided as to whether an AID child should be allowed only limited information regarding the donor's ethnic origin and genetic health,[66] or whether an AID child should have the right of access to the donor's identity, as does an adopted person. Here again there may be additional consequences following from full disclosure to an AID child, which may affect the desire of the community to encourage full and complete disclosure.

One major concern appears to be that disclosure of donors' identities may discourage semen donation. Available evidence on this is rather tentative at the moment.[67] Consequently, an AID child's right to know may be far from certain. But it is clear from the above discussion that openness with an AID child regarding the circumstances of his or her conception is generally regarded as desirable, and may avert the potential for harm associated with deception and accidential disclosure. Consistent with this valuing of openness, is the conclusion that people who resort to AID should be counselled about the issues which they will have to confront later regarding a child's understanding of his or her circumstances of conception.[68]

CONCLUSION

In this chapter, attempts have been made to collate the basic fundamental arguments against the use of artificial reproductive methods by the infertile to have children. Clashes on personal beliefs concerning the nature of procreation and whether artificial reproductive methods are consonant with one's basic belief are questions for the individual to resolve. Similarly, whether to accept third party intervention in procreation is a matter for the infertile couples concerned. The question of an individual's right to procreate does not stop here. What is in the best interest of the resulting child has always been one of the most cogent arguments which needs to be addressed and considered. This issue is closely tied up with eligibility.

The question of eligibility found a forum for discussion in Parliament recently in the debates to the Human Fertilisation and Embryology Bill. An amendment was moved to prohibit access to AID and IVF treatment by unmarried women. This was narrowly defeated.[69] The mover of the amendment doubted whether the position of those unmarried couples who were in a so-called 'stable relationship' was really as favourable as it sounded.[70] On the opposing side, it was argued that having children was a private area of human affairs and that it was not for the state to decide who should or should not be allowed to bear children. Furthermore there was no connection between marriage and the quality of parenthood.[71] The question of discrimination and enforcement was also raised. On the question of enforcement, it was said that 'if a marriage certificate had to be produced, a clinic would have to prove that a woman was not separated, divorced or widowed. Such a law would encourage marriages for convenience'.[72] Since AID can be self-administered, the effect of the amendment may force those who would otherwise obtain the treatment from a licensed clinic to by-pass the system introduced by the Bill; namely, that a patient should receive counselling before the treatment and that the donor's semen be screened for diseases which can be passed on to the recipient through semen, for example, the HIV virus.

The effect of the amendment, if passed, would be that a woman living apart from her husband might legitimately receive AID, whereas an unmarried woman living in a stable relationship would be prohibited from receiving the treatment. Such was the overt discrimination on the basis of marital status that Lord Hylton commented that 'the weakness of the amendment is that it seems to discriminate against the infertile unmarried woman or couple because those who are fortunate enough to be fertile will simply go ahead in the normal way'.[73] It was suggested that the amendment would infringe Article 12 of the ECHR. The Lord Chancellor, having taken advice on the matter, took the view that the amendment would not infringe Article 12.[74] This view is consistent with the status of Article 12 advocated earlier in Chapter 3. In other words, since the proposed prohibition does not prevent an unmarried woman from marrying, and since Article 12 does not confer a right to reproduce on the unmarried, national law prohibiting unmarried women from having children by using infertility treatment cannot contravene Article 12. However the question of the scope of Article 8 was brought up again when the right to treatment of the unmarried was discussed. The question was posed as to whether Article 8 might be wide enough to cover the right of an unmarried woman to receive treatment under the Bill – subject to counselling – as part of her right to private life.[75] No categorical answer was given, but grave doubts were expressed as to whether the scope of Article 8 extends to such questions.[76]

It can clearly be seen that the idea of reproductive freedom is seriously threatened when eligibility for infertility treatment to enable an individual to have children is on the agenda. Although eligibility can be examined from various angles – the interests of children, the sanctity of marriage and family life, equality and utilization of medical resources – individual rights nevertheless often tip the balance.

The Human Fertilisation and Embryology Act 1990, recognizes the problem of assessed to infertility treatment by the unmarried but does not provide any clear answers. Section 13(5) says:

> A woman shall not be provided with treatment services unless account has been taken of the welfare of any child who may be born as a result of the treatment (including the need of that child for a father), and of any other child who may be affected by the birth.

Section 13(6) also imposes counselling as a precondition to treatment. Section 13(5), however, can give rise to a number of difficulties.

> What does it mean to say that 'account has been taken' of the future child's welfare and that 'of a child who may be affected by the birth'? What must be shown in order to demonstrate that the statutory duty has been discharged? This gives rise to the additional difficulty, not addressed by the Act, of who takes account, and what is to happen if services are provided in breach of the duty. Similarly, the Act itself is silent on who may have *locus standi* . . . to challenge the account which has been taken and the conclusions arrived at.[77]

When the debate on artificial reproduction first started, academics and lawyers alike were all extremely apprehensive about the unknown and colossal legal implications of these techniques. The potential legal quagmire was, and still is, difficult to fathom. With all the possible genetic permutations in artificial reproduction, who are the parents of a resulting child? What about birth registration and the child's right to know? What about the parents' right to privacy and confidentiality of medical records? How about the child's right of inheritance? What about disposal of frozen embryos after the death of the infertile couple? What about their use after the death of the husband and the rule against perpetuity? These are all questions which need to be resolved to provide some certainty for those who are likely to be affected by artificial reproductive techniques. Thus far, consideration has been given to the moral and social arguments and issues which are inevitably linked to artificial reproductive techniques. In the next chapter, attention will focus on some of the immediate legal issues which these techniques engender.

NOTES

1 See generally, *Human Procreation, Ethical Aspects of the New Techniques, Report of a Working Party Council for Science and Society*, Oxford, Oxford University Press, 1984 (hereinafter cited as *Human Procreation*, CSS, 1984).

2 The question of the use of these techniques in surrogacy arrangements poses additional problems. This question is, therefore, considered separately, see Chapter 6.

3 See generally Singer, P. and Wells, D., *The Reproduction Revolution*, Oxford, Oxford University Press, 1984.

4 See the Vatican's disapproval of artificial reproductive techniques, *The Times*, 11 March, 1987, p. 3.

5 A theory which owed much to Aristotle and the Stoics. See Singer, P. and Wells, D., op. cit., pp. 39–41.

6 See *Report of the Committee of Inquiry into Human Fertilisation and Embryology*, London, HMSO, Cmnd. 9314, 1984, paras. 4.3 and 5.6 (hereinafter cited as *The Warnock Report*). See also the Vatican's rulings on the impropriety of artificial reproductive techniques, *The Guardian*, 11 March, 1987.

7 See Blustein, Jeffery, *Parents and Children: The Ethics of the Family*, Oxford, Oxford University Press, 1982, pp. 233–6; Cohen, Carl, 'Sex, birth control, and human life', in Baker, Robert and Elliston, Frederick (eds), *Philosophy and Sex*, New York, Prometheus Books, 1975, p. 150; Pope Paul vi, 'Humane Vitae', in *Philosophy and Sex*, op. cit., p. 131.

8 Singer, P. and Wells, D., op, cit., pp. 40–1.

9 See O'Donovan, Oliver, *Begotten or Made?*, Oxford, Clarendon Press, 1984, pp. 17–18.

10 Nor is it true that it is necessarily less meaningful. '[F]ertilisation achieved outside the bodies of the couple remains by this very fact deprived of the meanings and the values which are expressed in the language of the body'; see Vatican's ruling against artificial reproductive techniques, *The Times*, 11 March, 1987, p. 3.

11 See Mill, John Stuart, 'On Liberty', in Feinburg, Joel and Cross, Hyman (eds), *Philosophy & Law*, California, Wadsworth (2nd edn.), 1980, p. 180.

12 See Johnstone, Brian, 'The moral status of the embryo: two viewpoints', in Singer, Peter and Walters, William (eds), *Test-Tube Babies, A Guide to Moral Questions, Present Techniques and Future Possibilities*, Oxford, Oxford University Press, 1984, pp. 49–56.

13 See generally *The Warnock Report* and Harris, John, '*In vitro* fertilisation: the ethical issue', *Philosophical Quarterly*, (1983) **33**, p. 217. For a brief survey of the debates on embryo experimentation, see *The Warnock Report*; Warnock, Mary, 'Absolutely Wrong', *The Times*, 30 May, 1985; 'Why Warnock is wrong', *The Times*, 6 June, 1985; Editorial, *The Times*, 13 Febuary, 1985; 'The birthright that science deserves to lose', *The Guardian*, 6 June, 1985; *The Guardian*, 16 October, 1985.

14 *Vide supra*.

15 The Unborn Children (Protection) Bill, Session 1984–5, H.C. Bill No. 23, and the Unborn Children (Protection) (No. 2) Bill, Session 1985–6, H.C. Bill No. 220.

16   Clause 1(1) states, 'Except with the authorisation of the Secretary of State under this Act, no person shall. . . procure the fertilisation of a human ovum in vitro. . .'. Clause 1(2) says that authorisation is allowed only for an IVF procedure to be carried out for the purposes of enabling a specific woman to bear a child.

17   *Vide infra.*

18   See Govier, Trudy, 'What's wrong with slippery slope arguments?', *Canadian Journal of Philosophy* (1982) **12**, p. 303.

19   Ramsey, Paul, 'Shall we reproduce?', 'Rejoinder and future forecast', *Journal of the American Medical Association* (1972) **220**, pp. 1480, 1481.

20   *Vide supra*, Chapter 3.

21   See *The Warnock Report*, para. 13.3.

22   See *Voluntary Licensing Authority for Human In Vitro Fertilisation and Embryology; First, Second and Third Report*, London, Medical Research Council/Royal College of Obstetricians and Gynaecologists, 1986, 1987 and 1988.

23   For a detailed discussion of the ACT, see Morgan, Derek and Lee, Robert G., *Blackstone's Guide to the Human Fertilisation and Embryology Act 1990*, London, Blackstone Press Limited, 1990.

24   The statutory authority will take over the work of the Interim Licensing Authority, see ss 5–10.

25   See *The Warnock Report*, para. 4.10.

26   See, for example, in 1949, Pope Pius xii condemned AI as immoral. '. . . Artificial insemination in marriage, but produced by the active element of a third party, is equally immoral. . . . The husband and the wife have alone reciprocal right over their bodies in order to engender new life. . . .' See Finegold, Wilfred J., *Artificial Insemination*, Springfield, Illinois, Charles C. Thomas, 1964, p. 78.

27   In 1945, a Commission set up by the Archbishop of Canterbury to consider the practice of human artificial insemination concluded by majority that '. . . the act both of a married donor, and a married recipient constitute adultery'. According to the Commission, adultery involved the surrender of either reproductive powers or organs of generation whether capable of actual generation or not. The Report was published in 1948, and reprinted in 1952 by S.P.C.K. under the title *Artificial Human Insemination*, p. 37.

28   See *The Warnock Report*, para. 4.10.

29   *Vide supra*, Chapter 2.

30   Ibid.

31   *MacLennan* v. *MacLennan*, (1958) S.C. 105. *Vide infra*, Chapter 5.

32   *Vide infra*, Chapter 5.

33   *Vide supra*, Chapter 3 on marital privacy.

34   See *Legislation on Human Infertility Services and Embryo Research – A Consultation Paper*, HMSO, London, Cm. 46, 1986, para. 25 (hereinafter cited as the *Consultation Paper*); see now S13(6) of the Human Fertilisation and Embryology Act 1990.

35   Hugh Lafollette argues that for the protection of children, the state should require all parents to be licensed. By implication, the so-called right to have children and to rear children is not an unqualified right, and it is conditional on parents being able to demonstrate that they can meet certain minimal standards of child rearing; that they would not be likely to abuse or neglect their children and would be able to provide for the basic needs of the children. He argues that by analogy with adoption, 'our moral and legal systems already recognise that not everyone is capable of rearing children well. In fact, well-entrenched laws require adoptive parents to be investigated – in much the same ways and for much the same reasons as in the general licensing program advocated here'. See Lafollette, Hugh, 'Licensing parents', **9** *Philosophy and Public Affairs* (1980) 182, p.

193; Frisch, Lawrence E., 'On Licentious Licensing: A reply to Hugh Lafollette' and Lafollette, Hugh, 'A reply to Frisch', **10** *Philosophy and Public Affairs* (1981), pp. 175 and 181.

36 On the question of eligibility and surrogacy, *vide infra*.

37 Arguably the current anomaly between biological procreation and parenting without public scrutiny as opposed to in-depth investigation of prospective adoptive parents is based on a perceived difference between the nature of the rights in question.

38 See pp. 55–63 and Chapters 5–7.

39 See Somerville, Margaret A., 'Birth technology, parenting and "deviance"', *International Journal of Law and Psychiatry* (1982) **5** p. 123.

40 See Note 57.

41 See *Thake* v. *Maurice*, [1984] 2 All ER 513, p. 516; Peter Pain, J. loc. cit.

42 Somerville, op. cit.

43 The counter argument which may be put forward is that whether a person has no right to parenting depends on positive proof of incompetence to undertake the task. For the justification in differentiating natural parenthood and parenthood through the use of birth technology, see above.

44 See Chapter 8.

45 Para. 2.11. In the UK, there appears to be no uniformity of practice; thus St Mary Hospital's IVF Unit offers treatment to couples who have been living together for at least three years, whilst the IVF Unit at King's has no policy regarding the patient's relationships although where the relationship, or the lack of it, may present a problem, the case will be considered on an individual basis.

46 In the Act, the term 'a married woman' includes a woman who is 'living with a man as his wife on a *bona fide* domestic basis although not married to him'. See S3(2) (a)(i).

47 Golombok, Susan and Rust, John, 'The Warnock Report and single women: what about the children?' *Journal of Medical Ethics* (1988) **12**, pp. 182–6.

48 Ibid., p. 183.

49 See the similar view of Hanscombe, Gillian, 'The right to lesbian parenthood', *Journal of Medical Ethics* (1983) **9**, p. 33; see also Higgs, Roger, 'Lesbian couples: should help extend to AID?', *Journal of Medical Ethics* (1978) **4**, p. 91.

50 IVF Unit, St Mary Hospital, Manchester.

51 IVF Unit, King's Hospital, London.

52 *R.* v. *Ethical Committee of St Mary Hospital, ex parte Harriott, Family Law* (1988), p. 165.

53 *The Warnock Report* considered the question of eligibility and concluded that it is 'a very difficult one'. It believed that 'hard and fast rules are not applicable to its solution'. It said

> We recognise that this will place a heavy burden of responsibility on the individual consultant who must make social judgements that go beyond the purely medical. . . . We considered whether it was possible for us to set out the wider social criteria that consultants, together with their professional colleagues, should use in deciding whether infertility treatment should be provided for a particular patients. We decided it was not possible to draw up comprehensive criteria that would be sensitive to the circumstances of every case. We recommended that in cases where consultants decline to provide treatment they should always give the patient a full explanation of the reasons.

para. 2.12.

54 *Artificial Insemination*, explanatory information booklet to parents, London, RCOG, 1979.

55 See Snowden, R.S. and Mitchell, G.D., *The Artificial Family*, London, Unwin Paperbacks, 1981, pp. 82–5.
56 See *Human Procreation*, CSS, 1984, p. 47, 244.
57 See generally, Liu, A.N.C., 'Wrongful life: some of the problems', *Journal of Medical Ethics* (1987) **13**, p. 69.
58 See *Zepeda* v. *Zepeda* 41 Ill App. 2d 240; *Williams* v. *State of New York* 18 NY 2d 481 (1966); *McKay* v. *Essex Area Health Authority* [1982] 2 All ER 771.
59 *Vide infra.*
60 See Snowden, R. and Mitchell, G.D., *Artificial Reproduction: A Social Investigation*, Allen & Unwin, London, 1983, p. 106.
61 Snowden, R. and Mitchell, G.D., op. cit. *Artificial Reproduction: a Social Investigation*, pp. 97–123.
62 Ibid.
63 Clinical research suggests that in early adolescence, a genealogically bewildered child (that is, a child who either has no knowledge or only uncertain knowledge of one or both of his natural parents) will often begin searching for clues about his or her unknown parents from every direct or indirect shred of evidence. This sometimes amounts to an obsession. Genealogical deprivation may affect a child's sense of self-image, identity, belonging and security. The need to know one's biological origin is confirmed by a number of studies. See, for example, Sants, H.J., 'Genealogical bewilderment in children with substitute parents', in *Child Adoption*, Association of British Adoption and Fostering Agencies, London, p. 69. See McWhinnie, A.M., 'Who am I?', in *Child Adoption*, op. cit., p. 104.
64 See Sections 26 and 27 of the Children Act 1975. See generally, Cretney, S.M., *Principles of Family Law* (4th edn.), London, Sweet & Maxwell, 1984, pp. 473–5.
65 This provision was first made in Section 11 of the Adoption of Children (Scotland) Act 1930, now Section 45 of the Adoption (Scotland) Act 1978 and schedule 10, para. 20 of the Children Act 1989.
66 See *The Warnock Report*, para. 4.21.
67 The experience in Sweden suggest that fears of reductions in the frequency of semen donation prove to be groundless; see *Surrogate Motherhood, Report of the Board of Science and Education*, London, BMA, 1987, p. 19. The unpublished survey of Robyn Rowland in Victoria, Australia, also supports this conclusion, see Singer, P. and Wells, D., op. cit., pp. 74–5.
68 See the *Consultation Paper*, para. 25.
69 See *Hansard*, H.L., Vol. 516, Col. 787–804. The move was defeated by 61 to 60 votes.
70 Ibid., Lady Saltoun of Abernethy, Col. 788.
71 Ibid., Lord Ennals, Col. 789.
72 Ibid., Col. 791.
73 Ibid., Col. 796.
74 Ibid., Col. 800.
75 Ibid., per Lord Prys-Davis at Col. 1102.
76 Ibid., Col. 1106.
77 Morgan, Derek and Lee, Robert G., *Blackstone's Guide to the Human Fertilisation and Embryology Act 1990 – Abortion and Embryo Research – The New Law*, London, Blackstone Press Limited, 1990, p. 145.

5 Legal Issues in Founding a Family by Artificial Techniques

INTRODUCTION

There are a number of legal issues relating to the founding of a family by artificial reproductive techniques. For instance, what is the effect of artificial techniques on a marriage? Does the use of donated gametes constitute adultery in law? As will be seen, these issues are relatively unambiguous today. Issues concerning the legal status of children born as a result of artificial techniques are less exigent today.[1] The reason for this is that the policy of recent law has been to remove, as far as possible, the legal disadvantages pertaining to children born out of wedlock. In England and Wales, this has been effected by the Family Law Reform Act 1987 (FLRA) and, in Scotland, by the Law Reform (Parent and Child) Act (Scotland) 1986 (LRPCA 1986).[2]

Nonetheless, the question of parenthood is still pertinent in the context of founding a family through the use of artificial techniques. On the one hand, the traditional concept of parenthood cannot satisfactorily be applied to artificial reproductive methods.[3] On the other, since individuals resorting to artificial reproductive methods for the founding of a family are deliberately bringing children into the world for parenting, it is pertinent to ask, at least, who ought to have parental duties regarding such children.[4] The issue of parenthood and registration of birth engendered by the use of artificial techniques will be explored, and proposed solutions will be examined, in this chapter. Since these questions have been considered by *The Warnock Report*,[5] and its recommendations were intended to be applicable throughout the UK,[6] their recommendations and the Human Fertilisation and Embryology Act 1990 (HFEA) will be considered.

LEGAL ISSUES RELATING TO FOUNDING A FAMILY BY ARTIFICIAL REPRODUCTIVE TECHNIQUES[7]

Artificial Reproductive Techniques and Their Effect on Marriage

The legal effects of artificial reproduction (whether involving the use of donated gametes or not) on a marriage are relatively non-controversial today.[8] Nonetheless, it is worthwhile to mention them briefly, since they clearly concern founding a family and marriage. For instance, does AI amount to consummation of a marriage? Does it bar a decree of nullity? Is AID adultery? Although these issues are usually considered in relation to AI, and AID, and the following discussion will be conducted mainly in those terms, they have equal applications to IVF, and the use of donated gametes in general.

Consummation of Marriage

One legal issue raised in connection with AI is the question whether or not it constitutes consummation of a marriage. In both English and Scots law, what is required to establish consummation of a marriage is intercourse which is 'ordinary and complete' and not 'imperfect and unnatural'.[9] It follows from this definition that there is a clear distinction between consummation and conception. The former is achieved by sexual intercourse.[10] AI, therefore, cannot amount to consummation of a marriage. A number of English cases have considered this now settled legal issue.

In *R.E.L. (otherwise R.)* v. *E.L.*[11] a decree of nullity was granted on the ground of the husband's sexual incapacity, even though a child was born as a result of AIH. There was no consummation of the marriage.[12] Again, in *Slater* v. *Slater*,[13] AID was not considered to constitute consummation of a marriage. This was assumed in *Q* v. *Q*.[14] In the Scottish case of *A.B.* v. *C.B.*, [15] there was no question that AIH constituted consummation of a marriage. Equally, therefore, IVF cannot in itself constitute consummation of a marriage.

Approbation of Marriage

Since AI or IVF cannot amount to consummation of a marriage, can they amount to approbation of a marriage, barring a decree of nullity?

The essence of the doctrine of approbation of marriage in both English and Scottish law has been explained in the following terms:[16]

> . . . that in a suit for the nullity of marriage, there may be facts and circumstances proved which so plainly imply, on the part of the complaining spouse, a recognition of the existence and validity of the

marriage, as to render it most inequitable and contrary to public policy that he or she should be permitted to go on and challenge it with effect.

In England and Wales, the doctrine is now contained in Section 13(1) of the Matrimonial Causes Act, 1973, which provides that,[17]

The court shall not . . . grant a decree of nullity on the ground that the marriage is voidable if the respondent satisfies the court:

(a)   that the petitioner, with knowledge that it was open to him to have the marriage avoided, so conducted himself in relation to the respondent as to lead the respondent reasonably to believe that he would not seek to do so; and

(b)   that it would be unjust to the respondent to grant the decree.

First, Section 13(1) puts the burden of proof on the respondent to satisfy the court that the conditions in the section are fulfilled. Second, the petitioner's conduct can only be a bar to nullity if he or she knew at the time that it was open to him or her to obtain the relief. In *W. v. W.*,[18] the marriage was not consummated owing to the incapacity of the wife. The couple adopted a child. Later, the husband petitioned for a decree of nullity. The Court of Appeal set aside the decree, holding that the marriage had been approbated. The Court held that although there was no issue that the husband knew of his remedy in nullity at the date of the adoption, he must be taken to have known of such remedy having regard to all the facts and circumstances of the case.[19]

W. v. W. was distinguished in *Slater* v. *Slater*.[20] In that case, the Court of Appeal held that neither during the time of AID, nor at the date of the adoption of the child did the wife have knowledge of her remedy in nullity. Therefore, neither of these events amounted to approbation of the marriage by the wife. A decree of nullity was granted to her. Again, in *Q. v. Q.*,[21] it was held that the fact that the wife had given birth to a child as a result of AID did not amount to approbation of the marriage by her, since at the time of receiving AID, she had no knowledge of the legal remedy open to her as a result of the husband's incapacity; a degree of nullity was thus granted.

The third requirement of Section 13 is that it would be unjust to the respondent to grant the nullity decree. For instance, in *D. v. D.*,[22] the parties adopted two children at a time when the husband knew that he could have the marriage annulled on the ground of the wife's wilful refusal to consummate the marriage. Justice Dunn held that the case was even stronger than that of *W. v. W.* because the husband knew of his remedy. However, a decree of nullity was granted because, in this case, there was no injustice to the wife in doing so.

In Scotland, as in England, an action for nullity on the ground of impotence may be barred if it is shown that the pursuer has, with full knowledge of the fact and the law, approbated the contract, or taken advantages and derived benefits from the matrimonial relationship which it would be inequitable to permit him or her to treat as if it had never existed.[23]

Thus, in the case of *A.B.* v. *C.B.*,[24] a husband's action for nullity on the ground of the wife's impotence was dismissed. It was held that the husband had, with full knowledge of the facts and the law, approbated the marriage by cooperating in the wife's AIH, and agreeing to adopt a child.

In sum, although the doctrine of approbation in Scots and English law is slightly different, a UK court may refuse to grant a decree of nullity on the ground that the conduct of a spouse, in submitting to AI or IVF, has been such as to approbate the marriage. Each case, thus, depends very much on its own facts.

Adultery

One well-discussed legal issue in relation to AI is whether AID amounts to adultery.[25] In English law, the elements of adultery are clear. There must be voluntary or consensual sexual intercourse between a married person and a person (whether married or unmarried) of the opposite sex, not being the other's spouse.[26] In this context, some penetration, however slight, suffices.[27] Consequently, in English law, AID should, and would, almost certainly not be considered as adultery, although this point has never been directly examined by an English court.

In Scots law, AID is not adultery. This was decided in the case of *MacLennan* v. *MacLennan*,[28] where a husband petitioned for divorce on the ground that his wife had committed adultery. The wife denied adultery and explained that her child was born as a result of AID. The husband contended that this defence was irrelevant because AID without the consent of the husband amounted to adultery in law. It was held that AID did not constitute adultery whether it was undertaken with or without the husband's consent.

Lord Wheatley came to this conclusion after holding that, for there to be adultery in a legal sense, there must be two parties of the opposite sex engaging in a sexual act involving some degree of penetration. Consequently, AID cannot amount to adultery.

The decision in *MacLennan* is consistent with English law on the legal requirements necessary to establish adultery. From the point of view of common sense, as has been argued, it is sensible to distinguish between adultery on the one hand, and the use of donated semen in AI (AID) for the founding of a family, on the other.[29] These are acts of an entirely different nature, and they have different intentions and intended consequences. Moreover, it would be implausible to argue that where a married couple resort to IVF which involves the use of donated semen, the wife is committing adultery. An interesting point in this context is that there has been no suggestion that ovum donation is adultery, even though some regard the surrendering of one's reproductive powers as sufficient to amount to adultery.[30]

Currently, the question as to whether donation and use of donated gametes amounts to adultery is largely academic. Section 1 of the Divorce Law Reform Act 1969 (applicable to England and Wales) and Section 1 of the Divorce (Scotland) Act 1976 have made irretrievable breakdown of a marriage the sole ground for divorce.[31] Arguably, the conduct of a wife who undertakes AI without the consent of the husband, or that of a husband who donates semen without the consent of his wife, may be treated as behaviour or conduct evidencing breakdown of the marriage, and thus allowing a spouse to obtain a divorce. However, the fact that divorce may be available is insufficient to challenge the techniques themselves. If divorce is available in these circumstances, this is because of the manner in which the techniques were used and not due to the nature of the techniques themselves.

In the preceding section, the legal effects of AI, IVF and the use of donated gametes on a marriage have been considered. Consideration has been brief since they are now relatively settled and non-controversial issues. One may conclude that AI or IVF cannot amount to consummation of marriage. Further, whether AI or IVF may or may not amount to approbation of a marriage is a question of fact in each case. Finally, donation and use of donated semen for the founding of a family cannot amount to adultery on the part of either a recipient or a donor in Scots law. This is also the case in English law. However, the issue is largely otiose today since a divorce can be obtained by proving certain facts other than adultery. Consideration of these problems, therefore, may not any longer be the crucial focus of legal debate. However, a much more complex and potentially far-reaching area requires elaboration – that is, the question of parenthood. In the following section, the issue of parenthood in artificial techniques will be explored.

Parenthood and Artificial Reproductive Techniques: AI and IVF

The HFEA has finally made provisions on fatherhood and motherhood. However, the background leading up to these provisions and some of the unsaid assumptions need to be made explicit.

The complexities of interpersonal relationships and legal standing following the use of artificial reproductive techniques are such that some explanation is required of the way in which certain terms will be used. In the following discussion, 'parent', 'mother' and 'father' are terms used to denote a legal relationship between an adult and a child. The undernoted terms, however, are purely descriptive. 'Biological mother/father' refers to a woman/man who contributes an ovum/semen to the creation of a child. 'Ovum/semen donor' refers to a biological mother/father who donates her or his genetic gametes. 'Social mother/father' refers to a woman/man who intends to rear a child, regardless of her or his genetic link with the child.

In natural reproduction, the biological mother and father of a child, who are almost invariably also the social mother and father, are regarded by the law as parents. Both English and Scots law attribute to them parental duties (as opposed to parental rights)[32] regarding the child. Thus, it has been said that the existing English (and Scottish) definition of parenthood is based on genetics.[33] This mode of attributing parental duties, using genetic factors will hereinafter be called the *genetic mode*. Although the use of the genetic mode in natural reproduction for the attribution of fatherhood is not disputed, whether this is also the real basis for motherhood can be questioned. This, nonetheless, does not affect the argument in this chapter.[34]

In cases where people resort to artificial reproduction (AI and IVF) to reproduce and found a family[35] (that is, where neither donated gametes nor surrogacy is employed), there is no doubt that the genetic mode applies. This is so because the only difference between artificial and natural reproduction here is the way in which a child is conceived. The marital status of a person using AI or IVF is irrelevant; just as in natural reproduction, an unmarried couple who procreate will be the parents of the child. Therefore, if a male partner uses his semen to inseminate artificially his female partner, they are, and should be, regarded as parents of the resulting child, and consequently, they should have parental duties regarding the child. However, since the child may be born out of wedlock, the father's rights regarding the child differ from that of a married father.[36]

Where donated gametes (semen and/or ovum) are used in artificial reproduction, whether in AI or IVF, the obvious question is, who is the mother and/or father of a resulting child? Can the genetic mode be applied here satisfactorily?

Since fatherhood is often discussed in the context of semen donation and its use in AI (AID), this will be examined first. The principle which applies there will be equally applicable to IVF where donated semen is used. The question of motherhood in the case of a donated ovum will subsequently be analysed.

Semen Donation and Fatherhood

Where, for example, a husband is sterile and the wife receives AID, the unsatisfactory nature of using the genetic mode to attribute fatherhood is apparent. Until recently, English law regarded a semen donor as the father of the resulting AID child. Such a child was in the same position as that of a child conceived outside marriage. As a matter of legal theory, as the English Law Commission pointed out,[37] the donor might be liable as the child's father to maintain the child, and might indeed apply for access or custody.[38] As a corollary, the husband would have no parental rights or duties regarding the child. The social reality, however, was different. Because of the practice of keeping a donor's identity anonymous, neither the child nor the mother would be able to trace the donor. Hence, they would not be able to enforce any liability to maintain. The donor would know nothing about the child, and he would therefore not be in a position to seek access or custody. For the same reason, it was unlikely that any intestate succession rights existing between the donor and the child would have any effect. Even if the marriage between the husband and wife broke up, the husband would have treated the child as a child of the family and would thus effectively be under the same financial obligations to the child as if he or she were the husband's legitimate child.

This division between the law and social reality was caused by the inadequacies of present British law in dealing with the social reality of AID. In other words, there was no legal provision which recognized the legal rights and duties of a social father (the husband, as in the above case), and excluded a semen donor from having legal rights and duties regarding an AID child. If an AID child was to be given protection and standing, as near as possible to the equivalent of those children conceived by natural means, then the division between the law and reality would have to be resolved.[39]

Legal reform was effected by Section 27(1) of the FLRA 1987[40] which, accepting the Law Commission's recommendation,[41] says:[42]

(1) Where after the coming into force of this section a child is born in England & Wales as the result of the artificial insemination of a woman who (a) was at the time of the insemination a party to a marriage (being a marriage which had not at that time been dissolved or annulled); and (b) was artificially inseminated with the semen of some person other than the other party to that marriage, then, unless it is proved to the satisfaction of any court by which the matter has to be determined that the other party to that marriage did not consent to the insemination, the child shall be treated in law as the child of the parties to that marriage and shall not be treated as the child of any person other than the parties to that marriage.

This provision (which will hereinafter be called the *AID provision* and is sometimes called the 'deeming provision')[43] clearly reflects the wishes and intentions of both the semen donor and the married couple who resort to AID in order to found a family. A semen donor's intention is to help another to have a child, and he intends that his part in procreation ends with the donation, and does not extend to parenting, nor to the responsibilities and legal duties which are associated with it. Conversely, the intention of the married couple is that the husband will undertake parental rights and duties regarding the resulting child. The rationale (which will hereinafter be called the *donation rationale*) underlying the AID provision, therefore, is to recognize and acknowledge the reality of semen donation and its use (at least within marriage)[44] by presuming a husband to be the father of an AID child where his wife undertakes AID and by attributing to him parental duties (and rights). The corollary to the donation rationale is that a semen donor should have no rights or liabilities regarding an AID child (this will hereinafter be called the *corollary provision*).

The AID provision essentially represents an exception to the genetic mode, which is the general basis for attributing fatherhood, so as to reflect the reality of semen donation and its use. If the donation rationale is to achieve its real objectives, then a clear definition as to what amounts to gamete donation is necessary.[45] Otherwise, the wishes of the parties will be thwarted rather than promoted.

One point to be noted is that Section 27 is not retroactive in that it applies only to children born after the coming into force of the provision. A better approach might have been to give Section 27 retroactive effect in which case the legal status of all AID children could have been regularized to conform with the *de facto* situation of many such children. Since Section 27 applies only to England and Wales and there is no comparable Scottish provision, the place of birth of the child is significant (see later for Section 28 of the HFEA).

The Unmarried Couple

So far the discussion has concentrated on married couples. What is the position of those unmarried people who may resort to AID, given that the right to reproduce and the right to found a family are rights of an individual (irrespective of one's marital status)?[46]

The Law Commission did not consider this issue in full. It merely said,[47]

> Where the woman undergoing AID is living in a stable union with a man who is not her husband (whether she is herself married or not), the question whether that man should be permitted to become father of the AID child by consenting to the treatment raises complex issues

relating to the rights of unmarried cohabiting couples, which are
outside the scope of this Report.

Since neither *The Law Commission Report*, nor *The Warnock Report* has
considered this, the issue is an open one.

If one considers the situation as exemplified by the Law Commission – that is, where an unmarried couple resort to AID, one may
argue that if the law and society may legitimately disapprove of the
unmarried using AID – the conclusion in the preceding section that
the law should reflect the reality of AID may not apply with equal
force.

If, as the Law Commission suggested, it was unclear whether a
male cohabiting partner could be permitted to become the father of an
AID child, presumably the semen donor would be treated as the
father. Yet, it will evidently be unfair to hold a semen donor liable to
an AID child solely because a recipient woman is unmarried. Nor
would it be fair to hold him liable to an AID child because a medical
blunder has resulted in his semen being used for the artificial
insemination of an unmarried woman.

According to an intuitive understanding of what is entailed in
semen donation, as expressed by the donation rationale, the
unmarried male partner should be regarded as father of an AID child
if he consents to his partner undertaking AID, just as in the case
where a husband consents to his wife's AID. According fatherhood
to such a person does not mean that he will have the same rights
regarding the child as a married father.[48] He will, however, at least,
have parental duties regarding the child, and a semen donor will be
excluded from having rights or duties in respect of the child.

The Warnock Report clearly envisaged the availability of AID to an
unmarried couple in a stable union and not simply to married
couples.[49] The HFEA sets no limit to restrict infertility treatment only
to the married. If an AID child is not to be left in a legal vacuum,
where his or her legal father is not his or her social father, then the
existence or otherwise of a legal marriage should not be permitted to
affect the child's rights and expectations. In other words, extending
the AID provision to the unmarried will be in the best interests of the
child in that the legal mechanism which is thought to be appropriate
for determining fatherhood in an AID child born to a married couple
applies equally to an AID child born to the unmarried (see later
Section 28 of the HFEA).[50]

At the moment, Section 27 FLRA 1987 does not apply to the
unmarried and the position is that an AID child born to them will be
illegitimate. The argument is that a man should be regarded as the
father of an AID child if he consents to his partner's AID. Thus, the
AID provision should be extended to unmarried couples as well as to

married couples. This approach is taken in New South Wales and Victoria which provide that if a child is born to a married woman as a result of artificial insemination and if the semen used was not produced by her husband but the insemination was done with his consent, the husband shall be presumed for all purposes to have caused the pregnancy and to be the father of the child.[51] Similar provisions can also be found in South Australia and Western Australia.[52] All these statutes cover *de facto* spouses.[53]

Extending the AID provision to unmarried men does not necessarily have to be interpreted as an encouragement to the use of AID by the unmarried. After all, as will be seen,[54] *The Warnock Report* recommendations in respect of motherhood where a donated ovum is used made no distinction on the basis of the marital status of a woman. It merely tackles the undesirabilities of legislative inaction, which the law and society recognize and acknowledge. As past experience has demonstrated, the use of AID was not curbed or restrained despite the division between the legal theory of fatherhood and social reality.

The implication of the AID provision, and its proposed extension to the unmarried, is that before an AID child could be rendered 'fatherless', proof would be needed to establish that a husband or male partner did not consent to a woman's AID. In other words, this presumption of consent would render a child fatherless in some situations, for example, where AID is undertaken by a woman without the consent of her male partner.

Ovum Donation and Motherhood

The Warnock Report recommended that when a child is born to a woman following donation of another's egg, the woman giving birth should, for all purposes, be regarded in law as the mother of the child, and the egg donor should have no rights or obligations in respect of the child.[55] This would be the case regardless of a woman's marital status. This approach is widely accepted, and is apparently an application of the donation rationale, although as will be seen later, the real basis for motherhood may not be the genetic mode.[56] Section 27 of the HFEA gives effect to this approach; it says that a woman who is carrying or has carried a child is the mother regardless of her genetic connection with the child.

Embryo Donation

Once the question of parenthood regarding donated gametes is resolved according to the donation rationale and the corollary principle, parenthood in respect of a donated embryo is not complicated. Thus, *The Warnock Report* recommended that where a child is born to a married couple following embryo donation, the husband and the wife will be the parents.[57] In a case where a woman is unmarried, she will be the mother.[58] However, *The Warnock Report* did not consider who would be the father.[59]

Arguably, the man (if there is one) who consents to the mother having the embryo inserted in her womb should be regarded as the father, as this is similar to a man who consents to a woman undertaking AID.[60] In other words, the marital status of the parties should, as argued before, be regarded as unimportant for the purpose of parenthood (see later for Section 28 of the HFEA).[61]

Legal Provisions for Parenthood

[T]he question of status and parentage bears directly on a wide spectrum of legal rights and obligations respecting all parties involved, including support rights . . . and succession rights. And in turn, these legal consequences affect the social and psychological stability of the child, both in its family and in society . . .[62]

The question of parenthood in artificial reproduction presents a complex challenge for the law. The traditional mode of according parenthood does not deal with the intentions of the parties involved in artificial reproduction, which in such cases become crucial. Specific legislation tackling comprehensively the question of parenthood merely confronts the problems, which the law and society recognize and acknowledge following the use of gamete donation. The effective resolution of the question is desirable since it will provide legal certainty for the determination of parenthood for children born both through natural and artificial reproduction. The approaches suggested in this chapter in relation to children born through artificial reproductive techniques accord with our intuitive understanding of the nature of gamete donation and its use; they also reflect an individual's responsibility in founding a family through artificial techniques.

For the purpose of this discussion, adequate resolution of the question of parenthood in artificial reproductive techniques – to remove the potential legal handicaps a child born as a result may face – may be significant for reasons other than mere pragmatism. For instance, it might be argued that the deliberate creation of a child whose position is subject to legal and social discrepancies and is inferior to that of a child conceived naturally, may render the use of artificial reproductive techniques socially and morally unacceptable.

The argument being that the rights of the infertile have less significance than the rights or interests of children.

However, what is contended here is that a comprehensive resolution of the question of parenthood in artificial techniques, thus removing the discrepancies between the law and social reality regarding parenthood for a resulting child, is ideologically consistent with the assertion of the rights of the infertile. Thus, although concerns about the legal position of a child born as a result of artificial techniques may have weight, their resolution can be affected without interfering with the rights of the infertile.

The legal uncertainties resulting from lack of legal consideration directed specifically at artificial reproduction has been partially confronted by Section 27 of the FLRA 1987. Section 27 is however a limited stop gap measure. The Human Fertilisation and Embryology Bill 1989 goes a little further in dealing with the question of status. It will apply to England and Wales, Scotland and Northern Ireland. The sections on status (27–9) are not retroactive, and 'shall have effect only in relation to children carried by women as a result of the placing in them embryos or of sperm and eggs, or of their artificial insemination (as the case may be), after the commencement of those sections'.[63] Further, when those sections come into force, Section 27 of the FLRA 1987 will have no effect.

The HFEA provides a much more comprehensive approach to the question of parenthood. On the question of maternity of children born as a result of assisted reproduction, Section 27(1) says that,

> A woman who has carried a child as a result of the placing in her of an embryo or of sperm and eggs, and no other woman, is to be treated as the mother of the child.

This covers the procedures of AI, IVF and GIFT and thus settles the question of motherhood irrespective of marital status.

On the question of paternity, the effect of Section 28 is to make the husband of a woman who undergoes assisted reproductive methods – whether it is AID, IVF or GIFT with donated semen – father of the resulting child, unless it is shown that he did not consent to her treatment. Further, that the semen donor will not be treated as the father of the child.

Section 28 in effect extends the AID deeming provision in Section 27 of the FLRA 1987 to all other reproductive techniques, so that the question of fatherhood can only be rebutted if the husband can show that he did not consent. At one stage it was suggested that Clause 27 (now Section 28) should make it clear that the husband must consent in writing to the wife's treatment before he would be treated as father of the resulting child. However as the Act makes clear that, where there is any doubt as to the husband's consent, this ambiguity is resolved in favour of the child to avoid hardship to the child. This approach, it was said, is in line with the common law presumption of paternity which protects a child born within marriage. In any event the practice is that the written consent of the husband is always procured before the wife undergoes treatment. Therefore the problem is likely to be academic. Unless we envisage wives resorting to do-it-yourself AID at home without the consent or knowledge of the husband, the deeming provision is unlikely to create much hardship in reality.[64]

Where it could be shown that the husband objected, then the resulting child will be fatherless. Section 28 goes one step further. An unmarried man who consents to his partner's infertility treatment under the HFEA becomes father of the resulting child. This is by virtue of Section 28(3). This provision therefore gives legal effect to the argument made earlier, that the AID principle and the corollary provision should extend to the unmarried and cover all artificial reproductive techniques. At the time of writing, Sections 27 and 28 are not in force. When the Sections come into force, Section 27 of the FLRA will be superseded.

In the preceding section, it has been argued that most techniques of artificial reproduction for the purposes of creating children part company with natural reproduction. The mode of ascribing parenthood therefore needs to be modified to cater for these novel means. The law now recognizes 'social parents' (as opposed to genetic parents) as legal parents. This approach however creates its own difficulties which will have to be considered. It is convenient to adopt the approach that a husband consenting to the wife's AID shall be regarded as father of the resulting child. Legal recognition of the husband as father will not only give the child the status of legitimacy but will also mean that the husband can register as the child's father. As a corollary, the semen donor who is most likely to be the genetic father of the child will not be registered as such.

Registration of Birth

The issue of birth registration is often regarded as problematic in relation to AID. Consequently, the following discussion will be conducted in that context, but it can have equal application to ovum and embryo donation.

Given that a semen donor should not, as argued above, be regarded in law as the father of a resulting child, should the social father be allowed to register as such?

Prior to any legal recognition of the status of the husband, the situation of AID was that both the mother and her husband would want the name of the latter to appear in the register as father of the child. But since the child's father was most likely to be unknown, in declaring that the husband was the child's father, one might contravene the Perjury Act 1911 which applied to England and Wales.[65] Section 4 of the Act provided that if any person wilfully made a false answer to any question put to him or her by a registrar relating to particulars required to be registered concerning a birth with intent to have it inserted in a register of birth, such person would be guilty of a misdemeanour.[66] In Scotland, Section 53(1) of the Registration of Births, Deaths and Marriages (Scotland) Act 1965 provided for a similar offence.

The AID provision arguably allows a husband to be registered as the father of a child who is born in England and Wales as a result of his wife undertaking AID without contravening Section 4 of the 1911 Act. One major drawback to this AID provision is that it involves a statutory authorization to falsify birth registration, since in reality the donor is most probably the father of the child.

Two alternatives which will avoid falsification of the birth register have been suggested. Annotation of the birth register canvasses the idea that a husband's consent to his wife receiving AID in a prescribed form should have to be produced to the registrar who would then make a special note in the register to indicate that the entry of the husband's name as that of the father is by virtue of the AID provision. Another alternative is to utilize some kind of adoption procedure.[67] Neither of these alternatives appeared to be popular. The government took the view that the consensus of opinion was that the husband should be allowed to be registered as the father, and that an AID child should have a birth certificate which concealed the circumstances of his or her conception.[68]

This approach has been adopted by the HFEA. In the course of parliamentary debates to the Bill, Lord Teviot moved an amendment that parties who take advantage of medical advance in reproductive techniques, and are conferred the status of parents by Clauses 27 and 28 should only be able to register their status as such providing that the birth certificate of the child was marked so that the entry could be traced to the provisions of the Bill.[69] As Lord Teviot put it:

> The present Bill allows for the birth of a child following AID or as a result of any one of many modern techniques to be registered as if that child were a normal legitimate child. That is so not only where the legal father is not the genetic father or the legal mother is not the genetic mother but also where neither the legal father nor the legal mother is the genetic parent of the child . . . The birth certificate of such a child should indicate in some way the fact that it is not the genetic child of its legal parents . . . If we do not do anything to mark the certificates we are in effect abandoning any real claim that our birth certificates and birth registers show genetic relationships.[70]

It was said that annotation of the birth certificate will also have the effect of pressuring the parents to tell the child the truth concerning its circumstances of conception. Where the legislature confers parenthood without requiring the appropriate annotation, the parents, it was argued, might be inclined to keep this fact secret and this would not be in accordance with the child's right to know.

This proposed amendment was rejected by the House. No annotation won the day; this was seen to be an approach which struck a balance between the interests of the child in tracing his genetic origins, privacy of family life and confidentiality of personal information. The effect of annotation, other than enhancing the child's right to know, is that it would become part of the public record open to all to inspect. Any well-informed individual seeing the person's birth certificate would know that that person had been born following assisted reproductive methods and that his parents had undergone treatment. This, it was thought, was contrary to personal privacy both from the couple's and the child's point of view. Furthermore, the question of confidentiality of medical information would also be compromised. Finally, Lord McKay rationalized the gist of the debate and said that too much had been made of the argument that a birth certificate contains truthful information about the actual circumstances of birth.

> [I]n many cases where infertility treatment is not involved, the information about the child's father on the birth record may not reflect the true genetic position. That can arise for a number of reasons; for example, the mother may not know who the child's father is . . . After all, the birth certificate is a record not a legal statement about the reality of who the child's father is.[71]

Right to Know?

The gap between the social and legal reality of parenthood is to a large extent closed by Sections 27 and 28 of the HFEA. Family privacy and confidentiality of medical records are now protected because the law does not require annotation of the birth certificates. The child's right to know is therefore now completely left with, and at the discretion of, the parents. This again is perceived as a question of family privacy. Where the child does not suspect his or her circumstances of conception, no question of tracing one's genetic origins arises. Where it does arise, Section 31 of the HFEA[72] provides a limited right to know.

The Bill provides that the Human Fertilisation and Embryology Authority (HUFEA) shall maintain a register of information supplied to it by clinics providing treatment services. Information required for record keeping includes: the provision of treatment services for any identifiable individual; the keeping or use of the gametes of any identifiable individuals or of an embryo taken from any identifiable woman; any identifiable individual who was or may have been born in consequence of treatment services.

Section 31(3) provides that a person who has attained the age of eighteen (the applicant) may apply to the authority requesting it to furnish certain information. If the authority is satisfied that the information contained in the register shows that the applicant was, or may have been, born in consequence of treatment services, and if the applicant has been given a suitable opportunity to receive proper counselling about the implications of receiving it, the authority is under a duty to furnish certain information. Actually what sort of information the authority is under a duty to disclose under Section 31(4) (a) is unclear. Both *The Warnock Report*[73] and the White Paper[74] favoured non-identifying information. Alternatively, the applicant may request the authority under Section 31(4) (b) to give notice stating whether he and a person specified in the request (as a person whom the applicant proposes to marry) would or might be related. Further, a minor intending to marry may also request the authority to state whether he and his intended spouse would or might be related. The authority is under a duty to do so provided that the information contained in the register shows that the minor was, or may have been, born in consequence of treatment services, and provided the minor has been given a suitable opportunity to receive proper counselling about the implications of compliance with the request.[75]

CONCLUSION

Although the question of parenthood is the major legal concern of most people involved in artificial reproduction, ancillary questions on inheritance rights of the children born as a result of artificial reproductive techniques have also attracted attention. Doubts arise as to whether, say, an AID child who is not the genetic child of the husband (H) can inherit if the disposition is framed in terms of 'to X and the heirs of H'. Strictly speaking the child falls outside the ambit of the will. The difficulty here, of course, is that without any specific inclusory or exclusory language it is difficult to ascertain what the testator's intention would have been had he or she known of the biological origins of the child in question. One approach is to see inheritance rights concomitant to status and parentage. It seems to fly in the face of common sense to provide an AID child and his social father with the status of parent–child without according the child the legal benefits flowing from that relationship. Therefore, it has been suggested that unless the contrary is expressed by the testator, a child born as a result of artificial conception should acquire inheritance rights to the estates of those persons who are his parents, and to the estates of others as if he were the natural child of such parents. There should also be reciprocity in relation to inheritance rights. The effect of this is to use the parent–child relationship to determine the reciprocal rights of a child born pursuant to one of the artificial reproductive techniques for the purpose of determining testate or intestate succession in accordance with the relevant law. Section 29 of the HFEA provides the answer to the above situation, but does not affect succession to any dignity or title of honour.

The legal issues pertaining to the use of artificial reproductive techniques ae numerous and those considered in this chapter are only some of the obvious and immediate ones the resolution of which will help to put the use of such techniques on a sound legal footing. But the survey and discussion in this chapter of all the legal problems associated with the use of artificial conceptive techniques is by no means exhaustive. A recent Tennessee case, involving a dispute between a couple over seven frozen embryos, revealed the divergent and polemic nature of some of the issues pertaining to these techniques. In that case, Judge Dale Young was asked to rule on the question of custody of the seven frozen embryos which were constituted by the gametes of a couple who had since divorced.[76]

The wife in the case asserted that she should be allowed to use them for future implantation for the purpose of having children, whilst the husband argued that nothing should happen to them without his consent (the judgement noted that the embryos could not be preserved for more than two years and that the husband 'strenuously objects to the anonymous donation of the human embryos even for their survival').[77]

The uniqueness and novelty of the case did not present any difficulty to the attorneys who argued it. Questions such as are embryos property or human? whose reproductive rights prevail? should the husband be 'forced' to have a child? were all explored. The Circuit Court Judge ruled that the embryos created through IVF were human life and not property. He said that

> . . . from fertilisation, the cells of a human embryo are differentiated, unique, and specialised to the highest degree of distinction . . . human embryos are not property . . . Human life begins at conception.[78]

He asked 'What then is the legal status to be accorded a human being existing as an embryo, *in vitro*, in a divorce case in the state of Tennessee?'[79] The court took the view that,

> The age-old common law doctrine of *parens patriae* controls these children, *in vitro*, as it has always supervised and controlled children of a marriage at live birth in domestic relations cases in Tennessee . . . In the case at bar, the undisputed, uncontroverted testimony is that to allow the parties seven cryogenically preserved human embryos to remain so preserved for a period exceeding two years is tantamount to the destruction of these human beings. It was the clear intent of Mr and Mrs Davies to create a child or children to be known as their family. No one disputes the fact that unless the human embryos, *in vitro*, are implanted, their lives will be lost; they will die a passive death. Mr Davis strenously objects to the anonymous donation of the human embryos even for their survival; Mrs Davis wants to bring these children to term; the human embryos were not caused to come into being by Mr and Mrs Davis for any purpose other than the production of their family. Therefore, the court finds and concludes that it is to the manifest best interest of the children, *in vitro*, that they be made available for implantation to assure their opportunity for live birth; implantation is their sole and only hope for survival. The court respectfully finds and concludes that it further serves the best interest of these children for Mrs Davis to be permitted the opportunity to bring these children to term, through implantation.[80]

Temporary custody of the embryos was granted to the wife. Child support, visitation and final custody will be decided if one of the embryos results in a birth.

Anti-abortionists heralded Judge Dale Young's statement on the nature of an embryo as vindication of their cause towards reducing the impact of *Roe* v. *Wade*.[81]

With this judgement, the husband argued that he felt 'raped of his reproductive rights' and vowed to appeal to the Tennessee Court of Appeal.

On the question whether the wife should be allowed to have the embryos for implantation, there is certainly this strong argument that her right to carry a child to term has never been under supervision, at least not by the husband.[82] A man has never been, under US or UK law, given a say as to whether a child should be born after he has fertilized the egg of his mate and, had the decision of the case gone the other way, it would be the precursor to the erosion of a woman's right to decide whether to bear and beget, an argument which was categorically put away in *Roe*. However, there seems to be little consideration of the unique fact in this case. Although it is absurd to argue that a man should have a say in whether implantation should occur after fertilization (*in vivo*) has taken place between his sperm and his partner's ovum, or whether a woman should or should not have an abortion, the embryos in this case were extra-corporeal. Should the husband have the right not to have children? Or has he been committed irrevocably as soon as the embryo came into existence to have his child? Some may insist that an embryo that has been created must be accorded with an opportunity to fulfil its potential and that implantation is the only course of action consistent with the respect we ought to give to an embryo. However it has not been argued that it should be forcibly returned to the uterine environment. Had the couple agreed not to further their attempt to have children by IVF, the fate of the embryos depends on the practice of the IVF unit and whether there are any willing recipients in the absence of any legislative direction. However, the stage at which the husband objected to the implantation should be significant, and in this case it was circumvented by what was perceived to be the parties' intention at the outset and the question of the beginning of human life. At one point it was said that the parties participated in the IVF programme for one purpose; to produce a human being to be known as their child. Given the conclusion that human life begins at conception, the court held that Mr and Mrs Davis had accomplished their original intent to produce a human being to be known as their child. Once the parties had, according to the court, 'accomplished their intent', Mr Davis's objection became irrelevant. The best interest of the children is that they be made available for implantation to assure their opportunity for live birth – implantation being their sole and only hope for survival.

This case accords more protection to embryos *in vitro* than embryos *in vivo*. Further, a couple in an IVF programme may not perceive their intent to create a child for having a family as 'accomplished' at the stage of fertilization. Indeed, one may argue that the intent of the parties to add a child to their family unit had been frustrated by their divorce. Since the case involves embryos, pro-life value permeates the judgement and it was said that 'it is to the manifest best interest of the children, *in vitro*, that they be made available for implantation to assure their opportunity for live birth'.[83]

Disputes of this nature are not inevitable and could have been avoided by paperwork in advance. Lessons were learned from the *Rios* case in Melbourne in 1984 when two Californians left embryos in an Australian clinic and were killed in an aeroplane crash. A Melbourne judge decided that the embryos should be made available to other couples. Nobody wanted them and they have since 1981 remained frozen.[84] Since that case, Australian clinics insist on agreements on what should happen to embryos in the event of death or divorce. It has been claimed that there are 4000 frozen embryos lying around in American refrigerators,[85] and unless the question of control is clarified, more disputes in the nature of the Tennessee case may well arise in the future.[86]

The question of storage of embryos is now covered by the HFEA. On this question, some of the recommendations of the Warnock Committee are now in Section 14. For instance, it says that the maximum period for the storage of gametes is ten years and five years for embryos. There is a regulation-making power which would allow for the shortening or lengthening of these periods. Section 14 however, only deals with the issue of disposal in a very limited way. Therefore, were a frozen embryo case to occur in this country, no legal provision would give guidance as to how the dispute should be resolved. Section 14 stipulates that no gametes or embryos shall be kept in storage for longer than the statutory period and, if stored at the end of the period, shall be allowed to perish. This is consistent with the Warnock proposal that after the maximum storage period has expired, the authority has the right of disposal.[87] *The Warnock Report* further recommended that if one partner dies, then the right of disposal of any stored embryo by that couple should pass to the survivor. If both died, then that right passes to the authority. Where there is no agreement between the couple, as in the Sue Davis case, then the right of disposal should pass to the storage authority as if the maximum period for storage had expired.[88]

With the possibility of storage comes the possibility of children born after the death of the semen donor. Section 28(b) of the HFEA makes it clear that where a donor's semen or an embryo created with his sperm is used after his death, he is not to be treated as the child's father. This merely emphasizes the donation principle. This provision, however, is not confined to donations. It applies to cases where a husband's sperm is stored and used after his death by his wife. By that time the deceased's estate could be distributed so that children born after the death of the husband will be disregarded for the purposes of succession and inheritance.

As can be seen, there are myriad difficulties which flow one after another. But this in itself has not proved to be a fundamental obstacle to the fulfilment of the right of the infertile to have children and establish a family. Indeed, every effort has been made to ensure that infertility treatment continues to be provided for those who need it. Basically, it is the use of another person's body for the gestation of a child, namely surrogacy, which has kept the issue of artificial reproduction current and topical in the last decade.

NOTES

1   No UK court has considered the legal status of an AID child. For the US cases

which considered the question of legitimacy of AID children, see Cusine, D.J., 'Artificial insemination', in McLean, S.A.M. (ed.), *Legal Issues in Medicine*, Aldershot, Gower, 1981, p. 163.

2   See the *Law Commission's Working Paper on Illegitimacy*, No. 74, London, HMSO, 1982, para. 3.16 (hereinafter cited as *Law Commission's Working Paper, No. 74*); Levin, Jennifer, 'Reforming the Legitimacy Laws', *Family Law* (1978) **8**, pp. 35–9; Samuels, Alec, 'Illegitimacy: The Law Commission's Report', *Family Law* (1983) **13**, pp. 87–90; Eekelaar, John, 'Second thoughts on illegitimacy reform', *Family Law* (1985) **15**, pp. 261–3.

3   *Vide infra*, Chapter 5 and Chapter 7, pp. 73–81.

4   In natural reproduction, both English and Scots law accord automatic parental rights and duties to married parents and unmarried mothers. Unmarried fathers have parental duties once paternity is established, and parental rights can be obtained through a court order. See Section 4 of the Family Law Reform Act 1987, Sections 2 and 3 of the Law Reform (Parent and Child) Act (Scotland) 1986, henceforth FLRA, 1987 and LRPCA 1986, respectively. See also Section 4 of the Children Act 1989.

5   *The Report of the Committee of Inquiry into Human Fertilisation and Embryology*, London, HMSO, Cmnd. 9314, 1984 (hereinafter cited as *The Warnock Report*).

6   See para. 1.10.

7   Artificial reproductive techniques can raise many other legal issues, for example, the legal status of embryos *in vitro*, see Wright, Gerald, 'The legal implications of IVF', in *Test-Tube Babies, a Christian View*, London, Unity Press, Becket, 1984, pp. 39–44.

8   *The Warnock Report* did not discuss this legal aspect of artificial reproduction at all, except to mention that AID is not adultery in law; see para. 4.10.

9   D. v. A. (1845) 1 Rob. Ecc. 279, p. 299, *per* Dr Lushington; *Corbett* v. *Corbett* [1971] P 83; *J.* v. *J.* [1978] *SLT* 128.

10 A decree of nullity may be obtained on the ground of inability to consummate a marriage even if a child has been conceived by *fecunatio ab extra*, *Clarke* v. *Clarke* [1943] P 1.

11 [1949] P 211.

12 The wife's conduct in submitting to AIH was not held to have approbated the marriage; see pp. 70–1, on a discussion of the doctrine of approbation of marriage.

13 [1953] P 252.

14 *The Times*, 12 May, 1960.

15 1961 SC 347.

16 See *C.B.* v. *A.B.* (1885) 12 R. (H.L.) 38, *per* Lord Watson, p. 45. Approved in *A.B.* v. *C.B.* 1961 SC 347.

17 See Cretney, S.M., *Principles of Family Law* (4th edn.), London, Sweet & Maxwell, 1984, p. 84.

18 [1952] P 152.

19 Evershed, M.R. said, ibid., p. 158:
    A proceeding to adopt a child under the Adoption of Children Act, 1926, which was then in force, involved certain proposition and consequences. It involved that when two persons jointly adopted a child, they must proceed on the footing that they were spouses . . . The application was made on the footing that the applicants were parties to a valid marriage.

20 [1953] P 252.

21 *The Times*, 12 May, 1960.

22 [1979] 3 ALL ER 337.

23 *C.B.* v. *A.B.* (1885) 12 R. (H.L.) 36, *per* Lord Selbourne, approved in *A.B.* v. *C.B.* 1961 SC 347.

24 *Vide supra*.

25   Tallin, G.P.R., 'Artificial insemination', *Canadian Bar Review* (1956) **34**, pp. 1–27, 166–86, 628–31; Hubbard, H.A., 'Artificial insemination: a reply to Dean Tallin', *Canadian Bar Review* (1956) **34**, pp. 425–51; Bartholomew, G.W., 'Legal implications of artificial insemination', *MLR* (1958) **21**, p. 236. See also Cusine, Douglas J., *New Reproductive Techniques: a Legal Perspective*, Aldershot, Dartmouth, 1988, Chapter 6.

26   Accepted by *Dennis* v. *Dennis* [1955] P 153.

27   Ibid.,
> I do not think that it can be said that adultery is proved unless there be some penetration.

Ibid, at p. 160, *per* Singleton, L.J.
> . . . I can find no other sure ground upon which to base my decision. . . than that which was adopted by . . . my Lord, namely, the test of penetration; penetration not necessarily complete, but some penetration in order that the physical fact of adultery may be proved either directly or indirectly by inference. Ibid., p. 163, *per* Hodson, L.J.

28   [1958] *SLT* 12.

29   *Vide supra*, Chapter 4.

30   *Vide supra*, Chapter 4, on the view of the Archbishop of Canterbury's Commission on AID.

31   Lord Wheatley, in *MacLennan*, [1958] *SLT* 12, p. 14:
> It is almost trite to say that a married woman who, without the consent of her husband, has the seed of a male donor injected into her person by mechanical means in order to procreate a child who would not be a child of the marriage has committed a grave and heinous breach of the contract of marriage.

32   See the Children Act 1989.

33   Except in adoption, see *Legislation on Human Infertility Services and Embryo Research – A Consultation Paper*, London, HMSO, Cmnd. 46, 1986, para. 33 (hereinafter cited as the *Consultation Paper*). This appears also to be the underlying assumption of *The Warnock Report* when it recommended (para. 6.8.) that
> where a woman donates an egg for transfer to another the donation should be treated as absolute and that, like a male donor she should have no rights or duties with regard to any resulting child.

34   *Vide infra*, Chapter 7 on motherhood.

35   Neither the *Law Commission Report on Illegitimacy*, London, HMSO, Cmnd. 118, 1982 (hereinafter cited as the *Law Commission Report, No. 118*), nor *The Warnock Report* mentioned this, probably because it is not perceived to be an issue at all. See Appendix 1 for Lord Denning's move to amend Clause 1 of the Family Law Reform Bill [H.L.], Session 1986–7, H.C. Bill, 70.

36   See Section 4 of the FLRA 1987 and Sections 2 and 3 of the LRPCA 1986.

37   *The Law Commission Report, No. 118*, paras. 12.4–12.7.

38   See for example, *A.* v. *A.*, *Family Law* (1987) **8**, p. 170, High Court.

39   Attempts to resolve this issue were considered on more than one occasion. See the amendment (which was withdrawn) put down by Lord Kilbrandon to the Bill leading to the Children Act 1975: *Hansard* (H.L.) 20 February 1975, Vol. **357**, Cols. 511–522; and the AID Children (Legal Status) Bill which was given a First Reading in the House of Commons on 28 June 1977: *Hansard* (H.C.) Vol. **934**, Cols. 276–279; *The Law Commission Report, No. 118*, para. 12.8.

40   It came into force on 4 April 1988. See the Family Law Reform Act 1987 (Commencement No.1) Order 1988, SI 1988/425.

41   *The Law Commission Report, No. 118*, para. 12.8.

42   Similar provisions exist in some US states, Holland, Portugal and Switzerland. See Cusine, D.J., 'Artificial insemination', in McLean, S.A.M. (ed.), *Legal Issues in Medicine*, Aldershot, Gower, 1981, p. 163.

43 The LRPCA 1986 does not have a similar provision. Equally, the Act's forerunner, the Scots Law *Commission Report on Illegitimacy*, No. 82, Edinburgh, HMSO, 1984, did not consider the issue relating to children born as a result of artificial techniques at all, see para. 1.2.

44 On the question of fatherhood where AID is undertaken by the unmarried, *vide infra*.

45 See the discussion of the position of a commissioning father, *vide infra*, Chapter 7.

46 *Vide supra*, Chapters 3 and 4.

47 *Law Commission Report, No. 118*, paras. 12.9–12.10.

48 *Vide supra*.

49 See para. 4.16.

50 See legislation in New South Wales and Victoria which provides that if a child is born to a married woman as a result of either artificial insemination or the implantation into her womb of an ovum which has been produced by her and fertilized outside her body, and if the semen used was not produced by her husband but the insemination or implantation was done with his consent, the husband shall be presumed for all purposes to have caused the pregnancy and to be the father of the child, see Artificial Conception Act 1984 (N.S.W.), SS 5(1), (2); Status of Children Act 1974 (Vic.), SS10(c)(1), (2)(a), 10(D)(1), (2)(a). Similar provisions can also be found in South Australia and Western Australia. All these statutes cover *de facto* spouses, see S3(1),(2)(a) (N.S.W.); S10a (S.A.); S10A(1), (2)(a) (Vic.); S3(1), (2)(a) (W.A.).

51 See Artificial Conception Act 1984 (N.S.W.), S5(1), (2); Status of Children Act 1974 (Vic.), SS10(c)(1), (2)(a), 10(D)(1), (2)(a).

52 See Family Relationships Act 1975 (S.A.) and Artificial Conception Act 1985 (W.A.).

53 See S3(1),(2)(a) (N.S.W.); S10a (S.A.); S10A(1),(2)(a) (Vic.); S3(1),(2)(a) (W.A.).

54 *Vide infra*, Chapter 7.

55 Para. 6.8.

56 *Vide infra*, Chapter 7.

57 See para. 7.6.

58 Ibid.

59 Ibid.

60 *Vide supra*, Chapter 4.

61 See the Australian legislative provisions cited above. They provide that if a child is born to a married woman as a result of either artificial insemination or the implantation into her womb of an ovum which has been produced by her and fertilized outside her body, and if the semen used was not produced by her husband but the insemination or implantation procedure was carried out with his consent, the husband shall be presumed to be the father of the child. *De facto* spouses are also covered.

62 *Report on Human Artificial Insemination and Related Matters*, 2 Vols, Ministry of the Attorney General, Toronto, July 1985, p. 175.

63 Section 49(3).

64 A proposal to amend the Bill was not withdrawn. Baroness Warnock came up with an extraordinary revelation. She argued that such a positive requirement of consent would create hardship in some situations. She said that among Asian women, infertility was usually regarded as a female problem and it was a sufficient cause for divorce. Consequently, such women would be inclined to undergo infertility treatment (AID) without the knowledge of their husbands. This practice 'is one class of case that weighed with us [the Warnock Committee] when we decided that it was better to present the case [namely, the deeming provision] in this rather negative way'. See *Hansard*, H.L. Vol. **516**, Col. 1345.

65 Professor J.M. Thomson mistakenly thought that the Act applies also to Scotland; see *Family Law in Scotland*, London, Butterworths, 1987, p. 136.
66 No recorded cases have been decided under Section 4. Section 7 also provides that the offence extends to a person who aids and abets another person to commit the offence. This means that doctors or counsellors advising one to enter the name of the husband as the father of the child may contravene the 1911 Act.
67 See Law Commission Report, No. 118, para. 12.20 and Law Commission *Working paper*, No. 74, paras. 10.18–10.20.
68 See the *Consultation Paper*, para. 30.
69 *Hansard*, H.L. Vol. **516** Col 1306.
70 Ibid., Col. 1307.
71 Ibid., Col. 1317. According to the estimate of clinical geneticists, 'wrong paternity' occurs in 5% of the population, ibid. However, the entry in the birth certificate is a legal statement of the sex of a person. The only exceptions are where an aberration is made on recording or identification of the sex of a person.
72 See Morgan, Derek, 'The Human Fertilisation and Embryology Bill: regulating clinical practice', *Family Law* (1990), p. 122.
73 Para. 4.21.
74 *Human Fertilisation and Embryology: a framework for legislation*, Cmnd 259, London, 1987, para. 29–31.
75 Section 31(6) (7).
76 *Junior L. Davis* v. *Mary Sue Davis*. No. E – 14496, Circuit Court for Blount County, Tennessee, at Maryville, Equity Division (Division I) 1989 Tenn. App. Lexis 641. See also *The Times*, 10 August, 1989, 11 August, 1989, 22 September, 1989, 23 September, 1989.
77 Ibid.
78 Ibid.
79 Ibid.
80 Ibid.
81 *Vide supra*.
82 *Vide infra*, Chapter 7.
83 *Davis* v. *Davis*, op. cit.
84 See 'Embryos in the fridge', *The Economist*, 12 August, 1989.
85 Ibid.
86 See Ontario Law Reform Commission's recommendations on control of embryos, para. 27(1) that
    (a) A fertilised ovum outside the body, produced with the gametes of the intended recipient and her husband or partner, should be under the joint legal control of the man or woman. (b) Where one of the couple dies, legal control of the fertilised ovum should pass to the survivor. If both should die, control should pass to the physician, clinic, gamete bank, or other authority that has actual possession of the ovum. (c) Where the couple cannot agree concerning the use or disposition of the fertilised ovum, legal control should pass to the physician, clinic, gamete bank, or other authority that has actual possession of the ovum.
87 Para. 10.10.
88 Para. 10.12–10.13.

6 The Rights and Wrongs of Surrogacy

INTRODUCTION

Of all the artificial reproductive techniques debated in the last decade, surrogacy has been the most controversial. Surrogacy itself is not an artificial reproductive technique and it means no more than the employment of a woman by another person for the purposes of having children. As has been explained previously, the possible genetic permutation of a surrogate-born child suggests that the child may or may not have any genetic connection with either the surrogate or the commissioning parties. In this situation, the objective of the transaction for the commissioning parties is the production of a child for the purposes of parenting. Furthermore, since the surrogate has no genetic connection with the child (as in IVF and ET surrogacy), she is more appropriately described as using her gestation function for the purposes of bringing a child into being. However, it must be said that this way of perceiving the role of a surrogate is not necessarily indisputable as some may consider that the surrogate's rights and duties over the child in this case are no less than in a situation where she carries her own genetic child (for example, as in the case of partial surrogacy).

Complicated as it may be when artificial reproductive techniques are combined with surrogacy, one can see that, on the one hand surrogacy can be a viable solution to the problems faced by some infertile couples. It can also widen the sphere of choices for some women who have hitherto thought that career and motherhood are mutually exclusive because of the overbearing hindrance of pregnancy to one's career. On the other hand, surrogacy brings a number of people's interests into conflict. One claim is that the infertile have the right to use surrogates to have children (either to reproduce and/or to have a family). Further, since surrogacy may effectively be the only hope for some people who seek to exercise their right to found a family (whether through reproduction or not), its significance to these people cannot be denied. There is also the claim of potential surrogates that it is their right to decide whether to enter into a surrogacy contract with the commissioning parties. Implicit in these claims are the libertarian considerations that reproduction and creating family relationships are private matters in which the state has *prima facie* no right to interfere. Libertarians support this presumption for non-interference and contend that it is for the interventionists to demonstrate a convincing case which would give legitimacy to any form of intervention in the freedom of contract for the satisfaction of their respective rights between the commissioning parties and the surrogate. Opposing these views is the idea that there are inherent limits to freedom and liberty, and surrogacy – which is seen as an attack on fundamental moral values and social structures – should not be permissible. The debate therefore brings into sharper focus the limits of individual liberty, the role of women in reproduction, and society's values towards family and parenting. This chapter therefore examines the conflicts inherent in the debate on surrogacy. It considers the different approaches advocated and the different assumptions underlying views for or against surrogacy. Thus, analysis in greater detail of surrogacy is appropriate before any conclusion is reached as to whether an individual's rights to reproduce and/or to found a family are sufficiently broad as to include freedom of access to surrogacy.

In the UK, surrogacy is not illegal or unlawful.[1] Since the publication of *The Warnock Report*,[2] and the *Baby Cotton case*,[3] surrogacy has been consistently, and often passionately, debated.[4] *The Warnock Report*, by a majority of 16:14, rejected all forms of surrogacy,[5] asserting that 'the weight of public opinion is against the practice'.[6]

Although sentiment is insufficient to justify interference with rights, it is necessary to analyse the apparent public hostility to surrogacy in more depth, in order to assess whether or not fundamentally important reasons underpin it, and make interference in personal choice justifiable. In discussing the acceptability of surrogacy, the form of surrogacy (partial or full) is largely irrelevant.[7] At one time, before the question of motherhood was settled by the law,[8] it was argued by some that there was a difference between the two types of surrogacy; namely, whether the practice of surrogacy was objectionable depended on whether one was considering partial or full surrogacy.[9] In the former situation, the surrogate was the biological mother of the child whereas in the latter she was not (that is, she was carrying someone else's child). Partial surrogacy therefore might be questioned on moral, social and legal grounds but not full surrogacy. However, such a distinction failed to confront the thrust of the issue, that is, was the idea that a woman agreed to carry a child to term, with the intention that she should surrender the child to be brought up by a person or persons other than herself objectionable?

As will be seen later,[10] biological link with a child is not crucial in determining motherhood. Thus partial and full surrogacy cannot, and need not, be distinguished on the grounds of the biological link between the surrogate and the child. In any event, if the alleged difference between the two cases on genetic grounds is insisted upon, it can be blurred or removed if, for example, the surrogate in partial surrogacy agrees, before AI, to make a donation of her ovum so as to divest herself of the rights and liabilities which she would otherwise have as a result of her genetic link with the child.[11]

In the second place, the alleged distinction between the two cases may not be apparent, or vital, at all when one examines the arguments against surrogacy.[12] In other words, the arguments most commonly and most powerfully used against surrogacy centre rather on the nature of the agreement itself than on the genetic contribution made. For the above reasons, the following appraisal of some of the most common objections to surrogacy will be regarded as relevant irrespective of the form of surrogacy in question.

The discussion will therefore move from the lowest level – the alleged unacceptability of surrogacy in principle (if any) – and graduate to surrogacy for a fee. This kind of analytical approach is useful in that it helps in discerning the various types of argument against surrogacy, their directions and relative force. Thus, people may be sympathetic towards surrogacy in principle but hostile towards surrogacy for a fee. The underlying reason for this difference of attitude and approach can be explained and this understanding can assist legislators and society as a whole in formulating a course of action regarding this controversial issue.

SURROGACY IN PRINCIPLE

Surrogacy in principle (see Chapter 2, p. 16) is usually undertaken between sisters and friends. Exceptionally, it may be between strangers.[13] Although some may regard surrogacy as merely a logical extension of technological development, and its practice as being simply a logical corollary of the rights to reproduce and/or to found a family, to others, it is entirely unacceptable. Literature on the subject, however, sometimes presents a somewhat confused picture of what it is about surrogacy that is objectionable.

For example, in *The Warnock Report*, the objection to surrogacy in principle[14] seems to be that it is wrong to treat others as a means to an end.[15] In *A Question of Life*, surrogacy is said to be wrong because of the possible harmful consequences to the child.[16] But in an article, by Mary Warnock, it was said that,[17]

. . . [many] feel very differently if what they think of is surrogacy undertaken between sisters or friends. And this is because in such a case the mother who gives birth to the child, though she will not bring it up or count it as hers, will nevertheless be permitted to love it. . . . The child himself, if . . . told that his aunt is his mother, will in some sense have gained, not lost. He will have two mothers instead of one. No one has rejected him. He was born out of love and charity, not out of greed. And so it is clear that what is really felt to be *wrong is surrogacy not for love but for money* [emphasis added].

This quotation seems to suggest that surrogacy in principle (and perhaps even surrogacy with reasonable compensation) is not felt to be wrong at all. These confusions are in part due to the fact that, in discussing the acceptability of surrogacy, the often vital distinctions between the various financial dimensions of surrogacy are not clearly drawn.

In the following section, some of the arguments against surrogacy in principle will be identified and examined.[18] Notably there are two main types of argument. First, that surrogacy is an unnatural practice, and second, that surrogacy is harmful to both surrogates and surrogate-born children.

Surrogacy as an Unnatural Practice

This argument, to a large extent, mirrors that which is used against AI and IVF.[19] However, its application here has been slightly modified. The roots of conceptual thinking here relate to preconceived ideas of what a woman's role in procreation ought to be, rather than being based on a claim that artificial techniques for conception are unnatural. In other words, the meaning of unnatural, as used in arguments about surrogacy, has been extended beyond that employed as an objection against artificial techniques.

Thus it may be said that surrogacy is unnatural because it is contrary to a woman's natural post-natal 'instinct' to part with a child after parturition. However, it must first be pointed out that social scientists have indicated a number of reasons which cast doubt on this so-called instinct as either natural or universal female behaviour.[20] First, the widespread practice of infanticide for flimsy reasons, such as vanity, equalizing the sexes and discipline, in some societies, makes it hard for one to maintain that common post-natal behaviour is a natural human female 'instinct' as such.[21] Anthropologists have also found that, in some societies, mothers are willing to part with their babies without a pang.[22] Moreover, the practice of aristocratic families in England and France during the eighteenth and nineteenth centuries of placing children out to wet nurses from birth for a lengthy period (such as four or five years), throws profound doubt on whether maternal behaviour is 'instinctive'.[23] Indeed, it has been argued that maternal behaviour is in fact a kind of socially conditioned 'sentiment', the expression of which may vary from individual to individual, time to time and society to society.[24] Consequently, it may be an overstatement to suggest that surrogacy is 'unnatural' in the sense described above. In fact, surrogacy is an ancient practice.[25] One could, therefore, contend that the fact that it has long been practised makes it one of the most 'natural' (in the sense of customary) and obvious ways of dealing with certain types of infertility.

Admittedly, both English and Scots law render unenforceable agreements by parents to divest themselves of parental rights and duties,[26] except when transfer of parental rights and duties is achieved through judicial process, such as in the case of adoption or a court order. However, these provisions are clearly unconnected with the notion of maternal 'instinct' as such,[27] and if surrogacy is objected to on the grounds that it is a private agreement attempting to transfer parental rights and duties, setting up a legal mechanism for the transfer (as in adoption) would be the straightforward answer.

A variation of the argument that surrogacy is 'unnatural' may be based on the argument that it is a distortion of, and a threat to, the conventional pattern of child-bearing and child rearing.[28] While it may appear to be a distortion of the conventional way of procreation and parenting, it could hardly be regarded, for that reason alone, as a strong argument for the unacceptability of surrogacy. Novel practices often raise new problems and new concerns, but unless it is found that they not only undercut traditional norms but also threaten social structures and institutions, leading to the collapse of fundamental moral values and principles, where individual rights are at stake, they should not be rejected. In a pluralistic society where moral standards are not fixed and rigid, the threshold of tolerance allows deviation from accepted practices which do not harm others. This brings us to arguments of potential harm to the surrogate and surrogate-born child.

Harm to Surrogates and Surrogate-born Children

One factor which may have an important bearing on the moral and social acceptability of surrogacy in principle is the possible harm surrogacy may cause to both a surrogate and a surrogate-born child. Here it may be difficult to separate the two sets of potential harm as the parties are sometimes perceived to be linked in terms of potential harm and detrimental effects (if any). Thus, it has been said that surrogacy is unacceptable because bonds exist between a surrogate and the foetus *in utero* and their separation will be harmful to both parties.

Little is known about the effect of this alleged bonding on a child. Hence, it is prudent to avoid a conclusion one way or another as to whether, consequential to the separation of the surrogate and the child, either or both will be harmed. *The Warnock Report*, in fact, did not place great emphasis on this bonding theory in its conclusion against surrogacy.[29] Nor did the recent surrogacy report when it observed that

> There is no strong evidence for prebirth bonding of a child to the woman who gives birth to it. So if birth mother and child are separated soon after the birth there is little likelihood of direct psychological damage to the child. There may be indirect psychological damage in later years . . . But if surrogacy is like ordinary adoption in this respect (and there seems no reason to think that it is not), then such damage is likely to be neither serious nor common.[30]

This bonding theory, however, may become very important in a custody dispute.[31] Having said that, it must be added that although there is no direct scientific evidence which establishes that psychological and emotional harm are inevitable consequences for a surrogate who parts with the child, there is some evidence to the effect that a woman may, after surrendering the child, experience a deep sense of loss; something that would possibly remain with her for the rest of her life.[32] The analogy used here is often that of the experience of mothers who give up their children for adoption and who then regret, or feel the sense of loss, later on in their life. However, hardly anyone expresses reservations or scruples about the practice of adoption on the grounds of such possible harm. The obvious reason is that, in adoption, we are talking about the lesser of two evils, in circumstances where the child is already in existence and adoption is the better alternative for the child. Therefore, potential emotional upset to the mother, if it is not possible to avert, is considered an unfortunate, but possibly an inevitable, side effect. In surrogacy we are talking about a woman who enters into an arrangement, who, if properly counselled, is aware (if not fully) of the possible emotional distress resulting from giving up the child. Here we are in the realm of interpersonal relationships and the concomitant emotional difficulties and problems which may arise. Nonetheless, the employment of the harm argument in surrogacy is completely out of line in a society informed by libertarian values, where each individual is free to enter into personal relationships with another person involving a different degree of emotional commitment. There is no suggestion that this freedom should be curtailed simply because of the likelihood of severe emotional scarring of the parties involved on the breakdown of that relationship. Nor is it suggested that the possible effects of emotional split on innocent children is a valid ground for curtailing that freedom. In 1985, 191 000 petitions for divorce were filed in England and Wales[33] and the harmful effects thereby caused to adults and children are more obvious than potential harm likely to be caused to a surrogate and surrogate-born child in a surrogate arrangement. The harm argument, therefore, smacks of an extreme form of paternalism[34] and any such submission in the debate on surrogacy heralds a setback from liberal values which have been treasured and jealously guarded.

Still, from the point of view of the child, it may be unrealistic to suggest that a surrogate-born child will definitely not experience a confusion of personal identity similar to that known to be experienced by an adopted child.[35] A surrogate-born child may be just as anxious to know about the circumstances of his or her birth and/or his or her bearing and/or biological mother. It has been acknowledged that

> The child might also have psychological problems. Having been told, honestly and openly, that it was born of a surrogate arrangement, it might experience a sense of rejection based on the fact that a woman was prepared to give it up at birth. The child might yearn to meet its birth mother. The child may also feel guilt on behalf of its parents' problems with childlessness. It might wonder whether there was anything undesirable in its genetic background. It might be taunted by other children or fear rejection by its peers. All these are issues which the adopted child may also face, but the surrogate child might, for instance, feel uneasiness that a large amount of money had been paid for it or might feel that its parents have unrealistic expectations for it.[36]

In Chapter 4 the weight of this consideration as a factor against the use of artificial techniques for the founding of a family (whether through reproduction or not) was assessed. The conclusion reached was that the needs of children to know about the circumstances of their conception (and birth) can, and should, be facilitated by a policy of openness, proper record-keeping of births consequential to the donation of gametes, and counselling before access to birth records.

The issue in surrogacy is very similar. Although it is not much debated, there is no apparent reason why a similar approach could not be adopted.[37]

Again, from the perspective of a surrogate-born child, it is hardly feasible to contend that he or she could be so badly harmed by the circumstances of conception and birth that he or she should not have been born.[38] In many ways, therefore, the argument which relates to potential harm to a surrogate-born child can be accommodated by reference to similar criteria as were used in respect of AI and IVF,[39] since the argument does not seem to differ significantly from that which may arise from the employment of artificial techniques in general. Thus, a solution similar to that proposed in such cases may be employed in relation to surrogacy.

Consideration of the two groups of arguments against surrogacy does not, of course, exhaust the possible range of objections. It may be said, for example, that it is totally unacceptable for a woman to be treated as a machine for breeding purposes. Some may even go so far as to condemn surrogacy on the grounds that it resembles slavery. Since these two arguments are most commonly directed at surrogacy where money payment is involved, they will be considered in greater depth later.[40]

The contentions considered so far have not shown that surrogacy in principle is morally or socially reprehensible, thereby justifying its prohibition. Surrogacy in principle can be regarded as a noble undertaking, the essence of which is to help another to have a child. If this beneficent view is taken, then there need be no argument concerning the rights of an individual either to found a family (whether through reproduction or not) through surrogacy, or to use one's reproductive and/or gestational function. Where a willing surrogate is available, this method of generating life, and bringing it to fruition, cannot, therefore, be struck at. Moreover, although it is clear that a surrogate-born child may experience some disadvantages because of its circumstances of birth, and accepting the importance of this, it can be contended that the resolution of the problem – as with AI and IVF – lies not in banning surrogacy, but rather in regulating its use in a sensitive way.[41]

SURROGACY WITH MONEY PAYMENT – THE EVIL ELEMENT

It has been noted that the two main arguments already outlined do not cover exhaustively the range of the debate about surrogacy. Although surrogacy need not entail money payment, in some cases it does. The addition of money payment serves to add contentious fuel to the fire. In this context, surrogacy represents a challenge to our perception of a woman's role in reproduction and the family in particular, and more generally, it helps to focus sharply the issue of a woman's role in society – an issue which feminists have been debating over the last century. Underlying the deep rift between opponents and proponents of surrogacy is the conflict that surrogacy produces: it widens the choices pertaining to reproduction available to both men and women; at the same time it holds the possibility of a free market for baby buying in which a class of poor and indigent baby breeders will emerge, and in which both babies and breeders are treated as commodities whose values are assessed by reference to colour and physical characteristics. Surrogacy with money payment therefore has been regarded by some as sufficiently evil to justify its condemnation and prohibition.[42]

The question to be posed therefore is whether the involvement of money payment in a surrogacy arrangement changes the essential character of the agreement sufficiently to require its condemnation. Even accepting that surrogacy in principle is not objectionable, might the introduction of monetary considerations render a surrogacy arrangement sufficiently morally reprehensible as to justify inter-ference with an individual's freedom to found a family (whether through reproduction or not) by employing surrogacy, and a woman's use of her reproductive and/or gestational function?

When considering whether, and if so why, money payment is objectionable, it is important to distinguish between two kinds of payment: surrogacy with reasonable compensation and surrogacy for a fee. Whether a particular case falls into a particular category depends on the nature of the payment and the facts of the individual case.[43] Since the amount paid in a surrogacy arrangement may affect one's view as to its acceptability, this distinction between the two categories of payment will be maintained in the following discussion. However, where such a distinction is not apparent or necessary, the term 'money payment' will be used.

Surrogacy with Reasonable Compensation

Surrogacy with reasonable compensation differs from surrogacy in principle only insofar as reasonable compensation is paid to a surrogate. Although some may argue that surrogacy with reason-able compensation is a less altruistic act than surrogacy in principle, this may not inevitably be so. The mere fact of financial compen-sation does not necessarily indicate that a surrogate acts less altruistically than someone who is willing to bear a child for no financial reimbursement.[44] It may be that the former cannot afford to become a surrogate without being compensated. A surrogate may only bear a child at her own expense for the commissioning parties if she has the resources, for example, to pay for the costs of pregnancy, and to maintain herself during that period. In any event, since it is the commissioning parties who want to have a child by seeking the service of another, it seems only fair and reasonable that they should bear the costs of the pregnancy.[45] To that extent, reasonable compensation may indeed facilitate the expression of altruism which may otherwise not be possible. Consequently, it may be argued that surrogacy with reasonable compensation, like surrogacy in principle, is neither morally nor socially unacceptable. Its prohibition, therefore, which would deny to some infertile people their right to reproduce, limit the right of the infertile to found a family, and invade the right of potential surrogates to privacy, is not easily justified.

While the concept of 'reasonable compensation' may not be entirely lacking in complexity, two matters may be noted at this stage. First, the fact that out-of-pocket expenses are met by the commissioning parties has been argued not to affect the inherently altruistic nature of the arrangement. If surrogacy in principle is an acceptable method enabling the vindication of the rights of the infertile, then surrogacy with reasonable compensation must be too. Second, the problem as to what compensation is 'reasonable' need pose no fundamental difficulties for this assertion, since that is a matter which can be worked out by the parties concerned to their satisfaction.[46]

Surrogacy For a Fee

Although surrogacy with reasonable compensation may, therefore, be an acceptable method for founding a family, surrogacy for a fee (see Chapter 2, p. 16) often attracts strong moral condemnation.

The arguments against surrogacy for a fee have not been well analysed. They tend to be no more than simple assertions of belief. For instance, in the parliamentary debates on the Surrogacy Arrangements Act 1985, it was said that '. . . a financial transaction, to secure the lease of a woman's womb is repugnant',[47] Mr Harry Greenaway said, '[i]t is a very doubtful moral proposition for a woman to be asked to carry a baby for financial gain'.[48] No detailed reasoning was offered to support these contentions. Nonetheless, one can identify two general arguments against surrogacy for a fee. First, it may be thought to be contrary to a woman's dignity, and second, it may be seen to resemble baby-selling or baby-buying. These arguments will be discussed below.

Inconsistent With Human Dignity

It has been suggested that it is inconsistent with human dignity for a woman to lease her womb for a fee, and consequently to be treated as a machine for breeding.[49]

The first point which has to be made about this contention is that one must be cautious about the use of value-laden expressions which may preclude rational discussion as to what is inherently objectionable about surrogacy for a fee. 'Womb-leasing' and 'treating oneself or one's gestation function as a breeding machine' are expressions which are not purely descriptive of what surrogacy for a fee entails. Even if they were, no moral implications should, or could, be drawn at this stage about the rights and wrongs of the practice. Equally, no moral implication can be drawn if one chooses, albeit unusually, to describe decision-makers as primarily leasing their brain power, or typists as essentially leasing their fingers. The use of these expressions in respect of surrogacy for a fee is certainly value-laden, and indicates the underlying perception that it is worthy of moral condemnation. Yet, even though the description may seem to pre-empt an alternative conclusion, the arguments as to why surrogacy is inconsistent with human dignity merit consideration.

One argument which is not uncommon is that surrogacy for a fee is wrong because it is analogous to slavery.[50] Others argue that surrogacy for a fee is completely at odds with traditional female behaviour in relation to pregnancy and procreation, in that it is a situation where a woman allows the use of her gestational function in return for a fee.[51] Alternatively, surrogacy for a fee may be said to be degrading to a woman because it is thought to be a practice where she is being treated as a means to an end, that is, she is treated as a machine for the production of a child.[52] Finally, surrogacy for a fee may be considered wrong because it is potentially harmful to the surrogate. The emphasis here will be on the first three arguments, as the last has already been discussed.[53]

Slavery. Some may argue that surrogacy for a fee is unacceptable because it is analogous to slavery, in that a surrogacy arrangement will seek to exert extensive control over the personal daily activities of a surrogate.[54] However, this analogy can easily be defeated. As will be seen later,[55] it is very unlikely that either the English, or the Scots Courts, would enforce any of the essential parts of such an agreement. In effect, the surrogate can repudiate the agreement at any time. It may yet be argued that the surrogate may not lawfully terminate the pregnancy.[56] But the laws on abortion govern a surrogate in the same way as any other pregnant women. Consequently, if the inability of a surrogate to terminate a pregnancy lawfully is objected to, the complaint is directed at the abortion laws, not directly at surrogacy for a fee.

The slavery argument may, however, take a more subtle form. Although it does not imply that a master–slave relationship exists in surrogacy for a fee, in the sense that the master has the power of life and death over the slave, the substance of the slavery contention in surrogacy for a fee may be that since poor women are more likely to undertake paid surrogacy as a means of improving their financial situations, decisions taken under such circumstances could hardly be regarded as voluntary.[57] In other words, the rhetoric of free choice must be treated with caution if the range of choice is limited and social conditions are coercive of poor women to become surrogates for profit. As will be seen later,[58] this argument is hardly consistent with the general acceptance by liberal democratic societies, like the UK, that people sometimes earn money by undertaking jobs or tasks which they would not have chosen had there been other options. Indeed, such societies sanction voluntary trade-offs of physical or mental skill and labour in return for wages and protection to the extent that minimum wage legislation has been passed to make it unlawful for employers to under-pay workers. Furthermore, according to the libertarian principle espoused in this thesis, voluntary trade-offs between freedom of bodily function and the freedom which money may facilitate should not be prohibited unless there is something fundamentally and inherently objectionable about that particular type of trade-off. In other words, unless one distinguishes surrogacy for a fee from other trade-offs, or concedes that other paid jobs are also forms of slavery, then the analogy of surrogacy for a fee with slavery may be difficult to sustain.

Gestation for a Fee.   To say that particular behaviour or conduct is degrading to a person denotes that the behaviour is, or should be, a source of shame to that person. That is, since one's self-esteem is vested in the competent exercise of certain capacities, behaviour which fails to live up to that is seen to be degrading and undignified and to result in a lowering of status for that person. Surrogacy for a fee is said to be degrading to a woman because it is an activity which deviates from traditional and valued female behaviour in relation to pregnancy and reproduction. Obviously, those who hold such a view need not participate in such transactions. The relevance of the debate, however, as to what extent the law ought to, reflect and shape morality is limited in this context.[59]

Like prostitution and homosexuality, (which some people may regard as a deviation from the traditional form of sexual behaviour, and as immoral), gestation for a fee need not entail consequent illegality. Under both English and Scots law, prostitution *per se* is not illegal,[60] and homosexuality is not unlawful *per se* in English law.[61] Thus, there are strong precedents to support a cautious legislative approach in areas of reproduction and founding a family which are essentially aspects of an individual's privacy and liberty. In other words, whilst the morality or otherwise of surrogacy for a fee offers an interesting perspective on and approach to the issue, consistent with the formulation of the right to reproduce, the right to found a family, and a woman's right to use her reproductive and/or gestational function, a compelling interest (other than that some people regard it as a practice that is immoral) must be demonstrated to justify its prohibition. However, as will be seen later,[62] there may indeed be compelling reasons for the prohibition of surrogacy for a fee on other grounds.

Treating Another As a Means to an End and Exploitation. Some perceive surrogacy for a fee as an example of commissioning parties treating a surrogate as a means to an end. This argument is sometimes used even where no money payment is involved.[63] For example, *The Warnock Report*, by a majority of 16:14, concluded against surrogacy as a means to circumvent certain causes of infertility, making the following comment:[64]

> That people should treat others as a means for their own ends, however desirable the consequences, must always be liable to moral objection.

The philosophical position of *The Warnock Report* appears to reflect the Kantian principle that people ought to be treated as ends in themselves, rather than solely as a means to an end. The argument against surrogacy, therefore, is that, since surrogacy, by its very nature, involves the use of a person (presumably the surrogate) as a means to achieve the ends of another, it is morally objectionable.[65] Nonetheless, the principle that one should not treat another as a means to an end is not an absolute one; otherwise, many accepted daily activities and transactions, such as using blood donors, would be regarded as immoral.[66]

The Warnock Report further concluded that where 'financial interests'[67] were involved, presumably in a case of surrogacy for a fee, the transaction became 'positively exploitative'.[68]

Such treatment of one person by another becomes positively exploitative when financial interests are involved. It is therefore with the
commercial exploitation of surrogacy that we have been primarily, but
by no means exclusively, concerned.

But such a blanket statement is hardly sufficient to make out a strong
case against surrogacy. Is it being suggested that activities which
involve paying others to be a means to one's own ends are immoral?
If so, it is too sweeping a statement.

Most activities which involve paying others to be a means to one's
own ends are perfectly innocuous and acceptable. For instance, a
passenger who pays a taxi driver for a ride can hardly be said to be
acting immorally. Nor is the taxi driver likely to be considered
exploited by the passenger. In other words, not every situation in
which payment is made by X to Y, for the purpose of X achieving
something, and which involves Y in return in providing time,
physical presence, skill and so on, need be regarded purely and
simply as exploitative of either party. It may be that there is
something about the nature of what is either offered or provided in
surrogacy for a fee which renders this argument valid rather than
specious. If there is a real possibility of exploitation in this situation,
then the question must be asked, who is being exploited? If
exploitation of any, or all, of the parties is identified, does this render
the practice immoral? And if the practice is deemed immoral, does
this demand legal condemnation? This last question has been briefly
considered above; the first two questions will be considered here.

On the one hand, in a free-market system, it is possible that the
commissioning parties, desperate for children, may be subjected to
demands for unconscionably high fees from surrogates. A corollary
to this may be that those who wish to be assisted by a surrogate may
find that surrogacy is not an option available to them because they
cannot afford to pay the fee. In these circumstances, it may be argued
that, if exploitation is occurring, then it is the commissioning parties
who are its victims.

On the other hand, the attraction of payment may mean that low-
income women may be lured into becoming surrogates for those who
can pay. In one research study it was found that 40 per cent of
volunteer surrogates in the USA were unemployed, or in receipt of
welfare.[69] Here, money inducement may be so inviting to low-
income women – who may have few, or no, equally attractive
alternatives – that they will enter into surrogacy arrangements. The
spectre of poor women carrying babies for the rich may then arise.

However, unless there is something inherently different about the
use of the gestational function from the use of other body parts, it
may be argued that to offer a fee for services rendered is not only

entirely consistent with capitalist economies, but that *not* to make such a payment is exploitative. Nor does the likelihood that women of limited financial means would most commonly volunteer to become participants in surrogacy for fee transactions necessarily affect the morality of the transaction. Many men and women currently undertake dangerous and unpleasant tasks in return for (sometimes rather meagre) financial payment which they would not have undertaken had other options existed. Yet, it has not been suggested that society should ban, for example, coal mining, because people do it in order to earn an income.

From the perspective of the commissioning parties, it is perfectly possible that they would be willing to enter into a surrogate agreement even though the amount of the payment required by the surrogate is what others may regard as unconscionable. Therefore, whether to make a payment which others may regard as excessive, in order to satisfy a strongly-felt desire and to vindicate a right, is a matter which can be determined only by the person choosing to do so. This view is by no means radical or unusual, since much of what is paid by individuals in order to satisfy desires (for example, by purchasing a Picasso) is not susceptible to rational objective evaluation.

Two conclusions may be drawn at this stage. First, *The Warnock Report* has failed to establish why, and how, surrogacy for a fee is a 'positively exploitative' and unacceptable transaction. Condemnation of surrogacy for a fee, therefore, appears to have more to do with an in-built rejection of the practice rather than a conclusion arrived at after well-reasoned consideration of the issues involved. Second, there is legitimate deep concern and opposition to surrogacy for a fee – the sentiment that it heralds a new era where a woman's reproductive function will be available for purchase and be subjected to the harsh reality of the commercial world. The potential danger of exploitation in surrogacy for a fee, however, does not necessarily support prohibition. There are two main reasons for this. In cases where surrogacy for a fee is voluntary on both sides, prohibition would infringe the right of a surrogate to use her procreative and/or gestational function, as well as the right of the commissioning parties to found a family (whether through procreation or not).

In cases where surrogacy for a fee is potentially exploitative of either party, the right to procreate and/or to use one's gestational function, being negative in nature, does not require a state to ensure an environment which is non-exploitative, nor one which is favourable to the exercise of that right. The same conclusion applies as regards the commissioning parties' right to found a family. Indeed, prohibition of surrogacy for a fee on the grounds of possible exploitation can be regarded firstly as totally gratuitous and not justified by any legitimate claim for protection of any perceived legitimate interests of either potential surrogates or commissioning parties, and secondly, as defeating the rights of some of these individuals.

Baby-selling. One major argument against surrogacy with money payment is that it is tantamount to baby-selling. This has been regarded as a major obstacle to its acceptability.[70] The analogy often drawn is with adoption. The UK adoption laws generally prohibit money payment in connection with adoption.[71] The distaste which would be generally felt were babies bought and sold is instrumental in shaping the prohibition of money considerations in adoption.

However, the question must be posed as to the extent to which this analogy can appropriately be used. If surrogacy is not entirely on a par with adoption, then the value of the arguments against baby-selling could diminish. If, however, a sufficient link is perceived between the payment of a fee in surrogacy, and money payment in consideration of adoption, then the former may be objected to on the grounds of baby-selling and those commissioning parties who would wish to adopt a surrogate-born child in order to secure their relationship with the child could find that the adoption laws constitute a major legal impediment to this endeavour.

The question whether or not surrogacy with money payment can be equated to baby-selling has reached the UK courts. In the first reported English case, *A. v. C.*,[72] a woman agreed, for a sum of £500, to be artificially inseminated using the semen of a man who wanted a child. The surrogate changed her mind during pregnancy, and after the birth of the child, the natural (biological) father started wardship proceedings to obtain custody of the child.[73] Mr Justice Comyn, in the High Court, described the contract as a 'pernicious' agreement, saying that:[74]

> The agreement between the parties I hold as being against public policy. None of them can rely upon it in any way or enforce the agreement in any way. I need only to give one of many grounds for saying this, namely that this was a purported contract for the sale and purchase of a child.

In the Court of Appeal,[75] Lord Justice Ormrod described the case as a 'sordid commercial bargain'.[76]

The primary reason for these adverse comments on the surrogacy arrangement appeared to be the perception that it was equivalent to baby-selling. However, the strength of this argument, which essentially hinges on the contention that one is paid money for the surrendering of a child (whether in consideration of adoption or not), can be tempered if one views the £500 merely as reasonable compensation for the surrogate. Take, for instance, the practice in the USA for a surrogate to be paid approximately $12 000 (which, as suggested before, may be considered as reasonable compensation): 10 per cent of the money will be paid on confirmation of pregnancy, and the rest will be paid when she hands the child over.[77] Since a surrogate may change her mind by refusing to hand the child over to the commissioning parties, the money could be seen as being paid in return for her consenting to hand the child over. In other words, one may argue that the surrogate is selling the baby when she performs her part of the agreement in return for the commissioning parties' performing their side of the agreement. However, the argument for compensation is that money is paid to the surrogate not for her surrendering of the child but to recompense her for the cost or loss incurred during pregnancy and gestation on account of the commissioning parties. Where the surrogate changes her mind, the need to compensate her vanishes, since she did not bear a child for another; rather she has borne the child for herself.

Nonetheless, where surrogacy is for a fee, then the baby-selling argument can be applied most effectively to the profit element of the money payment which is seen to be coercive of the surrogate's surrendering of the child.

In the USA, state courts have come to different conclusions on the legal status of surrogate arrangements. In *Doe* v. *Kelley*, it was alleged that Jane and John Doe (pseudonyms) were a married couple. Jane was not capable of having children and the couple arranged that Mary Doe be their surrogate mother for the sum of $5000 plus medical expenses. The Wayne County Circuit Court stated that:[78]

> Baby-selling is against the public policy of this State and the State's interest in preventing such conduct is sufficiently compelling and meets the test set forth in *Roe*. Mercenary considerations used to create a parent–child relationship and its impact upon the family unit strike at the very foundation of human society and are patently and necessarily injurious to the community. It is a fundamental principle that children should not and cannot be bought and sold. The sale of children is illegal in all states.

The court proceeded to hold that the surrogate arrangement was void as it contravened the baby-selling statute and was contrary to public policy. In the Michigan Court of Appeals, it was alleged on behalf of the plaintiffs that the Michigan Adoption Code which prohibited the exchange of money or other consideration in connection with adoption infringed upon the plaintiffs' constitutional right of privacy. In refusing to declare that the Adoption Code was unconstitutional, the court said[79]

> While the decision to bear and beget a child has thus been found to be a fundamental interest protected by the right of privacy, we do not view that right as a valid prohibition of state interference in the plaintiffs' contractual arrangement. The statute in question does not directly prohibit John Doe and Mary Doe from having the child as planned. It acts instead to preclude the plaintiffs from paying consideration in conjunction with their use of the state's adoption precedures. In effect, the plaintiffs' contractual agreement discloses a desire to use the adoption code to change the legal status of the child, that is, its right to support, intestate succession, etc. We do not perceive this goal as within the realm of fundamental interests protected by the right to privacy from reasonable governmental regulation.

In New Jersey, in the controversial *Baby M case*, the Superior Court held that the surrogate arrangement was valid.[80] This landmark decision essentially gave the law's blessing to surrogate motherhood. Judge Sorkow held that according to the 'best interest of the child' principle, the biological father should have custody of the child and his wife was allowed to adopt the child. At the same time, the judge terminated the surrogate's parental rights. He took the view that this new social phenomenon, surrogate motherhood, was here to stay and that legislative regulation to govern it was the best way to approach the complicated issues raised in surrogacy, avoiding harm to society, the family and the child. Although in New Jersey, surrogacy was not governed by any law or statute, it was argued that a surrogacy arrangement was vitiated by state adoption laws which prohibited the payment of money as consideration for the surrendering of the child for adoption. This argument was rejected by Judge Sorkow who took the view that the biological father could not purchase his own child.

On appeal, the New Jersey Supreme Court unanimously held that the surrogate arrangement was void and contrary to public policy.[81] The court observed that[82]

> This [the surrogate arrangement] is the sale of a child, or at the very least, the sale of a mother's right to her child, the only mitigating factor being that one of the purchasers is the father. Almost every evil that prompted the prohibition of the payment of money in connection with adoptions exists here.

The Supreme Court, however, agreed with the conclusion reached by the lower court. It overturned the lower court's termination of the surrogate mother's parental rights (as there was no proof that the surrogate was unfit to act as a mother) and rescinded the adoption order of the father's wife. The surrogate was given visitation rights.[83]

But on the question of custody of Baby M, the decision of the trial court which gave custody to the father – a decision which was confirmed by the Supreme Court – evoked concerned comment from feminist quarters. Constitutional and legal issues aside, the case raised a number of social issues. It was said that surrogacy arrangements are discriminatory in nature. Only well-to-do couples can afford to hire a surrogate and only the poor are willing to give up nine months of their life for $10 000 in terms of monetary return. It was said that 'it works out at about 60-odd cents an hour before taxes'.[84] The facts in the *Baby M case* fit into the scenario which some have prophesied. The surrogate social background was that of a dropout from high school at 15, who married Mr Whitehead, a sanitation truck driver who had a serious drink problem and lost his job. Mrs Whitehead worked at one time as a bar dancer to help out financially. At the time the case came to court, the family was in serious financial difficulties. The family owed $8000 on the house in which they were living and the debt was due. When the surrogate decided to keep the child, she forfeited her $10 000 and eviction proceedings were instigated against the Whiteheads. Conversely, the Sterns were well-to-do professional middle-class people, one a doctor and the other a chemist. The class divide, some suspected, had influenced the court's decision on the question of custody, and Mrs Whitehead was bound to lose her case. Attack was centred on the nature of the details which were revealed to the court – details such as the way in which Mrs Whitehead played with the child – something which had a distinct middle-class bias,[85] and the characterization of Mrs Whitehead as being impulsive, self-centred and domineering, albeit not to the extent of being an unfit mother. Yet, when a comparison was made, the surrogate was found to be wanting and, in a way, less superior than the Sterns in terms of lifestyle, social advantage, way of life and the kind of love and care she could provide for the child.

However, it must be said that much of the heat of the debate in this custody battle was assuaged when Mrs Whitehead's parental rights were restored by the Supreme Court. Whether one agrees or disagrees with this decision, it must be said that in any custody dispute there is a 'losing' party and *Baby M* was no different, except that the battle was played in the full glare of international publicity elevating it to high drama.

In another surrogacy case in Kentucky, the court in *Surrogate Parenting Association* v. *Commonwealth ex. rel. Armstrong* distinguished between a baby-selling statute and surrogate arrangements and considered that the former does not apply to the latter which was an agreement entered into prior to the conception of the child.[86]

Thus, it can be seen that the US courts have come to different conclusions as to whether surrogacy with money payment falls within the baby- selling statutes. Attempts to argue that it is not baby-selling have not been particularly successful. One writer argues that:[87]

> . . . an agreement to have a baby for the purpose of giving it up for adoption is functionally different from selling babies already conceived. What the couple are doing is buying the right to *rear* a child by paying the 'mother'. The 'purchasers' do not buy the right to treat the child as a commodity since the child abuse and neglect laws still apply [emphasis original].

It is submitted that this argument is rather incomplete and, to a certain extent, flawed. Although it is correct that the commissioning parties are not buying babies as a commodity, and that they are within the ambit of the laws on child abuse and neglect, it seems unsound to suggest that the commissioning parties are merely buying 'the right to rear a child by paying the "mother"'. Even if there is such a 'right to rear a child', ought it be capable of being bought and sold? Will this be injurious to the interests of the child?[88] In other words, there may be other fundamental values which conflict with such a view of surrogacy for a fee. Consequently, this approach scarcely leads one closer to what is really regarded as objectionable about surrogacy for a fee.

Surrogacy, as a means of founding a family (whether through reproduction or not), may indeed be very close to the concept of adoption, except that adoption is usually the surrendering of a child in situations where parents find themselves unable or unwilling to undertake parental duties for one reason or another, whereas surrogacy is the deliberate creation of a child for the purpose of parenting by a person or persons other than the surrogate. Nonetheless, if one examines the legal position of money payment in connection with adoption, it may give some insight as to why surrogacy for a fee is often connected with the baby-selling argument.

The present UK law, and many US state laws, have reflected society's disapproval of any transaction that is seen as linked to baby-selling (or money payment connected with the creation of parent–child relationship). Thus, Section 50 of the Adoption Act 1958,[89] and Section 51 of the Adoption (Scotland) Act 1978,[90] generally prohibit payment of money in consideration for surrendering a child for adoption. Equally, US legislative provisions in various states prohibit payment of money or other reward to parents in consideration for adoption.[91]

There are two main reasons why public policy is against money payment in connection with adoption. First, a state has a legitimate interest in protecting mothers from being, as was said in one case:[92]

> . . . coerced, compelled, forced or pressured to feel constraint or obliged to yield up their infants whether by threats of violence, financial withdrawal, or derision regardless of how oblique or veiled the pressure might be.

Similarly, in the case of surrogacy for a fee, a state has a legitimate interest in ensuring that surrogates are not pressured by a fee to hand the child over to the commissioning parties.

This state interest can be reconciled with the argument made earlier, that the right to found a family is narrower in scope than the right to reproduce and/or to use one's gestational function, and that the state does have the power to interfere more readily with founding a family than in relation to an individual's right to procreate and/or to use her gestational function.[93] In other words, although the right of a surrogate not to be coerced into pregnancy is negative in nature, and thus does not demand the removal of social conditions which may be potentially exploitative,[94] the state can legitimately protect her right to found a family in the face of monetary inducement to give up the surrogate-born child. The converse of this is that a state may have a legitimate interest in preventing the founding of a family by the commissioning parties through payment of a fee.

Additionally, the use of money for the creation of family relationships may not always be in the best interests of a child. A person may pay for a child even though he or she is not suitable for parenthood. Admittedly, states do not generally intervene in natural reproduction to impose any conditions on fitness for parenting. Still, intervention is considered legitimate after birth, if there is evidence, for example, of abuse. Thus, it could be argued that if a state recognizes a certain method of founding a family (whether through reproduction or not) then it has an obligation to regulate it. The simple transfer of a child from one person to another, as in a private surrogacy transaction, without regulation is scarcely satisfactory.

The policy of the state – recognizing the undesirability of money in the creation of parent–children relationships – is one which prohibits, in general, money payment in people's endeavours to found a family.[95] At the same time, the state regulates, through close supervision, these endeavours, ensuring protection of the interests of adults and children. Hence, English law prohibits agreements to transfer parental rights and duties, and both English and Scots law render them unenforceable.[96] In the case of adoption, this state policy is expressed through stringent regulation and close supervision.

Since existing practice favours regulating people's endeavours in founding a family, rather than closing avenues to such endeavours altogether,[97] surrogacy should be regulated to ensure that (i) the childrens' best interests are not jeopardized, and (ii) where surrogates surrender children to the commissioning parties, they are not coerced, especially by monetary considerations. Indeed, judicial reactions to the recent English surrogacy cases may be cited as lending support to this view.[98] In these cases, judicial reaction towards surrogacy with money payment has been toned down. In the *Baby Cotton case, (Re A Baby)*,[99] a surrogate agreed, for £6 500, to carry a child for an infertile couple. The case finally led to the speedy passage of the Surrogacy Arrangements Act 1985.[100] Mr Justice Latey refrained from commenting on the morality of such an arrangement, considering that the best interests of the child were of paramount importance for the court in exercising its wardship jurisdiction.[101] The court ultimately granted the commissioning husband (also the biological father) care and custody of the child. In the *Adoption Application: Surrogacy case*,[102] Mr Justice Latey (again not commenting on the morality of the surrogacy arrangement) made an adoption order in favour of the commissioning parties. Again, in the *Surrogacy Twin Babies case*,[103] where the surrogate changed her mind (the amount paid was not disclosed), Sir John Arnold in the Family Division said that there was nothing 'shameful' about the arrangement.

These cases, however, do not connote judicial acceptance of surrogacy with money payment. As Mr Justice Latey said in both cases, the morality and acceptability of surrogacy is a question for Parliament (which has not taken any definitive stance),[104] not the courts. The task of the courts is to decide in a particular case what is in the best interests of the child. Nonetheless, in all three cases, the judges did not castigate the arrangements as immoral or shameful. Hence, one may infer a possible acceptance by the judiciary of surrogacy with money payment as a viable and acceptable means of founding a family.

These cases also demonstrated two further points. First, the public policy argument against, and the legal difficulty of, surrogacy with money payment may be overcome. Second, the role of the courts in cases of performed surrogacy arrangements can be similar to that which they perform in adoption.

Surrogacy and Adoption.   In the *Adoption Application: Surrogacy case*,[105] money payment of £5 000 was made to compensate the surrogate's loss of earnings and expenses.[106] The surrogate handed the child over to the commissioning parties as agreed, and the couple applied for an adoption order.

Section 50(1) of the Adoption Act 1958 says:[107]

Subject to the provisions of this section, it shall not be lawful to make or give to any person any payment or reward for or in consideration of (a) the adoption by that person of an infant; (b) the grant by that person of any consent required in connection with the adoption of an infant; (c) the transfer by that person of the care and possession of an infant with a view to the adoption of the infant; or (d) the making by that person of any arrangements for the adoption of an infant.

Statutory provision states clearly that the court shall not make an adoption order unless it is satisfied that the applicants have not contravened Section 50 of the Adoption Act 1958.[108]

Despite these provisions, the judge held that no payment had been made under Section 50(1), and he allowed an adoption order after considering that it would be in the best interests of the child.

The judge reasoned that 'it was only after the payments had been made and the baby born that any of [the parties] began to think about adoption and legalities. . . . [N]o payment or reward had been made within Section 50'.[109] This reasoning appears to imply that if the parties had not contemplated or intended the adoption of the child at the time of the payments, which might have been the case here, no payments had been made under Section 50(1) which covers any payment in consideration for the surrendering of a child, or for the granting of consent for the adoption of a child.

The outcome of the case is the only satisfactory conclusion. Section 50(1) was intended to tackle the problem of child trafficking, the possible objectionable features of which are (i) money inducement to mothers to give up their babies, and (ii) the possibility that the interests of the adults giving up or receiving children will take precedence over those of the children. Since the evidence in this case was that the surrogate was acting primarily for altruistic reasons, and that the payments were in fact for her loss of earnings and expenses – and were unconnected with payments for the surrendering of the child, or for granting of consent to the adoption of the child – it could legitimately be interpreted as not being a payment struck at by Section 50(1).

What is most interesting about the judgement is what was said *obiter*. The judge said that if he was mistaken about Section 50(1), that is, if there had been any payment within Section 50(1), he considered that Section 50(3)[110] permitted the court, in the exercise of its discretion in each case, to authorize payment not only prospectively, but also, retroactively.

This again is consistent with the spirit of Section 50.[111] It is not intended to be a bar to an adoption order in a case where payment was innocently made, where there was no evidence of coercion of the mother to give up the child, or irrespective of the child's welfare. It would, however, have such an effect if Section 50 was construed as limiting authorization solely to prospective payment.

The decision of the *Adoption Application: Surrogacy case*[112] is clearly satisfactory; it has effected the best result for all the parties. This liberal interpretation, if followed, may allow adoption of a surrogate-born child where the surrogacy is with money payment, whether the payment is for reasonable compensation, or as a fee.

The Role of the Courts in Performed Surrogacy Arrangements. The decision, and the *obiter dicta*, in the *Adoption Application: Surrogacy case*[113] indicate a possible role for UK courts in performed surrogacy arrangements.[114]

Where a surrogacy arrangement involves money payment, a court can assess the nature of the payment, and decide whether it was a case of surrogacy with reasonable compensation. If it was, as in this case, Section 50(1) will not apply, and an adoption order could be made in favour of the commissioning parties, providing that this is in fact in the child's best interests.

Where money payment to a surrogate is in fact a fee, that is, it is a payment within Section 50(1), the court may still exercise its discretion under Section 50(3) and authorize the payment retroactively if, and only if, adoption in the case is in the child's best interests.

In the *Surrogacy Twin Babies case*[115] custody was granted to the surrogate on the ground that it was in the best interests of the children since they had established a strong bonding with her. These two cases indicate that the court can play an important role in deciding what is in the best interests of a surrogate-born child; a similar role that they have long played in making adoption orders.

CONCLUSION

Surrogacy, a subject of intense and heated debate, raises many uneasy questions. The crux of these worries relates to the sort of society we wish to live in. The surrogacy debate reflects society's values towards fundamental issues such as individual freedom, women's reproductive function, children, family and parenting. *The Warnock Report*,[116] which is the major UK government document examining the issue, condemned it by a majority. The reasons behind this moral condemnation were, however – disappointing as it may be – largely attributable to the report's contentment with rhetorical arguments that surrogacy is a practice where one person treats another as a means to an end, and that it is positively exploitative. None of these really explore the complex, intricate and delicate issues raised in surrogacy. Above all, the report failed to distinguish or explore the nuances pertaining to the different possible financial elements of surrogacy each of which, as analysed above, is so vital in the debate regarding the acceptability of surrogacy.

As has been seen, one of the major arguments against surrogacy is the involvement of money payment which is capable of tainting the transaction with the evil elements of baby-selling. Where surrogacy is conducted in a free market economy, although the mere fact that a woman is paid a reasonable compensation for her gestation services does not automatically render the transaction immoral, it is difficult to dispel fears and feelings of uneasiness with such a transaction. Here we are in the realm of intuition, and it must be conceded that it is difficult to counter or dismiss the perception that surrogacy with money payment is, or is a modern mutated form of, baby-selling, and that this may be so perceived despite the fact that the intention of the commissioning parties and the surrogate is completely genuine, fulfilling their desires to have a child and to help the infertile respectively.

Given this fundamental objection to money in surrogacy, it appears to be proper for society to take steps to ensure that the exercise of the right to have children (whether this relates to the right to reproduce or the right to parenting) does not give rise to the ugly spectre of baby-selling, commodification of babies and women's reproductive function and the parent–child relationship at the expense of poor and illiterate women, child welfare and the erosion of social values regarding the family. Just as society is anxious to see that certain items ought not to be subjected to market forces, there is a realm of human relations which ought not to be the subject of buying and selling. This same argument has been used to oppose subjecting organs, blood, and regenerative materials such as semen to market forces.[117] The nearest UK society has come to this, in relation to regenerative materials, is to encourage donation by compensating donors for loss of time and travelling expenses by a token payment expressing appreciation for their donation. Similarly, profit from one's reproductive function or baby is utterly discordant with social values pertaining to these matters.

Although the fee element of surrogacy is unacceptable, a complete legal ban on surrogacy is no satisfactory solution. In the words of the Ontario Report,[118]

... given the relative accessibility of artificial insemination, pro-hibition would result in recourse to clandestine private arrangements that would realise the worst fears of those who oppose this practice. Dangers of exploitation of the weak by the powerful, pregnancies contracted by the irresponsible, and the introduction of infants into inappropriate, even dangerous circumstances would be seen to be accentuated if the practice were driven underground. At the greatest risk would be the child whose place in society would be uncertain. ...

Accordingly, we have rejected prohibition in favour of a form of regulation, in the belief that the latter best would protect the interests of all concerned . . .

What then should the law do? In 1985, the UK Parliament passed the Surrogacy Arrangements Act which outlaws the activities of commercial agencies as middle-men arranging surrogacy for prospective surrogates and commissioning parties. Besides this, there has been little legislative action on surrogacy (see later for Section 30 of the Human Fertilisation and Embryology Act). The judicial scene however is different. Comments about morality in recent English surrogacy cases have become somewhat subdued. This may be interpreted as a possible acceptance by the judiciary of some forms of surrogacy in the founding of a family. Furthermore, the *Adoption Application: Surrogacy case*[119] has removed one major legal impediment to surrogacy with reasonable compensation. The court in effect held that surrogacy with reasonable compensation did not amount to payment in consideration of adoption of a surrogate-born child. In any event, the court said that if it was payment, the court could authorize it, and allow an adoption order in the best interests of the child. The decision indicates that money payment in surrogacy does not necessarily create a legal obstacle to the adoption of a surrogate-born child.

Yet, the English law as it is may be far from satisfactory in a number of aspects.[120] As the case of *Adoption Application: Surrogacy case* has revealed, the courts, being the only forum which can examine and scrutinize the propriety of surrogacy with money payment, cannot attenuate or dilute the strength of the baby-selling argument. In other words, given that a court will make an adoption order if it is in the best interests of a child, and that the taint of impropriety in relation to money payment to a surrogate may have to be ignored, the baby-selling argument remains to be tackled. Unless the commissioning parties are obviously unfit for parenting, it seems unlikely that the court would refuse to make an adoption order in their favour, despite the fact that money payment was the dominant factor in inducing the surrogate to surrender the child. It is perhaps for this reason, and for the protection of the best interests of children, that proponents of surrogacy usually suggest the introduction of a regulatory scheme.[121]

Such a scheme is compatible with the argument in this chapter that surrogacy can be viewed as akin to adoption. Given that steps towards the creation of a parent–child relationship in surrogacy begin before a child is conceived, there is a strong case for the establishment of agencies – along the lines of the present adoption agencies – which will assess the suitability of commissioning parties and surrogates, and counsel and advise them to ensure that they understand the full implications of surrogacy. Such agencies can also regulate the question of payment to avoid the taint of baby-selling.

Again, by analogy with adoption, such agencies must have the skills necessary to deal with the issues involved in surrogacy, and should operate on a non-profit making basis. Legal prohibition of commercial surrogacies can be justified on the ground that their involvement in creating parent–child relationship has in the past proved to be deleterious to the interests of child and adult parties.[122]

If the skeleton of the above regulatory approach is accepted, then the state would be prescribing limits on the exercise of the right to found a family by surrogacy, and the right to use one's reproductive and/or gestational function.

The suggestion that surrogacy should be regulated[123] rather than banned has been made in other jurisdictions. In Ontario, the Law Reform Commission's study, *Human Artificial Reproduction and Related Matters* proposed legislative recognition of surrogacy.[124] In Michigan, House of Representatives Bill No. 5148 proposed detailed regulation of surrogacy.[125] The underlying philosophy of the regulatory approach is that while people do have rights in the areas of procreation and founding a family, some of the problems associated with surrogacy can best be tackled by a regulatory scheme.

A completely different approach to that advocated in this chapter was adopted by the state of Victoria, Australia. In response to *The Waller Report*[126] Section 30 of the Infertility (Medical Procedures) Act 1984 makes surrogacy, whether for a fee or not, an offence. This is accompanied by a penalty for contravention. Recently, a *Report of the New South Wales Law Reform Commission* also came down hard on surrogacy.[127]

Before looking in greater detail in Chapter 7 at the various legislative options outlined here, it must be said that regulation is not necessarily a straightforward task. In deciding and evaluating which option is preferred in terms of their desirability and efficacy (in achieving the goal of respecting the rights of individuals and avoiding the undesirable aspects of surrogacy), the nature of the obligations, which the various terms in a standard surrogate arrangement purports to impose on the parties involved, must be analysed and examined.[128]

NOTES

1   *Vide infra*, Chapter 7. Sections 2 and 3 of the Surrogacy Arrangements Act 1985 have criminalized the activities of commercial surrogacies and the advertising of, or for, surrogacy.

2   *Report of the Committee of Inquiry into Human Fertilisation and Embryology*, London, HMSO, Cmnd. 9314, 1984 (hereinafter cited as *The Warnock Report*).

3   *Re C (a Minor) (Wardship: Surrogacy)* [1985] 1 FLR 846.
4   See for example, *Surrogate Motherhood, Report of the Board of Science and Education* (hereinafter cited as *Surrogate Motherhood*, BMA, 1987); for the debates in other jurisdictions, see *Report of the Disposition of Embryos produced by IVF, the Committee to Consider the Social, Ethical, and Legal Issues Arising from IVF*, chaired by Professor Louis Waller, Victoria, Australia, 1984 (hereinafter cited as *The Waller Report*); and *Report on Human Artificial Reproduction and Related Matters* (2 Vols), Ministry of the Attorney General, Toronto, 1985 (hereinafter cited as *The Ontario Report*). For two more recent reports, see *The Final Report on Surrogate Motherhood*, The New South Wales Law Reform Commission (LRC 60), March 1989, and *The Surrogate Report*, The Working Party of the British Medical Association, 1989.
5   *The Warnock Report*, para. 8.17.
6   Ibid., para. 8.10.
7   For the distinction of full and partial surrogacy, *vide supra*, Chapter 2.
8   See Chapter 7.
9   See Page, Edgar, 'Book Review', *Journal of Medical Ethics* (1986) **12**, pp. 45–52.
10 See Chapter 7.
11 *Vide supra*, Chapter 5, on the 'donation rationale', and Edgar Page, on the suggestion of *in utero* donation, loc. cit.
12 *Vide infra*, pp. 96–119.
13 See Keane, Noel, *The Surrogate Mother*, New York, Everest House, 1981.
14 *The Warnock Report* did not make a distinction between surrogacy in principle, surrogacy with reasonable compensation, surrogacy for a fee and commercial surrogacies.
15 Para. 8.17.
16 See Warnock, Mary, *A Question of Life: The Warnock Report on Human Fertilisation and Embryology*, Oxford, Basil Blackwell, 1985, p. xii (hereinafter cited as *A Question of Life*, 1985).
17 'Legal surrogacy – not for love or money?', *The Listener*, 24 January, 1985, p. 2.
18 For other materials which provide a thorough survey of the rights and wrongs of surrogacy, see Freeman, Michael, 'Is surrogacy exploitative?' in *Legal Issues in Human Reproduction*, Roberts, Shelley, 'Warnock and surrogate motherhood: sentiment or argument?' in Byrne, Peter (ed.) *Rights and Wrongs in Medicine*, King's Fund Publishing Office, London, 1986, p. 80, and the reports cited above.
19 *Vide supra*, Chapter 4.
20 See Casler, Lawrence, *Is Marriage Necessary?*, New York, Human Science Press, 1974, Chapter 3.
21 Ibid.
22 Ibid.
23 See Badinter, Elizabeth, *Myth of Motherhood: An Historical View of the Maternal Instinct*, London, Souvenir Press, 1981.
24 See Badinter, Elizabeth, op. cit.
25 *Vide supra*, Chapter 2, p. 36.
26 *Vide infra*, Chapter 7.
27 Otherwise, there would have to be provisions to ensure that pregnant women care for their children.
28 See *The Warnock Report*, para. 8.11.
29 Paras. 8.17–9.20. Cf. Mary Warnock's article ('Legal surrogacy – not for love or money?' *The Listener*, 24 January, 1985, p. 3) in which it was said:
    [t]here is a deep and widely held belief that the relation of a child and the woman who carries it and gives birth to it is different from the relation

of that to its father. That is the centre of the moral objection to surrogacy.

30 See the *Surrogacy Report*, Appendix V, *BMA Annual Report of Council*, 1989–90, p. 39 at 42.

31 See the 'Surrogacy twin babies case', *The Daily Telegraph*, 13 March, 1987, p. 2. *Vide infra*.

32 See Elizabeth Kane who was an enthusiastic proponent of surrogacy and her account of the difficulties she encountered in coming to terms with surrendering the child. Kane, Elizabeth, *Birth Mother*, Melbourne, Macmillan, 1990.

33 See Hoggett, Brenda M. and Pearl, David S., *The Family, Law and Society: Cases and Materials* (2nd edn.), Butterworths, 1987, London, p. 206.

34 See Dworkin, Gerald, 'Paternalism', in Feinburg, Joel and Cross, Hyman (eds), *Philosophy and Law* (2nd edn.), California, Wadsworth 1980, p. 230; see also Mill, John Stuart, 'On Liberty', in *Philosophy and Law*, op. cit., p. 180.

35 *Vide supra*, Chapter 4.

36 See the Surrogacy Report, Note 4.

37 See *Surrogate Motherhood*, BMA, 1987, pp. 17–22.

38 *Vide supra*, Chapter 4.

39 *Vide supra*, Chapter 4.

40 *Vide infra*, Chapter 7.

41 *Vide infra*, for other reasons for regulating surrogacy.

42 See Radin, O., 'Market-inalienability', *Harvard Law Review*, **100**, 1849, pp. 1928–36 (1987) where he argues that surrogacy is oppressive 'commodification' either of babies or of women's reproductive services and argues for its removal from the market.

43 *Vide supra*, Chapter 2, pp. 6–7.

44 See *Adoption application: Surrogacy case* [1987] 2 All ER 826. *Vide infra*. pp. 114–16.

45 *Vide infra*, Chapter 8, for the argument that people should bear the cost of having children and that generally a state has no obligation to fund people in doing so.

46 *Vide infra*, p. 208, for the suggestion that a third party may participate in deciding reasonable compensation.

47 Bruinvels, Peter, *Official Report*, H.C., Vol. **77**, Col. 50.

48 Greenaway, Harry, *Official Report*, H.C., Vol. **77**, Col. 45.

49 See *The Warnock Report*, para. 8.10.

50 See Roberts, Shelley, 'Warnock and surrogate motherhood: sentiment or argument?' in Bryne, Peter (ed.), *Rights and Wrongs in Medicine*, King's Fund Publishing Office, London, 1986, p. 80.

51 See *The Warnock Report*, para. 8.11.

52 See *The Warnock Report*, para. 8.10.

53 *Vide supra*, Chapter 2.

54 See Roberts, Shelley, loc. cit.

55 *Vide infra*, Chapter 7, pp. 127–32.

56 Roberts, Shelley, loc. cit.

57 Roberts, Shelley, loc. cit., pp. 88–90.

58 *Vide infra*, 105 et seq.

59 For debates on the law's involvement in enforcing morality, see Devlin, P.D.B., *The Enforcement of Morals*, London, Oxford University Press, 1965; Hart, H.L.A., *Law, Liberty and Morality*, Oxford, Oxford University Press, 1982. See also *Report of the Committee on Homosexual Offences and Prostitution*, London, HMSO, Cmd. 247, 1957.

60   Although prostitution is not criminal *per se*, the criminal law steps in where other compelling interests are regarded as overriding. For instance, it is criminal to encourage others to become prostitutes, to allow premises to be used for prostitution, to live on the earnings of prostitution and to loiter or solicit for the purposes of prostitution. See the Sexual Offences Act 1956, Street Offences Act 1959, the Sexual Offences Act 1985, and the Sexual Offences (Scotland) Act 1976. For a detailed discussion of offences relating to prostitution, see Gordon, G.H., *The Criminal Law of Scotland* (2nd edn.), Edinburgh, W. Green & Son, 1978, pp. 914–19; Smith J.C. & Hogan, B., *Criminal Law*, London, Butterworths, 1978, pp. 425–35.

61   Section 1 of the Sexual Offences Act 1967 provides that homosexual acts between consenting adults in private are not a criminal offence. Compare Section 7 of the Sexual Offences (Scotland) Act 1976 which provides that conduct of gross indecency between males in private is a criminal offence; see Gordon, G.H., op. cit., pp. 905–6.

62   *Vide infra*, pp. 108–19, for a discussion of the baby-selling argument.

63   *Vide supra*, p. 96.

64   Para. 8.17.

65   *The Warnock Report* is unclear as to who it regards as being treated by whom as a means to an end. It may be that the commissioning parties are treating the surrogate or the potential child as a means to an end. Or, alternatively, it may be that the surrogate is treating the commissioning parties or the potential child as a means to an end.

66   See Marietta, Don E., 'On using people', *Ethics* (1971–2), **82**, 232.

67   *The Warnock Report* did not distinguish the different financial dimensions of surrogacy; it is possible that 'financial interests' referred also to surrogacy with reasonable compensation. This, however, does not affect the argument made here.

68   See para. 8.17.

69   See Winslade, W.J., 'Surrogate mothers – right or wrong?', *Journal of Medical Ethics* (1983) **9**, p. 153.

70   See generally, Wright, Moira, 'Surrogacy and adoption: problems and possibilities', *Family Law* (1986) **16**, p. 109.

71   *Vide infra*.

72   *Family Law* (1978) **8**, p. 170, High Court; *Family Law* (1984) **14**, p. 241, Court of Appeal.

73   The High Court granted access to the father, but not custody.

74   See *Family Law* (1978) **8**, p. 170.

75   The mother appealed to the Court of Appeal against the High Court judge's decision to grant access. The Court of Appeal denied access in the best interests of the child.

76   See 'Sordid commercial bargain', *Family Law* (1984) **14**, p. 241.

77   See Parker, Diana, 'Surrogate mothering, an overview', *Family Law* (1984) **14**, p. 140.

78   *Family Law Report* (BNA) 3011, 3013 (1980).

79   106 Mich. App. 169; 307 N.W. 2d 438 (1981).

80   No. FM–25314–86E, Superior Court of New Jersey, Chancery Division, 217 N.J. 313; 525 A 2d 1128 (1987).

81   In *dicta*, the Supreme Court said that it would find no legal impediments to a surrogate arrangement in certain instances: where the surrogate agreed to serve for no consideration and the agreement allows her to change her mind about the child after birth and asserts her legal rights as the mother of the child.

82   109 N.J. 396; 5337 A.2d 1227 (1988) (Lexis p. 20). For the details of the Supreme

Court's decision, see Appendix 5; for a sample of the surrogate contract in the case, see Appendix 3.

83 *225 N.J. Super.* 267; 542 A.2d 52 (1988).

84 See *The Observer*, 5 April, 1987.

85 One psychiatrist criticized Mrs Whitehead for giving Baby M four cuddly pandas to play with and thought that she would have done better to offer more stimulating toys.

86 704 S.W. 2d 209 (Ky, 1986); see also in the *Matter of Adoption of Baby Girl*, L.J., 132 Misc. 2d 972, 505 N.Y.S. 2d 813 (Sur, 1986).

87 Davies, Iwan, 'Contracts to bear a child', *Journal of Medical Ethics* (1985) **11**, pp. 61, 62.

88 *Vide infra*, pp. 188–213.

89 For the terms of the Section, *vide infra*.

90 The terms are the same as Section 50 of the Adoption Act 1958.

91 See Rushevsky, Cynthia, 'Legal recognition of surrogate gestation', *Women's Rights Law Reporter* (1982) **7**, p. 107.

92 *Galison* v. *District of Columbia*, 420 A 2d 1263, 1268 (D.C. 1979).

93 *Vide supra*, Chapter 3.

94 Ibid.

95 See Section 50 of the Adoption Act 1958 which applies to England and Wales, and Sections 51 and 24 of the Adoption (Scotland) Act 1978.

96 *Vide infra*, Chapter 7.

97 *Vide supra*, Chapter 4 on the current practice of not prohibiting the use of artificial techniques which allow people to found a family.

98 See *Re C (a Minor) (Wardship: Surrogacy)* [1985] FLR 846; *Adoption Application Surrogacy Case*, [1987] 2 All ER 826, and *Surrogacy Twin Babies Case*, *Daily Telegraph*, 13 March, 1987, p. 2.

99 *Re C (a Minor) (Wardship: Surrogacy)* [1985] FLR 846.

100 See Sloman, Susan, 'Surrogacy Arrangements Act 1985', *N.L.J.* (1985) **135** (2) p. 978.

101 He said that the '. . . moral, ethical and social considerations are for others and not for this court in its wardship jurisdiction', op. cit.

102 Op. cit. There was no written agreement in this case. Nor were lawyers consulted. The agreement was one based on trust. Surrogacy was achieved through natural intercourse between the surrogate and the commissioning husband.

103 *The Daily Telegraph*, 13 March, 1987, p. 2.

104 See the *Consultation Paper*, para. 41–3.

105 [1987] 2 All ER 826.

106 The payment originally agreed between the commissioning married couple and the surrogate (who was married with two children and had to give up her job to have the child) was £10 000. The surrogate refused to accept the balance of £5 000 after the birth of the child on the grounds that she had already made some money through publishing her story in a book. The payment of £5 000 was said by the judge to be an amount that did not in fact cover the surrogate's loss of earnings and expenses.

107 Contravention of Section 50 is a criminal offence for which the local authority may prosecute; see Section 50(2) and Section 54(2) of the Adoption Act 1958.

108 Section 22(5) the Children Act 1975.

109 [1987] 2 All ER 826.

110 Section 50(3) says 'This section does not apply to any payment . . . authorised by the court to which an application for an adoption order in respect of an infant is made.'

111   Section 50(1) and Section 50(3), taken together, state plainly that payment is unlawful unless authorised by the court. See also an accompanying section in the Adoption Act 1958, Section 7(1)(c). It states that before making an adoption order, the court should satisfy itself that the applicant 'has not received' and that no person 'has made' to the applicant, any payment in consideration of adoption except such as the court 'may' sanction.

112   *The Times*, 12 March, 1987, p. 27.

113   *Vide supra*.

114   Although as will be seen in Chapter 7, where a surrogacy agreement is breached, the law is an inadequate tool in regulating the behaviour of the parties.

115   *Vide supra*.

116   For other criticisms of the report, see Freeman, Michael, 'After Warnock – whither the law?' in *Current Law Problems*, (1989) **39**, p. 33; Freeman, Michael, 'Is surrogacy exploitative?', in McLean, Sheila A.M. (ed.), *Legal Issues in Human Reproduction*, Aldershot, Dartmouth, 1989, p. 164; Lee, Simon, 'Re-reading Warnock' in Bryne, Peter (ed.), *Rights and Wrongs in Medicine*, King's Fund Publishing Office, London, 1986, p. 37.

117   See the proposed Human Organ Transplant Bill which makes it a criminal offence to be concerned in payment for the supply of human organs for transplantation. The Bill however, does not prevent the reimbursement of reasonable expenses incurred in the supply of transplant organs, including loss of earnings by a living donor, see *British Medical Journal* **298**, 1989 p. 1670.

118   *Report on Human Artificial Reproduction and Related Matters* (2 Vols), Ministry of the Attorney General, Toronto, July 1985, p. 232.

119   *Supra cit*.

120   For other aspects of a surrogacy arrangement and the legal status of the various provisions, see Chapter 7.

121   See *The Warnock Report*, 'Expression of Dissent: A. Surrogacy', pp. 87–9.

122   See the *Report of the Departmental Committee on Adoption Services and Agencies*, B.P.P., 1936–7, Cmnd 5499. para. 30 (or *The Horsburgh Report*) which highlighted the unsatisfactory state of the English adoption law caused by the operation of unregulated intermediaries which operated on either a profitable or non-profitable basis. Today, the operation of adoption agencies in the England and Scotland is stringently regulated by the Adoption Act 1958 (as amended) and the Adoption (Scotland) Act 1978, respectively.

123   See others with the same view, for instance, 'The dissenting minority' in *The Warnock Report*, Freeman, Michael, 'Is surrogacy exploitative?' and 'After Warnock – whither the law?', op. cit.

124   *Report on Human Artificial Reproduction and Related Matters*, 2 Vols, Ministry of the Attorney General, Toronto, July 1985, p. 232.

125   See Rushevsky, Cynthia, 'Legal recognition of surrogacy gestation', *Women's Rights Law Reporter* (1982) **7**, pp. 107–142.

126   *The Waller Report*, op. cit.; see generally, 'Current Topics', *Australian Law Journal* (1984) **58**, p. 683.

127   See 'Surrogate motherhood', *Report of the New South Wales Law Reform Commission*, March 1989, p. 39. The commission took the view that,

>   . . . the disadvantages of the practice [of surrogacy] to be so great as to outweigh even the needs of the infertile. We cannot accept that it is in the child's interests to be conceived and born for this purpose. The process degrades the position of women in society and the process of childbirth. It lends credence to the view that children may be used as a means to an end and employs the services of professional medical practitioners and health care workers to assist.

For a brief discussion of the report, see 'Current Topics' *Australian Law Journal*, (1899) **63**, p. 303.

128   For a sample of a surrogate arrangement, see Appendix 3.

7 Legal Issues in Surrogacy

INTRODUCTION

It has been concluded that, even where money payment is involved, surrogacy is an acceptable method of exercising one's right to reproduce and the right to found a family. However, this mode of exercising one's rights can legitimately be regulated in order to ensure that the interests of children and surrogates are adequately protected.[1] The legal problems involved in a surrogacy agreement are complex; a virtual legal minefield for lawyers. But contracts have been drafted and utilized stipulating the rights and duties of the parties involved in such an agreement. What the surrogate is supposed to do in such a contract is to carry a baby to term (in accordance with the artificial reproductive techniques prescribed in the contract) and then surrender the child to the commissioning parties. This appears to be simple and straightforward. But there are many unforeseen issues that could arise. What if the surrogate fails to become pregnant after many months of AI; is she compensated for her effort? Can the commissioning parties repudiate the contract and find someone else? What if the commissioning parties die after the surrogate mother gets pregnant; is she to have an abortion?

The legal issues involved in a surrogacy arrangement are legion. In this chapter, only the fundamental salient issues which go to the heart of a surrogacy arrangement will be considered. In a nutshell, they can be formulated in terms of two questions: first, what is the legal status of some of the fundamental terms in such an arrangement, and is the arrangement lawful and enforceable? And second, both connected and separate from the first question, parenthood in surrogacy.

VALIDITY AND ENFORCEABILITY OF A SURROGACY ARRANGEMENT

The 'Transfer Term'

The Surrogacy Arrangements Act 1985 which outlawed the operation of commercial surrogacies left the issue of the lawfulness of a surrogacy arrangement open. Section 1(9) of the 1985 Act states,

> This Act applies to arrangements whether or not they are lawful and whether or not they are enforceable by or against any of the persons making them.

According to current English and Scots law, a surrogacy arrangement (whether for money payment or not) is not illegal or unlawful.[2] The Surrogacy Arrangements (Amendment) Bill 1986, Clause 1, which attempted to make a surrogacy arrangement unlawful, was lost through lack of parliamentary time.[3]

As was said in parliamentary debates on the Bill, the objective of Clause 1 was to ensure that a money payment made in a surrogacy transaction was irrecoverable.[4] Thus, in the case of breach by a surrogate, the commissioning parties could not sue to recover a payment which had already been made to her. This would not be the case if a surrogacy arrangement is merely void and unenforceable.

Nonetheless, under both English and Scots common law, an agreement to transfer or surrender parental rights and duties is contrary to public policy, and is unenforceable.[5] The English statutory provision which restates the common law rule is found in Section 85(2) of the Children Act 1975:

> Subject to section 1(2) of the Guardianship Act 1973 . . . a person cannot surrender or transfer to another any parental right or duty he has as respects a child.

And Section 1(2) of the Guardianship Act 1973 says,

> An agreement for a man or woman to give up in whole or in part, in relation to any child of his or hers, the rights and authority referred to in subsection (1) above shall be unenforceable, except [a separation agreement between husband and wife] . . .[6]

Similarly, the Scots common law rule has received statutory force in Section 10(2) of the Guardianship Act 1973.[7] In other words, under both English and Scots law, an agreement to transfer parental rights and duties is unenforceable. Section 36 of the Human Fertilisation and Embryology Act (HFEA) makes this clear.[8]

The obvious legal problem arising from using a surrogacy arrangement to found a family relates to one of its fundamental terms, namely, that which states that a surrogate is to surrender the child to the commissioning parties (hereinafter called the *transfer term*).

The law prohibiting an agreement to transfer parental rights and duties would apply to a surrogacy agreement depending on who was considered to be the mother, and therefore, who had parental rights and duties regarding the surrogate-born child. The 'transfer term' in a surrogacy arrangement would not contravene any statutory provisions if (in the most unlikely eventuality) a surrogate was considered not to be the mother of the child. The HFEA,[9] now makes it clear that the surrogate should be considered the mother.[10] In such a case, the 'transfer term' in a surrogate arrangement would be void and unenforceable.

Evidently, if a dispute were to arise between a surrogate and the commissioning parties regarding the custody of a surrogate-born child, the decision would be based on the child's best interests.[11] Otherwise, the court would be allowing a contractual term to pre-empt its investigation into the best interests of the child.

Given this understanding of the law as it is – that the 'transfer term' in a surrogacy arrangement cannot be enforced – the endeavour to found a family (whether through reproduction or not) is likely to be a haphazard and precarious enterprise. Nonetheless, since the right to found a family (whether through reproduction or not) is essentially a negative claim-right, there is no obligation on the part of the state to enforce a surrogacy arrangement or to ensure that it has a good prospect of succeeding.[12] However, as has been argued, there is a case for regulating the practice of surrogacy.[13] This, nonetheless, is to be distinguished from enforcement of surrogacy arrangements.

Although unenforceability can be a substantial obstacle to the commissioning parties endeavours to found a family (in the event of a surrogate refusing to surrender the child), surrogacy may still be regarded by some as a realistic and meaningful way of founding a family. It was reported in 1987 that in the US, since the late 1970s, some 500–600 children have been born through surrogacy arrangements. Of these cases, there had been three reported instances where surrogates changed their minds.[14] This being the case, it is necessary to examine and consider the legal status of other fundamental provisions in a surrogacy agreement before considering the shape which a regulatory scheme may take.

In a surrogate agreement, a surrogate will usually agree to carry a child to term (this will be referred to as the 'carrying term'), and to seek proper medical attention to ensure foetal health, not to smoke or consume food and beverages which may be harmful to the child (this will be referred to as the 'pre-natal care term'). These are clearly vital aspects of a surrogacy arrangement. Ordinarily, these goals and objectives would not only be unobjectionable but desirable as they will ensure, as far as possible, that any child born is healthy. However, legal enforcement of these terms is fraught with difficulties.

The 'Carrying Term'

Where a surrogate wishes to abort the foetus, contrary to the 'carrying term', the interests which commissioning parties have in enforcing the carrying term gate's non-abortion appear to be insufficient to prevent the operation. In *Paton* v. *British Pregnancy Advisory Service Trustees*,[15] the English courts first came across a case where the plaintiff (a husband and father) sought an injunction to restrain his wife from having an abortion intended to be carried out under the Abortion Act 1967, without his consent. Sir George P. Baker held that, in law, the husband had no legal right to stop his wife from having an abortion.[16]

> The Abortion Act gives no right to a father to be consulted in respect of a termination of a pregnancy. . . . The husband therefore has no legal right enforceable in law or equity to stop his wife having this abortion.

Paton was considered in *C.* v. *S.*[17] where a father sought an injunction to prevent his girlfriend from terminating an 18–21 week pregnancy. Although the case was not based on the right of a father to be consulted about an abortion – a point which was not argued[18] –it has nonetheless revived the whole debate in Britain.[19]

Cases in the USA since *Roe* v. *Wade*[20] are much more clear on whether a husband–father has a right to prevent his wife's abortion. In *Planned Parenthood of Central Missouri* v. *Danford A-G.*,[21] the Supreme Court held that,[22]

> [the state] may not constitutionally require the consent of the spouse . . . as a condition for abortion during the first twelve weeks of pregnancy. . . . Since the state cannot regulate or proscribe abortion during the first stage, when the physician and his patient make that decision, the state cannot delegate authority to any particular person even the spouse to prevent abortion during that same period.

The Supreme Court's view emphasizes a woman's right to decide whether to terminate a pregnancy and her right to self-determination. That is, since it is the woman who physically bears the child, and since she is most directly affected by the pregnancy, she should have, within certain limits, the right to make the final decision.[23]

A similar conclusion was reached in the Australian case of *K.* v. *T*:[24] Mr Justice Williams, of the Supreme Court of Queensland, held that a *de facto* father has no legal right to restrain the wife from having an abortion. On appeal to a full court of the Supreme Court of Queensland, three judges upheld that decision.[25]

In a more recent Canadian case of *Tremblay* v. *Daigle*[26] (or the

Chantal Daigle case), the court similarly found against the father. In that case, a potential father obtained an injunction to prevent his girlfriend from having an abortion. The Supreme Court of Canada set aside the injunction holding that the substantive rights which are alleged to support it – the rights accorded to a foetus or a potential father – do not exist. The court held that a foetus is not included within the term 'human being' in the Quebec Charter of Human Rights and Freedoms, and therefore does not enjoy the right to life conferred by Section 1.[27] On the alleged father's or potential father's rights, the court said that

> [T]his argument would appear to be based on the proposition that the potential father's contribution to the act of conception gives him an equal say in what happens to the foetus. Little emphasis was put on this argument in the appeal. It was alluded to by several of the parties in an indirect fashion, although it does appear to have been accepted [by the lower courts].
>
> There does not appear to be any jurisprudential basis for this argument. No court in Quebec or elsewhere has ever accepted the argument that a father's interest in a foetus which he helped create could support a right to veto a woman's decisions in respect of the foetus she is carrying. A number of cases in various jurisdictions outside Quebec have considered this argument and explicitly rejected it. . . . We have been unable to find a single decision in Quebec or elsewhere which would support the allegation of 'father's rights' necessary to support this injunction.

If a father–husband or a father cannot prevent a woman from having an abortion, it is difficult to envisage how the commissioning parties would be able to prevent a surrogate from having an abortion by reason of a surrogate agreement. The Abortion Act 1967, which applies to England, Wales and Scotland, lays down the circumstances under which an abortion can be legal. As long as an abortion is legal, that appears to be the end of the matter.[28]

In the USA, since a woman has a limited right to abortion, the relevant question is likely to be whether a surrogate can waive her (limited) right to abortion by an agreement, and further, whether such a waiver should be irrevocable. This question should not, however, overshadow a more important issue: how can the commissioning parties enforce this waiver without unacceptably infringing the liberty of a surrogate to decide whether or not to continue with the pregnancy?[29] Furthermore, should the commissioning parties have the right to enforce a surrogate's waiver? Given the importance of a woman's freedom to choose in relation to procreation and/or the use of her gestational function, it appears extremely unlikely that a court would hold that a surrogate has legally bound herself to continue her pregnancy. Consequently, where a surrogate wishes to have an abortion within the ambit set by the law, no other party can prevent her. The 'carrying term' in a surrogate agreement appears, therefore, to be unenforceable.

The 'Pre-natal Care Term'

The enforceability of a 'pre-natal care term' through the judicial process is also questionable.

The principles governing contractual equitable remedies in the UK courts are that specific performance of a personal service contract will not be ordered, not only because it may amount to an unacceptable infringement of one's liberty, but also because such an order may be futile (in that involuntary performance may result in something that is far from satisfactory). Nor will the courts issue an injunction if the result is directly or indirectly to order the specific performance of a personal service contract.[30] Thus, it appears extremely unlikely that a court will use its equitable remedies to order a surrogate to adhere to the 'pre-natal care term'.

However, since the 'transfer term' is unenforceable, the question really is, will a court use its equitable remedies to enforce a contractual term to undertake pre-natal care?

There are no UK precedents suggesting that the court would be willing, or ought, to take on such a task irrespective of contract.[31] In the recent English case of Re D (a Minor)[32] the House of Lords upheld the care order of Berkshire Social Services respecting a heroin addict's baby who was born with drug withdrawal symptoms. The decision was based on the interpretation of 'is being' in Section 1(2) of the Children and Young Persons Act 1969, which says:

> If the court before which a child . . . is brought . . . is of opinion that any of the following conditions is satisfied . . . (a) his proper development is being unavoidably prevented or neglected or his health is being unavoidably impaired or neglected or he is being ill-treated and that he is in need of care and control . . . then . . . the court may if it thinks fit make such an order . . .

It was held that, in deciding whether any of the conditions in Section 1(2) were satisfied, the justices were entitled to have regard to the fact that the mother had persisted in taking excessive drugs against medical advice during her pregnancy. Furthermore, in this context, the court could take into account the hypothetical future of the situation.[33] To that extent, the case was primarily concerned with what were the relevant factors in determining suitability for parenting.[34] It may have an indirect impact on the behaviour of pregnant women, but it is far from suggesting that the courts supervise, or will supervise, the conduct of a pregnant woman. Consequently, the 'pre-natal care term' in a surrogacy arrangement is unlikely to be enforceable in courts.

Some preliminary observations can be made from the above analysis of the legal status of various vital terms in a surrogate arrangement. First, the 'transfer term' is unenforceable and although the commissioning parties may wish to have a child for parenting via surrogacy, the practical reality of the usefulness of surrogacy is limited to the extent that the surrogate will not renege on the agreement. In the unfortunate event that she does, the contract cannot be the basis upon which the commissioning parties found their claim for the custody of the child. Second, the 'carrying term' and the 'pre-natal care term' are also unenforceable although not contrary to public policy or void. The implication of this is that the commissioning parties' attempt to enforce these terms will be futile and the better alternative may be to provide for the automatic termination of the arrangement on the surrogate's breach of a fundamental term.

As mentioned earlier, the question of parenthood has an important bearing on the question of the legal status of the 'transfer term', but it is also important to children born as a result of surrogacy.[35] *The Warnock Report* considered the question of motherhood (but not fatherhood),[36] notwithstanding its recommendation which, if accepted, would render criminal, the 'actions of professionals and others who knowingly assist in the establishment of a surrogacy pregnancy'.[37]

In the following section, the question of parenthood in surrogacy will be considered. As in Chapter 5, similar terminology will be used to describe what may possibly be complex human relationships. Thus, 'parent', 'mother' and 'father' are used to denote a legal relationship between an adult and a child. The undernoted terms, however, are purely descriptive, 'biological mother/father' refers to a woman/man who contributes an ovum/semen to the creation of a child. 'Ovum/semen donor' refers to a biological mother/father who has donated her or his genetic gametes. 'Social/commissioning mother/father (or parties)' refers to a woman/man who intends to rear a child regardless of her or his genetic link with the child. 'Surrogate/ bearing mother' refers to a woman who bears a child regardless of her genetic link with the child. As will be seen,[38] a commissioning father who is also a biological father will not be regarded as a semen donor.

PARENTHOOD AND SURROGACY

As has been noted,[39] the question of parenthood in natural pro-creation, is based on genetics – a biological mother and father are parents of a child, and are accorded parental duties regarding the child. Surrogacy, as implemented by artificial reproductive techniques, is a completely novel concept, and one major legal problem it engenders is, who are the parents of a surrogate-born child (and thus have parental duties regarding the child)? Who is the father? Is he the commissioning father (who may or may not be the biological father), or is he the semen donor? Is the mother the commissioning mother (who may or may not be the biological mother), or the ovum donor? Since all these permutations are technically possible, it should be clear that an attempt to rationalize the situation is needed.

Fatherhood

Here again, as in the case of artificial reproduction without the involvement of surrogacy (see Chapter 5), the HFEA has unexpectedly made an important provision on this point, and therefore resolved the difficulty to a certain extent. It is, however, worthwhile to examine the backgrounds to the problems in this area, and the solution in the HFEA, in greater detail.

A surrogate-born child has two possible candidates as his or her father: the semen donor (where, for example, the commissioning father is sterile), or the commissioning father (who may be the biological father, as in the case of partial surrogacy).

As has been argued before,[40] according to the 'donation rationale' a donor should have no rights or liabilities regarding a resulting child. The 'donation rationale', as exemplified by the 'AID provision', (which suggests that where a wife receives AID the husband should be considered the father of the child unless non-consent is proven, and that a semen donor will have no rights or liabilities regarding the child born as a result) can cause at least two problems in partial surrogacy. For instance, in California, the AID law deems a husband irrefutably to be the father of an AID child.[41] This can have application to partial surrogacy, where a surrogate has a husband, and she undertakes to be artificially inseminated using the semen of the commissioning father. The result will be that the surrogate-born child will be regarded, irrefutably, as the child of the surrogate and her husband, even if the husband had nothing to do with the surrogate arrangement, and the purpose of the surrogacy was to enable the commissioning parties to have a child. This result is undesirable for a number of reasons.

First, the husband becomes the father for no logical reason. Fatherhood is attributed to him on a purely fortuitous basis, that is, he happens to be the husband of the surrogate. Second, this is totally contrary to the intention of the parties.

Even if an AID law is framed in a less rigid form (for example, if it allows a husband to prove his non-consent to his wife's AID, and consequently, he is not regarded, under the AID law, as the father of the resulting child),[42] the commissioning father, who is the biological father, could be excluded by the 'corollary principle' because he would be treated as a semen donor?[43] If so, who is the father? This discussion shows that if an 'AID provision' is not to have unintended consequences in partial surrogacy, it has to be very carefully framed.

Where the commissioning father is the biological father, for instance, in partial surrogacy, he should be distinguished from a semen donor, since unlike the standard case of semen donation, he never intends to divest himself of his responsibilities and liabilities regarding a surrogate-born child who is born as a result of a surrogate's artificial insemination using his semen. Consequently, he should not be excluded from being the father of a surrogate-born child by use of the 'corollary principle'.

In the case where the commissioning father is not the biological father of a surrogate-born child, the 'donation rationale' should apply since an anonymous semen donor should not be regarded as the father. As argued before,[44] the 'donation rationale' which is an exception to the 'genetic mode', will when applied regard a man who is not the biological father, as the father of a child, where he consents to a woman's pregnancy through AI or IVF.

The same principle could equally apply in surrogacy, although the nature of the consent in respect of the two men involved has to be distinguished. In the case of the commissioning father, his consent is to a surrogate carrying a child created using semen from a donor so that he can found a family. Where a surrogate has a husband, his consent will relate to the wife's participation in the surrogacy. This distinction is necessary to avoid the situation of attributing fatherhood to the surrogate's husband, and depriving the commissioning father of fatherhood – a result which would be totally contrary to the intention of all parties.

In sum, in surrogacy, where a commissioning father is the biological father, he should be regarded as the father of a surrogate-born child. In other words, he should not be treated as a semen donor. Where he is not the biological father, he should be regarded as the father on the ground that he has consented to the surrogate's pregnancy, whether through AI or IVF, for the founding of a family by him. Here, his consent should be distinguished from that of a surrogate's husband (if she has one). A surrogate's husband should not be regarded as father of a surrogate-born child, because if he had consented to his wife's pregnancy, the nature of his consent would relate only to his wife's surrogacy. This caveat should apply equally to a surrogate's male partner who consents to her surrogacy if what has been argued previously about extending the application of the 'AID provision' to unmarried couples is accepted.[45]

Motherhood

The Warnock Report, as has been noted,[46] recommended that when a child is born to a woman following donation of another's egg, the woman giving birth should, for all purposes, be regarded in law as the mother of the child, and that the egg donor should have no rights or duties in respect of the child.[47] Similarly, it recommended that a woman carrying a donated embryo should be regarded as the mother of the child.[48] These recommendations are apparently the result of a consistent application of the 'donation rationale'.[49]

In relation to surrogacy, *The Warnock Report* recommended that whether in a case of partial or full surrogacy (that is, irrespective of whether the surrogate is the biological mother), the surrogate should be regarded as the mother of the child.[50] This will hereinafter be called the 'surrogacy recommendation'. The Report considered that the two types of surrogacy could be covered by its recommendations regarding egg and embryo donation, even though it acknowledged that 'the egg or embryo has not been donated'.[51]

This 'surrogacy recommendation', although widely accepted, and is now embodied in Section 27(1) of the HFEA,[52] is rather curiously expressed.[53] If there is no donation of ovum or embryo to a surrogate, why then should a surrogate become the mother in a situation where she is not the biological mother, given that the 'genetic mode', presumably, is the basis for motherhood?

Analysis of the issue of motherhood in surrogacy reveals that the real basis for attributing motherhood is that a woman has borne a child – which will hereinafter be called the 'bearing factor' rather than the use of the 'genetic mode'.

The 'bearing factor' as a basis for defining motherhood is, in fact, consonant with the attribution of motherhood in both natural and artificial procreation. For instance, although motherhood in cases of natural procreation, AI and IVF (whether donated ovum is used or not) may be explained, as it has been,[54] in terms of the 'genetic mode' and the 'donation rationale', there is no case where the application of these principles does not invariably accord motherhood to a bearer of a child.[55]

The 'bearing factor' as a basis for motherhood is entirely different from the 'genetic mode' for fatherhood. Nonetheless, they can both be logically justified according to the different role men and women play in natural and artificial procreation.

The 'bearing factor' suggests that bearing a child is both a necessary and a sufficient condition of the attribution of motherhood. The role played by the woman who carried and gave birth to a child is so significantly different from the role played by the male partner that the 'genetic mode' has less significance in determining motherhood.

Summary: Parenthood in Surrogacy

The above recommendation in respect of fatherhood is realistic. It reflects the intention of semen donors, and men who wish to found a family through the use of donated semen. As suggested earlier, if the 'donation rationale' operates to negate the parental rights and duties of a man who donates semen, cases of donation must be distinguished from cases where there is no donation of semen. The importance of this can clearly be seen by reference to the position of a commissioning father in partial surrogacy. In the case of a woman, the 'bearing factor' determines motherhood. Consequently, the question of ovum donation has no real importance.

The question of parenthood or status is dealt with by the HFEA Section 27(1), it says[56]

> A woman who is carrying or has carried a child as a result of the placing in her of an embryo or of sperm and eggs, and no other woman, is to be treated as the mother of the child.

On the question of fatherhood, Section 28 says that,

(1) This section applies in the case of a child who is being or has been carried by a woman as a result of placing in her of an embryo or of sperm and eggs or her artificial insemination.
(2) If –
    (a) at the time of the placing in her of the embryo or the sperm and eggs or of her insemination, the woman was a party to a marriage, and
    (b) the creation of the embryo caused by her was not brought about with the sperm of the other party of the marriage,
then, . . . the other party of the marriage shall be treated as the father of the child unless it is shown that he did not consent to the placing in her of the embryo or the sperm and eggs or to her insemination (as the case may be).

Some Final Remarks

It is now almost seven years since the publication of *The Warnock Report* and if surrogacy is as unacceptable as depicted by it, surrogacy should have been barred. Legal developments, judicial and legislative, however, indicate to the contrary.

Section 28 is wider in scope than Section 27 of the Family Law Reform Act 1987 (which will be overtaken by Section 28 of the HFEA when it comes into force). Whereas Section 27 only covered artificial insemination, Section 28 covers AI, IVF and GIFT. The effect of Section 28(2) is that if the surrogate is married, she will become the mother of the surrogate-born child, and her husband will become the father, unless he can show that he did not consent to his wife's surrogacy by AI, IVF or GIFT. The commissioning parties, therefore, will have no rights over the child except through adoption. This problem was drawn to the attention of Parliament during the debate on the Human Fertilisation and Embryology Bill by *Re W (Minors)*. *Re W* involved a surrogate mother (married with her own children) who bore the twins of the commissioning parties and was willing to relinquish them to the latter. During debates on the Bill, it was observed that according to Clauses 26 and 27, the commissioning parents would have to adopt the twins. Section 30 now provides the solution to situations such as this, and the commissioning parties may apply to the court for a parental order within six months of the birth of the child, or in the case of a child born before the coming into force of this Act, within six months of such coming into force. The court, before the making of the order, must be satisfied with a number of conditions. They include the fact that (i) both the father of the child (including a person who is a father by virtue of Section 28 of the Act), where he is not the husband, and the woman who carried the child have freely, and with full understanding of what is involved, agreed unconditionally to the making of the order, (ii) no money or other benefit (other than for expenses reasonably incurred) has been given or received by the husband or the wife for, or in consideration of, the agreement to hand over the child unless authorized by the court. Since Section 30(7) allows payment of reasonable expenses, this subsection therefore empowers the court to authorize payment of money or other benefit other than for expenses reasonably incurred. In the *Adoption Application: Surrogacy case*,[57] the Judge said *obiter* that retrospective authorization is possible. As there is no mechanism for prospective authorization under Section 30, one can only construe the power to authorize as retrospective in nature. This raises the interesting point that Section 30 becomes not only the first statutory provision which paves the way for informal surrogacy arrangements when out-of-pocket expenses are paid, but also surrogacy for a fee. Section 30, however, has its limits; it applies only to a married couple where they need full or partial surrogacy.

In Chapter 6, where the question of fundamental objections to surrogacy was addressed, the solution proposed was some form of regulatory scheme for surrogacy to meet both the objections of baby-selling and unregulated private transfer of parental rights for the creation of a parent–child relationship. Here some of the fundamental legal issues pertaining to a surrogacy arrangement and the question of parenthood have been considered, and it is appropriate now to examine possible regulatory schemes which deal with these issues.

Forms of Regulation

Model Human Reproductive Technologies and Surrogacy Act

Various forms of regulation have been mooted, some more stringent than others, for example, the Model Human Reproductive Technologies and Surrogacy Act.[58] This is an Act governing the status of children born through reproductive technologies and surrogate arrangements and it envisages the lawfulness of a surrogate arrangement provided that it conforms to certain requirements. These requirements are outlined below.

1. A licensed person performing the procedure [the licensed person] receives written certification that the parties successfully completed the medical and nonmedical evaluation and counselling.[59]

COMMENT
The standard used in the nonmedical evaluation of the suitability of the parties (to be parents) is the minimum standard. In other words, the parties should not be subjected to a more stringent standard than would normal parents simply because they are biologically incapable of having their own children through conventional methods. The minimum standard therefore would be set at the level where the state could justify interfering with parenting by taking the child into care in cases of abuse or neglect. This would mean that most individuals would pass the standard test and would have the right to have children.[60]

The alternative, and more stringent, test is that used in selecting prospective adoptive parents. There the standard is the likelihood of being good parents, rather than whether they are unlikely to abuse or neglect the child. More intrusive measures are taken to ascertain whether the parties would be good parents, and investigation into the parties' family, educational and employment background, character and personality, etc., will be necessary. As argued before,[61] the first test is more appropriate as the stringency of the test used in adoption is a reflection of the practical reality of adoption. The substantive test of suitable parents should not be artificially raised when circumstances do not so dictate.

2. The arrangement has received judicial preauthorization; parties to a surrogate contract shall jointly petition to the court for judicial preauthorisation of the arrangement, the court will only validate the arrangement if it is satisfied that,

(i)   the parties have given their informed consent;
(ii)   it contains no prohibited or unconscionable terms; and
(iii)   evaluations and counselling have been completed indicating that the parties qualified to enter into the arrangement.

The effect of a judicial order validating the surrogacy arrangements shall be the automatic termination of parental rights of the surrogate and her husband (if any) 72 hours after the birth of a child born as a result of the arrangement and the vesting of those rights in the commissioning parties unless the surrogate exercises her rights to keep the child, in which case parental rights shall be vested solely in the surrogate and her husband (if any).[62]

COMMENT

If the agreement is not validated, it will be void and therefore unenforceable.[63] One advantage of this proposal is that the court will be involved in determining whether the arrangement is fair and reasonable. Further, as a precondition for authorization the court will be required to satisfy that evaluation and counselling have been properly performed and that both parties are not found to be unsuitable to enter into such an arrangement. In *Baby M*,[64] although the surrogate went through a form of evaluation, the finding that she might experience difficulty in parting with the child was not disclosed to the parties – a piece of information which, had it been disclosed, would have put the Sterns on their guard and they might well have refused to go ahead with the arrangement. It is however unclear how the court will assess whether the terms are conscionable or not and what standard the court will apply to make that assessment. On the other hand, no clear all-embracing guidelines can be set for such an evaluation, and judgement must therefore depend on the facts of each case.

3. All parties to the surrogacy contract provide the licensed person with written indication of their informed consent to the arrangement.[65]

4. The procedure to impregnate a surrogate shall be performed only in accordance with regulations issued by the State Department of Health.[66]

There are other miscellaneous provisions governing a surrogacy arrangement and they are as follows:

(i) The Act confines eligibility of the commissioning mother to a married woman who is 'medically determined to be physiologically unable to bear a child without serious risk to her health or to the child's health'. This confines surrogacy to married couples and excludes them from using surrogacy for convenience. It also restricts the genetic permutations of the child to: (1) either of the commissioning parents must provide a gamete, and (2) either the commissioning mother or the surrogate must provide the ovum. In other words, the resulting child must be biologically related to at least one of the commissioning parents.[67]

COMMENT

This provision contains further restrictions on the circumstances in which surrogacy will be regarded as lawful or permissible. It excludes 'surrogacy for convenience'. There is no definition of the term surrogacy for convenience. But it refers to the use of surrogacy on grounds other than infertility, disease or genetic impairment making pregnancy undesirable or impossible. One view, of course, is that surrogacy for convenience is a misnomer. It assumes that pregnancy and motherhood are not, or at least are not capable of being perceived as, an inconvenience. However, it can be argued that if the right to reproduce involves the right to choose the means of reproduction, there should be no *prima facie* case for excluding surrogacy for convenience. But as will be seen later,[68] the consensus of opinion is that surrogacy for convenience is an unacceptable progression or extension of surrogacy. As the strength of the argument of this book, advocating a liberal approach to the use of artificial reproductive methods, is heavily based on the plight of the infertile and the importance of the satisfaction of a fundamental desire to have children and to found a family, surrogacy for convenience as a means of satisfying other goals or desires is an issue which is outside its ambit. According to this view, there is nothing inconsistent in restricting the use of surrogacy to where a woman is 'medically determined to be physiologically unable to bear a child without serious risk to her health or to the child's health'.

Another restriction on the circumstances where surrogacy is permissible is that the surrogate-born child must be genetically linked to one of the commissioning parties. This excludes IVF and ET surrogacy where the child is constituted genetically by the gametes of an ovum and sperm donors.

(ii) There are also some mandatory terms which must be inserted in the surrogacy arrangement and this will be supervised by the court which preauthorizes surrogacy arrangements. The terms are:

(i) consent of the surrogate that she will surrender custody of the child or accept the obligations as mother of the child if she gives notice to keep the child;

(ii) consent of the husband of the surrogate, if any, that he will surrender custody of the child or accept the obligations of parenthood if the surrogate gives notice to keep the child;

(iii) consent of the commissioning parents to accept the obligations of parenthood unless the surrogate gives notice of her intent to keep the child;

(iv) the right of the surrogate to keep the child if, at any time prior to 72 hours after the birth of the child, she gives notice to that effect;

(v) provision for adequate coverage through insurance of health care expenses of the surrogate and the child for the term of the pregnancy and 6 weeks after the termination of pregnancy for pregnancy-related complications;

(VI) surrogacy fee to be deposited into an escrow account which the surrogate will receive on:

  (a) the relinquishment of parenthood to the intended parents; or
  (b) where the contract is terminated before live birth by means other than a breach by the surrogate.[69]

COMMENT

These are the terms that must be provided for in the contract. In addition, the contract may include others such as those that relate to the lifestyle of the surrogate during pregnancy. Although the lifestyle provisions may not be enforceable, a breach by the surrogate of important terms of this nature would entitle the commissioning parents to treat it as a breach of the agreement on the part of the surrogate. The 72-hour rule effectively means that the custody of the child will be determined, at the latest, 72 hours after its birth. This rule will be in the best interests of the child as it will avoid protracted custody litigation. The best interests of the child and the 72-hour rule are supported by the requirement that all parties involved in the arrangement must undergo a nonmedical evaluation to determine their suitability to parent a child. This includes both the surrogate and her husband (if any) and the intended parents. The nonmedical evaluation is intended to ensure that whoever ultimately has custody of the child will be suitable parents. Apart from protecting the interests of the child, the 72-hour rule also protects the interests of the surrogate by giving her an option to change her mind and retain custody of the child. Although an effective screening procedure will probably screen out women who are likely to change their minds, the requirement that a surrogate must have had one uncomplicated previous pregnancy and delivery is an additional safeguard against a surrogate who might not fully realize the impact of giving up the child.[70]

The above mandatory terms do not prohibit payment to the surrogate for reasonable medical or living expenses before completion of the contract. But an ideal contract ought to provide for a pro rata payment to the surrogate in the event that the pregnancy is terminated before birth in circumstances that do not constitute a breach of contract on her part. For example, the surrogate may have to undergo several unsuccessful inseminations before the contract is terminated by either party, or an abortion may be required for the surrogate's health. In either situation the surrogate should receive some compensation for her time and services. A surrogate contract should indeed provide for these eventualities.

(iii) There shall be no specific performance of terms relating to impregnation of the surrogate or restriction on abortion other than that provided for by the relevant law.[71]

COMMENT
This provision is intended to safeguard the surrogate's right to privacy in matters that affect her own body and is consistent with the current state of the law.

(iv) The intended parents may recover only health care expenses and the fee if

(a) the surrogate refuses to become impregnated; or
(b) the surrogate has an abortion that is not medically necessary without the consent of the commissioning parents; or
(c) the surrogate elects to keep the child.

Where, within nine months after the surrogacy contract has been judicially approved, the surrogate fails to become pregnant through no fault of either party, the contract is voidable at the option of either party.

If the commissioning parents breach a material term of the contract, the surrogate may recover health care expenses that the intended parents were required to pay, collect the fee that is provided for in the contract and, if the breach is the refusal to accept the child, the surrogate may file a notice of her intention to keep the child and the intended parents may be liable for support.[72]

COMMENT
These provisions suggest that commissioning parents cannot sue for damages for emotional injuries if the surrogate has an abortion which is not medically necessary without the consent of the intended parents, or if she decides to keep the child. This is partly because it is difficult to measure the actual harm that the commissioning parents may have suffered. The loss of a child cannot be measured in monetary terms. Further, the possibility of the surrogate being liable for an uncertain amount of damages may interfere with her right to make a decision regarding keeping the child. It may indirectly be injurious to the child if the mother is made liable in damages. Precluding the possibility of obtaining damages in these circumstances will also present an incentive for the commissioning parents to seek out a properly evaluated and counselled surrogate.

Ontario Law Reform Proposal

The Ontario Law Reform Commission considered the question of surrogacy and recommended that legislation should be enacted to establish a regulatory scheme governing surrogate arrangements.[73] In many ways, the various aspects in the scheme proposed are very similar to that of the scheme mentioned above. And insofar as their major suggestions differ, they will be enumerated.

1. There is the requirement of approval by the court of the proposed arrangement and scrutiny by the court of the fairness and reasonableness of the terms. However, there is no mandatory requirement that the surrogate shall appear before the court. This envisages that the parties may wish to remain anonymous. The court can however, request the surrogate's attendance in the absence of the commissioning parents.

2. The court is required to assess the suitability of the commissioning parents and the prospective surrogate mother. But on the question of eligibility of the prospective surrogate, the Commission took the view that there should be no restriction. The Commission summarized the arguments in these terms:[74]

> It has been suggested that the opportunity to participate as a surrogate mother should be restricted to certain categories of women. It has been argued that, for example, such participation should be limited to women who already have given birth to children, because only they can truly appreciate the risks associated with pregnancy and the implications of surrendering a child upon birth. Alternatively, it has been said that women with children in their care should not be allowed to be surrogate mothers because these children may be traumatized upon surrender of the infant, fearing that they too will be given away. In addition, some commentators have suggested that married women are to be preferred, in the expectation that their husbands will be bulwarks of emotional support; others have taken an opposite view, in the belief that husbands will be potential sources of conflict. We consider that there is no theoretical or empirical basis upon which to adopt a categorical approach to the eligibility of women to serve as surrogate mothers. This conclusion is, however, subject to a single exception. Under no circumstances whatsoever do we believe that a minor should be permitted to participate in a surrogate motherhood arrangement as a surrogate mother.

3. On the possible genetic permutation of the child, the Commission took the view that there should not be any restriction on this.

4. Most importantly, it recommended that a child born pursuant to an approved surrogate arrangement should be surrendered immediately upon birth to the commissioning parents. There is to be no period of time in which the surrogate can reflect on her decision to enter into the arrangement. If she refuses to surrender the child after its birth, the court is to order the delivery of the child to the commissioning parents. It is also recommended that the court should be empowered to order the transfer of custody of the child upon birth if it is satisfied that the surrogate intends to refuse to surrender custody.

COMMENT

As the Ontario Law Reform Commission admitted, whether there should be statutory enforcement of a surrogacy arrangement 'is one of the most emotionally charged issues involved in surrogate motherhood'.[75] The alternatives are either statutory enforcement or permitting the surrogate to rescind the agreement unilaterally within a period of time after birth. 'In the first case, the risk of disappointment and trauma rests on the surrogate, while, in the second, it is placed on the commissioning parents.'[76] As stated:[77]

> The crucial question, however, is not where the risk of disappointment should lie, but which resolution will serve the best interests of the child. Unfortunately, the available scientific literature would appear to indicate no clear answer to this question. However, the Advisory Board that assisted the Commission, which included a child psychiatrist and a social worker, favoured requiring immediate surrender of the child to the approved social parents. It was thought that immediate surrender would serve to prevent bonding with the surrogate mother and facilitate bonding with the person – social mother – who, in the vast majority of cases, would be the ultimate recipient of the child and who, would be the primarily influence in its life during the neonatal period and infancy.

This draconian provision goes to the very heart of this regulatory scheme. It amounts to statutory authorization of judicial enforcement of surrogacy contracts. The major criticism of this provision, of course, is that it alters the common-law rule that an agreement to transfer parental rights is unenforceable and creates a statutory rule to the effect that an approved arrangement to transfer becomes enforceable on the birth of the child. The provision therefore places relatively little weight on the feelings of the surrogate who carries the child for nine months, during which time human bonds and attachment can sometimes transcend legal niceties. The bluntness of this provision appears to have been based on the views of two members of the Advisory Board and is contrary to the prevailing view that the surrogate should be given a breathing space to decide whether to rescind the contract.

5. The Commission recommended that the parties should be encouraged to come to an agreement about the following issues:

(i)   life and health insurance for the prospective surrogate mother;
(ii)   arrangements for the child should the intended parent(s) die or become separated before the birth of the child;
(iii) the right of the surrogate, if any, to have contact with the child; and
(iv)   the surrogate's lifestyle during pregnancy and the conditions under which pre-natal screening of the child may be justified.

6. The Commission considered the point as to whether intermediaries should be permitted to function within the context of the proposed regulatory scheme and whether profit-orientated private agencies could be tolerated. The belief was that surrogate motherhood arrangements should not be tainted by an offensive commercialism, and that the unregulated operation of private agencies may undermine efforts at rejecting commercialism by allowing its introduction through the back door. It was therefore suggested that private agencies should be allowed to operate only under supervision similar to that exercised over adoption agencies. Provision will be made to regulate the credentials of operators of agencies, number of personnel, advertisement and recruitment practices, services offered and fees charged.

7. One final recommendation of the Ontario Law Reform Commission which is worth noting is that a penalty of a fine be attached to surrogate arrangements outside this statutory scheme. The rationale is that, given the stringent requirements of the scheme, people may prefer not to be governed by it. Concerned with the possibility that people may seek to evade the regulatory scheme, the Commission proposed that a provincial offence be created imposing a liability on all persons involved in the impugned arrangement. This, according to the Commission, is an important provision in the regulatory scheme.

The Warnock Report recommendation which was given effect by the Surrogacy Arrangements Act 1985 took a different approach. It criminalized the activities of commercial agencies and 'the actions of professionals and others who knowingly assist in the establishment of a surrogacy pregnancy'.[78] The Victoria Infertility (Medical Procedures) Act 1984 imposes criminal liability on both intermediaries and parties to the arrangement. Thus, Section 30(2) says:

A person shall not–

(a) publish, or cause to be published, a statement or an advertisement, notice or other document that –

    (i) is intended or likely to induce a person to agree to act as a surrogate mother;

    (ii) seeks or purports to seek a woman who is willing to agree to act as a surrogate mother; or

    (iii) states or implies that a woman is willing to agree to act as a surrogate mother;

(b) make, give or receive, or agree to make, give or receive, a payment or reward for or in consideration of the making of a contract, agreement or arrangement under which a woman agrees to act as a surrogate mother; or

(c) receive or agree to receive a payment or reward in consideration of acting, or agreeing to act, as a surrogate mother.

COMMENT

Of all the above-mentioned approaches, the Victoria Act uses criminal law to its fullest extent. It makes it a criminal offence to facilitate, or participate in, a surrogate arrangement. The Ontario proposal however is both more extensive and more restrictive. It is much more extensive in its operation than the Warnock approach in that it covers the primary, as well as the secondary, parties who would be fined for operating outside the regulatory scheme; it is more restrictive than the Warnock approach in that it does not ban the activities of agencies but proposes regulation of their activities and a penalty if they circumvent the regulatory scheme. Such a regulatory scheme is therefore comprehensive in that it covers surrogacy and its agency-related activities.

Having said this, it seems that there can be no guarantee that all surrogate arrangements will be governed by the regulatory scheme. The positive nature of the scheme is that from the commissioning parents' point of view there is a high degree of certainty that the arrangements will provide them with a child for parenting. But besides the penalty for non-compliance, there is no other disincentive to comply. Intended parents whose surrogate arrangements are outside the statutory scheme can still secure a parent–child relationship with the surrogate-born child provided that the surrogate is willing to surrender the child. Comparing on the one hand, the risk of arrangements outside the scheme (that is, the surrogate refusing to surrender the child) – which according to statistics is minimal[79] – and the severity of the consequences when it materializes (as can be seen in *Baby M*)[80] and, on the other hand, the cumbersome nature of the scheme, people may still opt for the former.

CONCLUSION

Having considered in great depth the provisions of the two proposed regulatory schemes, it is appropriate here to consider their respective merits. It is important to bear in mind the objections to surrogacy as well as the aims of legislation. The latter ought to be twofold: first to protect women, particularly poor women, from being lured by money into surrogacy and being coerced into surrendering the children, and second, that children should not be bought and sold, or at least, transferred from one person to another, irrespective of their interests.

While there are minor variations in the two schemes, these are not significant to the operation of the schemes themselves. Some ancillary suggestions in the two surrogacy regulatory schemes are complementary to each other. But in relation to certain fundamental issues relating to surrogacy, the two schemes are essentially different. One such issue is the irrevocability of the surrogacy arrangement. What is argued here is that there should be no legal requirement that the surrogate be irrevocably bound by the contract and that there ought to be a grace period after the delivery of the child during which she should be able to rescind the contract. This is to cover the possibility (despite prior counselling) that the surrogate might not fully realize the implication of the pregnancy and her attachment to the child. As much as the intended parents would like to have the child, society, in accepting surrogacy as a means for the infertile to found a family, must also respect the right of the surrogate to choose to keep the child whom she has borne. The provision of a grace period is also consistent with the law of adoption where consent of a parent to the adoption of the child is revocable until an adoption order is made.[81]

In order to secure the best interests of a surrogate-born child, the law should try to discourage protracted legal custody disputes by stating that where the surrogate changes her mind within the grace period, she should have parental rights and that no order for specific performance is permitted. These provisions address the argument that there is potential for the exploitation of surrogates who may be forced to surrender the child by both the lure of money and the threat of legal proceedings. The Ontario Law Reform Commission's recommendation on enforcement of a surrogate arrangement is therefore not favoured because it has inflated the right of the infertile to have children at the expense of the right of the surrogate to have and to keep her child. Thus as the New Jersey Supreme Court in *Baby M* states,

> The right to procreate very simply is the right to have natural children, whether through sexual intercourse or artificial insemination. It is no more than that. Mr. Stern has not been deprived of that right. Through artificial insemination of Mrs. W, Baby M is his child.[82]

The court took the view that the right to procreate is separate from the right to parenting although it expressed it in a rather clumsy manner:[83]

> The custody, care, companionship, and nurturing that follow birth are not parts of the right to procreation; they are rights that may also be constitutionally protected; but that involves many considerations other than the right of procreation. To assert that Mr. Stern's right of procreation gives him the right to the custody of Baby M would be to assert that Mrs. Whitehead's right of procreation does not give her the right to the custody of Baby M; it would be to assert that the constitutional right of procreation includes within it a constitutionally protected contractual right to destroy someone else's rights of procreation (*sic*).

As the court has often observed, the question of parenting must be determined in accordance with the 'best interest of the child' principle. However where everything is equal, and this one assumes except where evidence shows otherwise, it seems that the mother's right to keep the child would prevail over the father's and the suggestion that the mother should be forced to surrender the child in accordance with an agreement is far from acceptable. Thus, in connection with the argument that the *ex parte* order in *Baby M*[84] had jeopardized Mrs Whitehead's custody claim, it was said that

> when father and mother are separated and disagree, at birth, on custody, only in an extreme, truly rare, case should the child be taken from its mother *pendente lite*. . . .[85]

This conclusion – that the mother should have the right to keep a child whom she has borne – is also consonant with the argument throughout this book that the commissioning parties have no right to positive assistance in their endeavour to have children. This effectively is the statutory enforcement proposal of the Ontario Law Reform Commission. If all goes well, the commissioning parties will secure their child, but if the surrogate changes her mind, her rights must prevail. Surrogacy as a means of having children, must be a choice for those who want to participate in the exercise. Having said that, a statutory scheme which provides for the screening of both parties, judicial consideration of the arrangements, and statutory regulation of the operation of agencies should go a long way towards meeting the needs of the commissioning parties in that informed consent, nonmedical evaluation and counselling of the surrogate are ensured.

In the foregoing chapters, the acceptability of artificial reproductive methods for the founding of a family (whether through reproduction or not), and some of the major legal difficulties associated with them, have been considered. In the penultimate chapter, the question of funding for artificial reproductive techniques will be examined.

NOTES

1   *Vide supra*, Chapter 6.
2   See H.C., Vol. **79**, Col. 118–19.
3   Surrogacy Arrangement (Amendments) Bill [H.L.] 1986, No. 169.
4   See the debates on the Surrogacy Arrangements (Amendment) Bill 1986, H.L., Vol. **473**, Col. 160–4; H.L. Vol. **475**, Col. 363–6.
5   See *Walrond* v. *Walrond* (1858) Johns 18; *Vansittart* v. *Vansittart* (1858) 2 De G. and J. 249; *Hope* v. *Hope* 8 De G.M. and G. 731; *Re Andrew* (1873) L.R. 8 Q.B. 153; *R.* v. *Smith* (1853) 22 L.J. (Q.B.) 116; *Humphrey* v. *Polak* [1901] 2 K.B. 385; for Scottish cases see *MacPherson* v. *Leisham* (1887) 14 R. 780; *Sutherland* v. *Taylor* (1887) 15 R. 224; *Campbell* v. *Croall* (1895) 22 R. 869, *Kerrigan* v. *Hall* (1901) 4 F. 10.

6 Now see Section 2(9) of the Children Act 1989.
7 Note: in Scotland, there is no statutory equivalent of Section 85(2) of the Children Act 1975. See Cusine, D., 'Womb-leasing': some legal implications', *N.L.J.* (1978) **128** (2), pp. 824, 825.
8 Human Fertilisation and Embryology Act 1990, Section 36.
9 Cited above.
10 See Section 27.
11 See *Baby M*, 225 N.J. 396; 5337 A 2d 1227 (1988); *The Baby Cotton case*, or *Re C (a Minor) (Wardship: Surrogacy)* [1985] FLR 846; *Adoption Application: Surrogacy Case* [1987] 2 All ER 826; 'The Surrogacy Twin Baby Case', *Daily Telegraph*, 13 March, 1987, p. 2.
12 Compare the approach of the Ontario Law Reform Commission which proposes statutory enforcement of a surrogacy agreement. See *Report on Human Artificial Reproduction and Related Matters* (2 Vols), Ministry of the Attorney General, Toronto, July 1985, p. 252.
13 *Vide supra*, Chapter 6.
14 See 'The lessons from Baby M', *The Economist*, 21 March, 1987, p. 18.
15 [1979] Q.B. 276.
16 Ibid., p. 281. Note that the 1976 Act gives no right to a mother either. Compare,

> . . . but the Abortion Act 1967 has given mothers the right to terminate the lives of their unborn children and made it lawful for doctors to help to abort them.

per Stephenson, L.J., in *McKay v. Essex AHA* [1982] 2 All ER, 771, 780e.
17 [1987] 1 All ER 1230.
18 The father's argument in *C. v. S.* was based on the interpretation of the term 'capable of being born alive', in the Infant Life (Preservation) Act 1929. The Court of Appeal upheld the interpretation of Mrs Justice Heilbron, in the High Court, that the proposed abortion was not in contravention of the 1929 Act in that the foetus was not 'capable of being born alive'. The House of Lords, at an emergency appeal committee, decided unanimously not to allow a challenge to the Court of Appeal's decision because there was 'no arguable point of law'.
19 See *The Guardian*, 25 February, 1987, p. 12 (Editorial Comments), and the introduction of the Infant Life (Preservation) and Paternal Rights Bill 1987, H.C. Bill 113. Clause 2 of the Bill proposed to amend Section 1(1) of the Abortion Act 1967 by inserting after Section 1(1) (b) the words '(c) that the father of the unborn child had been consulted about the mother's intention to terminate the pregnancy and that, where he is the mother's husband his consent as to the termination has been obtained.'
20 410 US 113 (1973).
21 428 US 52 (1976).
22 Ibid., p. 69.
23 Compare Teo, Wesley D.H., 'Abortion: the husband's constitutional rights', *Ethics* (1974–5) **85**, p. 337.
24 [1983] 1 Qd. R. 386.
25 *Attorney General (ex rel Kerr) v. T.* [1983] 1 Qd. R. 404. Note that judges in both cases consider their decisions as in accordance with legal principles rather than concerning themselves with the conflicting moral and religious views on abortion. See also *Paton v. British Pregnancy Advisory Service Trustees* [1987] 2 All ER 987.
26 Yet unreported, quotation from unedited judgement.
27 Section 1 of the Charter says: 'Every human being has a right to life, and to personal security, inviolability and freedom'. The Supreme Court took the view that the Charter, as a whole did not consider the status of a foetus. The lack of an

intention to deal with a foetus's status is, in itself, a strong reason for not finding foetal rights under the Charter. If the legislature had wished to accord a foetus the right to life, it is unlikely that it would have left the protection of this right in such an uncertain state. The difficult issue of whether a foetus is a legal person cannot be settled by a purely linguistic argument that the plain meaning of the term 'human being' includes foetuses. Like a purely scientific argument, a purely linguistic argument attempts to settle a legal debate by non-legal means. What is required are substantive legal reasons which support a conclusion that the term 'human being' has a particular meaning. The more plausible explanation is that different terms (human being and persons) were used in order to distinguish between physical and moral persons.

28   On the abortion law in England, Wales and Scotland, see Mason, J.K. and McCall Smith, R.A., *Law and Medical Ethics*, London, Butterworths, 1983, Chapter 5.

29   *Vide supra*, Chapter 3 on the right to privacy and the right to reproduce.

30   See generally, Treitel, G.H., 'Specific performance and injunction', in *Chitty on Contract, General Pinciples*, Vol. 1 (24th edn.), London, Sweet & Maxwell, 1977, p. 1631; Walker, D.M., *The Law of Contract and Related Obligations in Scotland* (2nd edn.), London, Butterworths, 1985, pp. 540–4.

31   Some US cases do suggest that the court may intervene in some extreme circumstances in the interests of the child, but not continuing supervision of the progress of a pregnancy to ensure foetal health, see Weinberg, S.R., 'A maternal duty to protect fetal health?, *Indiana Law Journal* (1983) **58**, p. 531.

32   [1987] 1 All ER 20.

33   That is, would the condition that existed have been likely to continue had the move of protecting the child not been commenced.

34   It has been a controversial decision in this respect. See *The Guardian*, 9 December, 1986, p. 12.

35   *Vide supra*.

36   Para. 8.20.

37   Para. 8.18.

38   *Vide infra*, p. 234.

39   *Vide supra*, Chapter 5.

40.   *Vide supra*, Chapter 5.

41   See Parker, Diana, 'Surrogate mothering: an overview', *Family Law* (1984) **14**, pp. 140, 141.

42   See *Syrkowski* v. *Appleyard* 420 Mich. 367 (1985). In this case, a married surrogate was artificially inseminated using semen from the commissioning father. The AID statute in Michigan was similar to the 'AID provision' (*vide supra*, Chapter 5). The surrogate's husband had signed an affidavit of non-consent to his wife's AID. The Supreme Court of Michigan held that the circuit court had jurisdiction under the Paternity Act to identify the father of a surrogate-born child despite the statutory presumption of the AID statute.

43   In fact, the 'corollary principle' cannot exclude the commissioning father because by the very definition of the term as used here, he is not a semen donor, *vide supra*, p. 133.

44   *Vide supra*, Chapter 5.

45   *Vide supra*, Chapter 5.

46   *Vide supra*, Chapter 5.

47   See para. 6.8.

48   See para. 7.6.

49   *Vide supra*, Chapter 5.

50   See para. 8.20.

51   Para. 8.20.

52   *Vide supra*.
53   The 'surrogacy recommendation' is widely accepted. See for example, Lord Denning's attempt to amend the Surrogacy Arrangements Bill 1985 to make a surrogate the mother of the child whom she has borne. *Hansard*, H.L. Vol. **465**, Col. 927. See also the Surrogacy Arrangements (Amendment) Bill 1986, sponsored by the Earl of Halsbury. Clause 2 seeks to make a surrogate the mother of the child.
54   *Vide supra*, Chapter 5.
55   *Vide supra*, Chapter 5.
56   Clause (2) excludes the application of Subsection (1) to an adopted person.
57   [1987] 2 All ER 826.
58   'Model Human Reproductive Technologies and Surrogacy Act', *Iowa Law Review* (1987) **72**, p. 943. This is the product of seminar work by students at the University of Iowa College of Law. See Appendix for parts of the Act.
59   Ibid., A6–101, 7–101.
60   *Vide supra*, on test and standard of eligibility for infertility treatment.
61   *Vide supra*.
62   A6–101; A6–103.
63   *Vide infra*.
64   See Appendix 5.
65   A6–101.
66   A6–101.
67   A6–102.
68   *Vide infra*.
69   A6–104.
70   A6–102(e).
71   A6–105.
72   A6–106.
73   *Report on Human Artificial Insemination and Related Matters*, 2 Vols, Ministry of the Attorney General, Toronto, July 1985, pp. 236–73; 280–5.
74   Ibid., p. 240. On the first argument, that only women who have had one uncomplicated pregnancy would truly appreciate the risk and complex emotional feelings involved in surrendering the child and would be able to give an informed consent, see A6–102 of the Model Human Reproductive Technologies and Surrogacy Act, loc. cit.
75   Note 74, p. 250.
76   Ibid., p. 251.
77   Ibid., p. 252.
78   Para. 8.18.
79   *Vide supra*.
80   109 N.J. 396; 5337 A 2d 1227 (1988).
81   See *Re F (an Infant)* [1957], All ER 819.
82   *Baby M.*, op. cit., p. 1253.
83   Ibid., at p. 1253.
84   Ibid., at p. 1261.
85   Ibid., at p. 1261.

8 State Funding of Artificial Reproduction

STATE FUNDING AND HAVING CHILDREN

It is one thing to say that people have the right to reproduce and the right to found a family, and that these rights may, in some circumstances entail the right to use artificial reproductive techniques and surrogacy. It is quite another thing to say that the state should fund and bear the costs of people's endeavours to have children in the exercise of their rights. The state may legitimately regulate the practice of surrogacy because it has a clear interest in seeing that surrogates and potential surrogate-born children are not exploited; it is however not implicated in funding for an individual's endeavours to have children. The basis of concern in regulating the practice of surrogacy is the same as state involvement in adoption: the state steps in to ensure that the consent of the mother to give up her child for adoption is genuine and that the child is placed with a suitable family. But if people have the right to decide for themselves whether and when to have children and how many children they would like to have, it seems curious that they should, at one and the same time, claim that the state should fund their endeavours to have children. This, of course, can be admitted if the right to reproduce and the right to found a family are seen as positive claim-rights, or if other arguments favour funding people's endeavours to exercise their rights. This is the issue to be examined in this chapter.

Obviously, the question of public funding is most relevant to the poor who otherwise would not be able to afford the cost involved in this activity; the UK's NHS provision of various health-related services may be of little interest to those who can afford private treatment. In the context of procreation or non-procreation, this trite observation operates with equal force. If the NHS were to withdraw its services relating to pregnancy, childbirth or termination of pregnancy, the poor would be hardest hit because some might not be able to afford contraceptives, abortions, or medical care relating to carrying a child to term and childbirth. Similarly, it is one thing to say that the infertile have the right to reproduce by using artificial reproductive techniques, but the value of such a conclusion will be extremely limited if only the rich can afford the substantial cost of private IVF treatment. Thus, the question of funding will be considered here.

STATE FUNDING FOR HAVING CHILDREN – A POSITIVE RIGHT TO REPRODUCE?

Is there a positive right to reproduce, so that individuals then have a claim against the state for assistance in their efforts to have children?

At the beginning of the discussion, one must assume that people have children because they want them (for a wide variety of reasons). Some people want to have many children, some want to have a couple, some want none. This freedom to choose is the very significance of the negative nature of the rights analysed earlier. Having children or not is a way of life; a chosen way of ordering one's life and spending one's money. The significant value of this freedom of choice will be dramatically reduced if everybody ends up in roughly the same financial position irrespective of their choice of procreation or otherwise. This will be the case if the community in general has to bear the financial burden of individual projects to have children. The argument is that freedom can be maximized if people are to be responsible for their own decision as to whether to have children, and those who choose not to have children will be able to spend their life and money in other pursuits. *Prima facie*, therefore, one has no claim for state funding for the provision of services which may render one a child of one's own.

State Neutrality on Procreation

In a society which treasures the freedom of its citizens, there should be no coercion for either choice (procreation or non-procreation). People should be free to choose either to have or not to have children and if the consequence of that freedom generally coincides with the state's interests in its population size (that is, there is no danger that the growth is so drastic as to lead to the lowering of the standard of living for everyone, hindering or impeding economic growth; or conversely, that there is insufficient birth to replace and sustain its current population), the state should have no part to play in people's reproductive behaviour.

Nonetheless, social values have always been inclined to favour having children. Childless couples are seen to be 'abnormal' and may be required to explain their childlessness. Worse, voluntary childless couples are sometimes seen to be selfish, mindful only of their own pursuits and not interested in contributing to the creation and upbringing of the next generation.[1] And if procreation is a chosen way of life, and children are desirable and valuable to their parents, the tax system has not failed to impress upon people, albeit in a token manner, that it is also a preferable way of life in which subsidization is available in the form of child tax allowances and child benefits. (This seems to be the only plausible explanation or rationalization of the universal nature of child benefits irrespective of need.)

Although social values may be tipped towards having children, this is not the same as saying that the state will fund, or is required to fund, people's endeavours to have children, or that potential parents have a justifiable claim against the public purse. Certain state provisions, such as day nurseries and universal free education, are capable of being interpreted as enabling people to have children, if not also encouraging them to do so, by lessening the burden and disadvantages associated with having and rearing children. But to what extent people are actually encouraged to have children because of the existence of these provisions is unclear. In fact, these provisions are probably motivated not by such considerations, but by the belief that children are an important asset to society which, in turn, has a duty to provide for their basic health care and education. Furthermore, the belief that mothers should have a choice either to stay at home or undertake employment is also an important and relevant consideration.

So far, the conclusion must be that it is difficult to find support for the proposition that there is a right to state funding towards the fulfilment of one's right to reproduce and/or to found a family. A sharper focus on the role of the state in reproduction is appropriate here.

If individuals are free to decide whether to have children, they should, *prima facie*, be responsible for the implementation of that decision. But this does not appear to be the practice at the moment in relation to implementing one's desire relating to procreation.

Not Having Children

In the UK, the NHS provides free contraceptive advice and abortion, while supplies of contraception are available at the standard pre-scription fee. Although there is no legal recognition of the right to an abortion, and abortion depends on certification by two practitioners that one of the grounds stipulated in the Abortion Act 1967 exists; the stringency of their interpretation varies from one practitioner to another, from region to region, and thus the availability of abortion varies.[2] However it must be added that since both contraception and abortion are part of the NHS programme, the choice not to have children can be, and is, affected by the public fund, and the state is clearly prepared, within the confines of the Abortion Act and the NHS contraceptive supply, to support an individual's attempt not to have children. It is difficult to be definitive about the complex motivations behind these policies. They are probably a combination of the following considerations: recognition of individual choices in fundamental matters relating to procreation or non-procreation, its possible health impact on both the mother and her existing children, and the well-being of children-to-be.

Having Children

The pecuniary costs most directly related to having children are ante-natal and childbirth medical care (and possibly lost earnings resulting from pregnancy and childbirth). The former is free on the NHS for those who need it and this makes sense in a welfare state. Rarely would it be disputed that pregnancy and childbirth are medical conditions both from the point of view of the mother, pregnant woman and the child. Insofar as pregnancy is health-related and in that advanced pregnancy and childbirth involve a certain degree of confinement, the need for work leave is seldom disputed. Statutory requirements for paid maternity leave and reinstatement can be seen as comparable to sick leave and as protection against discrimination against pregnant women at work.

The argument based on the role of the state in current reproductive practice is therefore thus: although there is no obvious and direct relation between funding of the various aspects associated with reproduction or non-reproduction and no recognition of a positive obligation to provide funding deriving from the right to have children or not to have children, if fertile people's desire to have, or not to have, children is facilitated by NHS funding, why should the same not apply to the infertile who desire to have children?

The obvious difference between the fertile and the infertile, of course, is that the former's dilemma is not with getting pregnant, but with whether, in the event of conception having taken place, to carry on with the pregnancy or to seek its termination; whereas for the infertile it is a question of getting to the stage of pregnancy. Nonetheless, there seems to be no logical reason to distinguish funding for procreation on the basis of whether it relates to (i) procuring, as opposed to (ii) preventing, terminating, or continuing pregnancy. In the final analysis, efforts to have children or procreate have only two outcomes – birth of a child or no child – and there is no other possible intermediate outcome. If the NHS is prepared to fund either outcome more or less in accordance with the wishes of the individual, there is no *prima facie* reason why it should not also fund the desired outcome of the infertile. Just as continuation of an unwanted pregnancy can cause a tremendous amount of distress or be detrimental to the woman's life and health, inability to have a child which is fervently desired can have an equally detrimental impact on one's psychological and mental health. The claim of the infertile for funding, however, must be examined separately. This is so because the circumstances in which the infertile find themselves are different from the normal scenario of fertile individuals whith whom we are familiar.

Fundamental Right to Have Children

Various declarations of human rights suggest that the right to marry and to found a family (that is, to have children) are fundamental human rights. Whether the latter right is based on the almost universal practice of procreation (thus seen to be a basic human need or desire), or whether it is based on the prevalent view that having children is an important personal goal as well as an essential human good – genuinely necessary for satisfactory individual self- development, or indeed the combination of both – is unclear. The assumptions of a basic human right to have children and that having children is a fundamental human good, are seldom challenged except in the context of population-control debates where it has been argued that urgent need to monitor and control population growth may justify qualification or deprivation of the right to decide freely the number of children one would like to have.

However, as Suzanne Uniacke rightly pointed out:

> Something's being a basic human need or desire – whether it be interpersonal sex, reproduction, or even the struggle for life – does not thereby create a substantial right to the assistance of other people who have competing and more weighty needs and rights of their own. For example, another person's consent is crucial to the permissibility of using parts of his or her living body, in what would otherwise be highly intrusive ways, in meeting any of these ends. And one's need or desire does not itself oblige others to have such consent.

Discussion in the preceding section also pointed out the fact that there is no direct correlation between state funding of the various aspects of procreation and non-procreation and thus it is difficult to admit a positive claim to assistance for reproduction on the basis of right. A positive right to reproduce may entail the sterile being rendered fertile, something which is clearly impracticable, or mean that the state has a duty to provide a procreational partner for those who are single.

ALLEVIATION OF DISTRESS GENERATED BY THE INABILITY TO FULFIL A FUNDAMENTAL HUMAN DESIRE

In a world with finite resources, every expenditure represents a choice between alternatives. Although unanimity on the value of a particular expenditure is rarely possible, assessment of a proposed expenditure, if it is seen to be legitimate or justifiable, must involve an appraisal of the nature of the good to be achieved, the importance of the good in the priority of our value system. It is therefore appropriate to examine in greater detail the nature of the problem of infertility, the seriousness of the problem, the kind of 'good' that assisted-reproductive techniques aim to achieve, the importance of the good, the likelihood of success of these techniques, the existence or otherwise of an alternative approach to the problem, and the kind of demand these techniques impose in the context of an existing health-care system.

Some authors have equated IVF procedures with plastic or cosmetic surgery, say to rectify an ugly-shaped nose which may be a source of distress to the individual concerned. But as suggested earlier on, there is a significant difference between the two procedures in that the former is to achieve what is almost universally regarded as a fundamental good (both to society and the individual concerned) and the latter not quite as obviously so.

The cost of IVF presents a substantial claim on the public fund which needs to be examined carefully.[3] The birth of a recent 'test-tube' baby was said to have cost £5 000.[4] This, however, is not the average cost for a successful IVF baby. IVF treatment has a relatively low success rate, and some couples may need to go through a number of treatments without successfully becoming pregnant or having the chance of a giving birth to a child. Thus, the cost of artificial reproductive techniques to assist people to reproduce could present a substantial demand on public resources,[5] even if confined to assisting those who have physical impediments which prevent reproduction. Is that justifiable even for the fulfilment of a fundamental right to have children?

Infertility is not a life-threatening condition, but coupled with the desire to have children, it can generate a tremendous amount of human distress and suffering, to the extent of overshadowing one's normal daily life.[6] Given this fact, there may be a prima facie utilitarian-based argument that artificial reproductive techniques should be part of a state-funded medical service. Further, infertility may cause serious psychological and mental illness. It may, there-fore, be illogical to treat the symptoms rather than deal with the causes at an early stage, for example, by the use of artificial techniques to alleviate infertility. The case for state-funded treatment of the infertile may thus arguably be anchored on utilitarian considerations.

Nevertheless, utilitarian considerations for state funding of arti-ficial reproductive techniques may not be simple. There are two aspects to this. In the first place, assuming that state funding of artificial reproductive techniques is currently the best option to alleviate the distress caused by infertility, artificial reproductive techniques themselves may not be the best long-term solution to the problem. A more cost-effective strategy in spending public resources to tackle distress caused by infertility may be to reduce the prevalence of infertility, for example, by prevention and education.[7] If so, utilitarian arguments may merely support temporary, rather than permanent, state funding of artificial reproduction to alleviate distress to those for whom prevention of infertility has come too late.

In the second place, there may also be utilitarian arguments against state funding on a temporary basis. For instance, state funding of artificial reproductive techniques may be anti-utilitarian, if the expectations of infertile couples are raised and then dashed because of the low success rate of IVF. The degree of disappointment, of course, may be less intense if, for example, infertile people are warned about this. Nevertheless, one may argue that since infertility treatment can be highly taxing emotionally, money spent on such treatment may be more cost effectively employed in assisting people to cope with the fact of infertility, and assisting them to develop and pursue other interests or avenues for a fulfilling life. Further, utilitarian arguments may better support spending what limited public resources there are in areas which cause more acute distress and suffering than that caused by infertility, for example, in improving provision for the handicapped or for those suffering from kidney failure.

The inability to assert a positive claim-right to reproduce and to found a family does not have to be seen as exhausting arguments for the state funding of the efforts of the infertile to have children. In the complex web of the system of rights, the claim for state provision for the satisfaction of what is regarded as a fundamental aspect of human life can be pursued in more than one way. Thus, although it may sound odd to claim the right to have a healthy functioning heart, it is in fact embraced within the right to health care which is provided for in both the International Covenant on Economic, Social and Cultural Rights (Article 12) and the European Social Charter (part 2, Article 11). The former speaks of 'the right of everyone to the enjoyment of

the highest attainable standard of physical and mental health . . . and
the creation of conditions which would assure to all medical service
and medical attention in the event of sickness'. The latter speaks of
the obligation of the contracting party 'to remove as far as possible the
causes of ill-health'. The concepts of 'health', 'ill- health' and 'highest
attainable standard' are obviously problematic, but protracted
discussion of these concepts for the ascertainment of the minimum
state obligation under these provisions is unnecessary and is
superseded by the fact that it is commonly accepted that infertility
and its associated conditions may become a health concern.[8]

> [I]nfertility may be the result of some disorder which in itself needs
> treatment for the benefit of the patient's health . . . . In addition, the
> psychological distress that may be caused by infertility in those who
> want children may precipitate a mental disorder warranting treatment.
> It is . . . better to treat the primary cause of such distress than to
> alleviate the symptoms.

It may therefore be contended that an affluent society, like the UK,
does not, and should not, ignore the plight of the infertile. Indeed,
when the claim to state funding of artificial techniques is compared
with (i) current spending on treatment that alleviates other causes of
distress, such as the misfortune of scarring which can be corrected by
plastic surgery or simple dental treatment for what some may regard
as purely aesthetic reasons, and (ii) current spending on non-artificial
infertility treatments, some expenditure on artificial techniques does
not seem entirely out of place.[9] On this point, *The Warnock Report*
came to the same conclusion.[10]

> There are many other treatments not designed to satisfy absolute
> needs (in the sense that the patient would die without them) which are
> readily available within the NHS. Medicine is no longer exclusively
> concerned with the preservation of life, but with remedying the
> malfunctions of the human body. On this analysis, an inability to have
> children is a malfunction and should be considered in exactly the same
> way as any other.

For instance, the NHS currently spends a certain amount of its
budget on various kinds of infertility treatment, from general
practitioners' advice to specialist diagnosis to relatively inexpensive
hormone injections (clomiphene pills and gonadotrophin therapy) to
expensive surgery aimed at re-opening blocked Fallopian tubes. Such
non-artificial treatment clearly facilitates having children one way or
another. One may therefore argue that existing expenditure does
support funding of artificial reproductive techniques which attempt
to overcome impediments to having children.

Thus, the question of funding for artificial reproductive techniques can be concluded in this way: although current expenditure on infertility-related treatment provides the practical reality of funding, the funding argument can be buttressed by a number of other arguments. First and foremost is the contention that there is possibly a direct correlation between state financial assistance for people's endeavours to have children and infertility treatment, in that, procreation and pregnancy-related expenditure are as much health-related as infertility treatment. Moreover, the desire to have children ranks relatively high in the order of social values and the fulfilment of one's personal goals and development is assisted by the utilitarian contention favouring the alleviation of distress caused by infertility. However, it is not argued here that surrogacy should be funded. According to the earlier argument, payment should be compensatory in nature. The inability to compensate another woman for being a surrogate is therefore seen as much as inability to afford to have a child oneself. Since there is no suggestion of subsidizing the poor who find having children too expensive an undertaking and, therefore, refrain from procreation, the question of state funding for surrogacy does not arise.

NOTES

1   According to Suzanne Uniacke 'IVF and the right to reproduce', *Bioethics* (1987) **1**.
    [If]reproduction is a basic need or desire it is certainly augmented in our own and similar societies by prevailing attitudes towards, in particular, women and childless couples. The childless, like the unmarried, are not simply in the minority amongst adults. They are also frequently considered odd and objects of pity, or else selfish, often irrespective of the way in which they themselves view their lives.
2   See *Report of the Committee on the Working of the Abortion Act*, Vols I, II & III, HMSO, London, Cmnd 5579, 1974.
3   The cost of AID will not be considered here because it is relatively inexpensive.
4   See *The Times*, 24 April, 1987, p. 3.
5   'The average cost of IVF treatment at Bourn Hall, a private facility, is estimated to be about £10 000 per delivered baby'; see Morgan, Derek, 'Technology and the political economy of reproduction', in *Medicine, Ethics and the Law*, Freeman, M.D.A. (ed.), London, Stevens & Sons, 1988, p. 31. See also Bromwich, Peter, *et al.*, 'In vitro fertilisation in a small unit in the NHS', *BMJ* (1988) **296**, p. 759, where the cost quoted per each cycle treatment is said to be £400. However the chance of a successful pregnancy is much better with larger units; see the *Third Report of the Voluntary Licensing Authority for Human In Vitro Fertilisation and Embryology*, 1988, or *BMJ* (1988) **296**, p. 1542.
6   See Pfeffer, Naouri and Wollett, Anne, *The Experience of Infertility*, London, Virago Press, 1983; Mazor, Miriam and Simons, Harriet (eds), *Infertility: Medical, Emotional and Social Considerations*, New York, Human Sciences Press, 1984.
7   Given that a substantial number of people become infertile as a result of avoidable damage. See Suzanne Uniacke, op. cit.

8   *The Warnock Report*, para. 2.4.
9   See Singer, P. and Wells, D., *The Reproduction Revolution*, Oxford, Oxford University Press, 1984, pp. 64–6.
10 Ibid.

9 Conclusion

Consistent with the characterization of the right to have children, the Human Fertilisation and Embryology Act has to a certain extent, endeavoured to provide a legal framework for those participating in artificial procreation. The provision of infertility treatment services will be the source of discussion no doubt in the future, and the operation of Section 13(5) will be the focus of further debates. Society's approach to this thorny issue will reflect its characterization of the right to reproduce as reproduction is becoming increasingly a public concern rendering the recognition of private rights all the more important. One observation which can be made is that although Parliament has, until recently, loathed to signal its approval to, or recognition of, surrogacy, the Human Fertilisation and Embryology Act has, to a large extent, resigned to its practical usage. Surrogacy by natural intercourse or self-administered AID can be done without medical intervention and Section 30 does not confine parental orders to situations where artificial insemination was achieved through treatment services provided under the Act. The tug-of-war between proper legislative regulation (as argued earlier) and the need to be seen to disapprove surrogacy resulted in ambivalence.

The question of funding and allocation of resources will always be difficult to resolve. But from an organizational point of view the present provision of infertility services within the NHS is far from satisfactory. This is ultimately detrimental to those who seek infertility treatment. *The Warnock Report* commented that:[1]

> . . . we are surprised at how few data there were on the prevalence of infertility, the extent of available services, their location and the numbers treated. Where figures were available, they were often out of date and of dubious relevance. Quite often, people with an infertility problem seek professional advice about other symptoms. Thus any estimate of the extent of infertility treatment within the NHS understates the present level of provision . . . We believe that these data deficiencies should be remedied so that policy makers and planners can make decisions against a background of objectively-assessed facts. We recommend that funding should be made available for the collection of adequate statistics on infertility and infertility services.

Indeed, very little information is available either on infertility or the extent of available services. Collection of accurate statistics and the formulation of an overall strategy for the provision of infertility treatment must therefore be the first steps in grappling with this genuine problem. The lack of accurate data is compounded by the present haphazard provision of the services which is inadequate, patchy and unevenly distributed. Some regions, such as clinics in the south of England, are better equipped than the north or Wales. But even in the best-provided regions in the south, 40% of the District Health Authorities have little or no special provision for infertile people.[2] *The Warnock Report* has endorsed the importance of separate clinics to deal with infertility:[3]

> We recommend that each Health Authority should review its facilities for the investigation and treatment of infertility and consider the establishment, separate from routine gynaecology, of a specialist infertility clinic with close working relationships with specialist units, including genetic counselling services, at regional and supraregional level. Where it is not possible to have a separate clinic we recommend that infertility patients should be seen separately from other types of gynaecological patients wherever possible.

Separate infertility clinics would make it easier to keep records to help fathom the size of the infertility problem. They would also facilitate the training of doctors in this field. According to a 1986 survey, only one-third of District Health Authorities had separate infertility clinics.[4]

With the lack of separate infertility clinics or separate provision for those seeking infertility treatment comes another common complaint: that investigation into infertility and the attendant treatment are bewildering experiences. The long waits during and between visits to clinics serve only to exacerbate feelings of frustration and helplessness. Because there are very few separate infertility clinics, patients sometimes find themselves waiting amongst others who are pregnant or seeking abortion. The lack of counselling services means that patients have to rely on self-help groups for information and exchanges of personal experience. How the requirement of counselling under the Human Fertilisation and Embryology Act will work remains to be seen.[5]

In terms of provision for infertility treatment, the present picture is far from satisfactory. The 1986 survey found that the three basic facilities required to provide a minimum comprehensive service – ultrasound scanners, rapid radioimmune assays and micro surgery – were available in only 40 Districts.[6] The inadequacy of the infertility service means that people can expect to wait a long time to get any kind of treatment. The problem was highlighted in the 1986 survey:[7]

Depressing as the waiting time figures are at first glance, even they are of limited value because they disguise the awful reality of the situation which awaits most infertile people who seek treatment. The causes behind infertility are often complex and difficult to diagnose; thus patients are frequently sent to more than one consultant or centre in the search for a cure, so the miserable experience of waiting for months to see a specialist can be repeated many times over. Nor is there any guarantee that the first referral will be to a consultant with an interest in the subject because most District Health Authorities do not hold separate infertility clinics.

The unsatisfactory aspects of current provision and funding strategy mean that infertility treatment is like a lottery. Those who live in the 'right' areas will get the benefit of advances in medical techniques and the appropriate treatment, whereas those who live elsewhere will either have to go private or not get treatment at all. The current organization of infertility services therefore is not only inadequate and wasteful, but does not give infertile people the assistance which they are entitled to expect.

The perception of the nature of the right to reproduce explicated in this book demands government action. Such characterization of the right to reproduce, though the prevalent view in Western democratic societies which uphold the values of liberty and privacy, is not necessarily given the same priority as other reproductive issues in societies where circumstances differ. In China, for example, there is perceived a pressing need to curb the domestic population growth. Since the One-Child Policy[8] was introduced in 1978, the government has imposed stringent economic incentives and distincentives to contain the population, aiming to restrict population growth to under 1.2 billion by the end of the century. Although the One-Child Policy has received considerable propaganda backing, reports of people disregarding it are not uncommon. This is only to be expected in a culture where the number of children one has is not only an indication of prosperity but also a source of manpower and thus an economic strength. Further, having a male offspring to carry on the family line is still considered important. Amidst these tough measures, however, is the recognition of the fundamental human desire and need to have children. Thus One-Child Family propaganda must appeal not only to loyalty to the Party but also to the need to save China's modernization programme from being jeopardized by over-population. In this wider perspective, the question of the right to have children is correlative to the duty to practise family planning: the right to reproduce should not be to the detriment of the general living standard of the community as a whole. Where circumstances are urgent and desperate enough, reproduction can accordingly be restricted.

To a large extent, this resembles the views expressed in the 1960s population debate[9] to the effect that people had no right to reproduce without limit. Demographers, biologists and nutritionists, joined by conservationists, called for the reduction of the human population.[10] Reproduction, it was said, had social consequences and to the extent that one's right to reproduce affected other people's well-being and liberties, it had to be qualified and redefined as a kind of privilege. Indeed, it was advocated that over-population, an issue of extreme exigency, would justify various coercive measures[11] to curb over-reproduction, the effect of which was predicted to be disaster on a global scale, famines and wars. Nonetheless, the PRC government does recognize the importance of having children and, when the right to have children is removed from this difficult interface of personal liberty and pressing public interest, artificial insemination and IVF are available for the infertile.

NOTES

1   Para. 2.14
2   Mathieson, David, 'Infertility Services in the NHS: what's going on?' (1986), a report prepared for Frank Dobson MP.
3   Para 2.16
4   Ibid.
5   Section 13(6).
6   Ibid.
7   Ibid., p.28.
8   On literature on the One-Child Policy, see Burns, Ailsa, 'Family policies in China', in *Australian Journal of Law and Society* (1983) **1**, p. 78; Kane, Penny, *The Second Billion: Population and Family Planning in China*, Penguin Books, London, 1987; Croll, Elisabeth, et. al., *China's One-Child Policy*, St Martin's, New York, 1985; Luk, Bernard H.K., 'Abortion in Chinese Law', *American Journal of Comparative Law* (1979) **25**, p. 327 and Salvage, Mark, 'Soviet and Chinese Abortion Law', *Standford Law Review* (1988), p. 1027.
9   See for example, *The Growth of US Population*, National Academy of Sciences National Resource Council, Pub. 1279 (1965); *Report of the President's Committee on Population and Family Planning: the Transition from Concern to Action* (Government Printing Office, Washington, D.C., 1968); Borgstrom, Georg, *The Hungry Planet*, New York, Collier Books, 1972; Ehrlich, Paul, *The Population Bomb*, New York, Ballantine Books, 1971; Paddock, William, *Famine–1975*, Boston, Little, Brown and Company, 1967.
10 See ibid.
11 See for example, Chasteen, E., 'The case for compulsory birth control' in *The American Population Debate*, Callahan, Daniel (ed.), Doubleday, NY, 1971 p. 276:
    Just as we have laws compelling death control, so we must have laws requiring birth control – the purpose being to ensure a zero rate of population increase. We must come to see that it is the duty of

government to protect women against pregnancy as it protects them against job discrimination and smallpox, and for the same reason – the public good. No longer can we tolerate the doctrinaire position that the number of children a couple has is a strictly private decision carrying no social consequences. There is ample precedent for legislation limiting family size; for example, the law which limits a married person to only one spouse.

Appendix 1 Guidelines – Regional IVF Unit, St Mary's Hospital, Manchester

1. We are only able to offer treatment to couples who have been living together for at least three years.
2. We only *treat* women less than 40 and/or couples where the male is less than 50 years old.
3. We are only able to accept couples who reside within the geographical boundaries covered by the North Western Regional Health Authority.
4. If you are overweight, it is difficult to see the ovaries on the scan and dangerous to undertake a laparoscopy or have a general anaesthetic. We treat women who are close to their ideal body weight for height.
5. Once accepted (that is, after the clinic visit), each couple is offered a *maximum* of three complete courses of treatment. A complete IVF course is one ending in the replacement of one or more embryos or the transfer of eggs and sperm into the tube with GIFT. Completed courses of treatment at other centres are included in this calculation.
6. Only childless couples are accepted onto the waiting list for possible treatment. Since October 1984 we are unable to accept couples who have a child living with them by the current or previous relationships or by adoption.
7. If you adopt a child whilst on the waiting list we will be unable to offer you treatment. If you adopted after having been accepted we would wish to discuss any further treatment with you and the social worker responsible for the adoption.

SOME QUESTIONS AND ANSWERS – IVF TREATMENT AT KING'S ASSISTED CONCEPTION UNIT

1. *Is there a long waiting list for IVF treatment in our unit?*
   The wait is about 10 months to 1 year from registration.

2. *Are there any criteria for selecting which patients to treat first?*
   Treatment is strictly in chronological order from the date of registration.

3. *Are there any criteria for selecting patients on the basis of likelihood of successful outcome?*
   No. All patients who are found to need IVF are registered for the waiting list.

4. *Are there any age criteria?*
   We do not have an age criterion *per se*. However, we explain to anyone over the age of 35 that they have a reduced chance of success, and that they may be well advised to have immediate treatment as private patients rather than wait on the non-paying waiting list. We continue to treat patients as long as their ovaries continue to respond to stimulation, even if they are over 40.

5. *Must the patient be married, or in a stable heterosexual relationship?*
   We have no policy regarding our patients' relationships. Where it is envisaged that a patient's relationship, or lack of relationship, may present a problem, then the case is discussed with all the staff of the Unit. Thus, decisions regarding treatment are made on an individual basis.

Appendix 2   Surrogate Parenting Agreement[1]

This AGREEMENT is made this 6th day of February, 1985, by and between MARY BETH WHITEHEAD, a married woman (herein referred to as 'Surrogate'), RICHARD WHITEHEAD, her husband (herein referred to as 'Husband'), and WILLIAM STERN (herein referred to as 'Natural Father').
RECITALS   THIS AGREEMENT is made with reference to the following facts: (1) WILLIAM STERN, Natural Father, is an individual over the age of eighteen (18) years who is desirous of entering into this Agreement. (2) The sole purpose of this Agreement is to enable WILLIAM STERN and his infertile wife to have a child which is biologically related to WILLIAM STERN. (3) MARY BETH WHITEHEAD, Surrogate, and RICHARD WHITEHEAD, her husband, are over the age of eighteen (18) years and desirous of entering into this Agreement in consideration of the following:
NOW THEREFORE, in consideration of the mutual promises contained herein and the intentions of being legally bound hereby, the parties agree as follows:

1. MARY BETH WHITEHEAD, Surrogate, represents that she is capable of conceiving children. MARY BETH WHITEHEAD understands and agrees that in the best interest of the child, she will not form or attempt to form a parent–child relationship with any child or children she may conceive, carry to term and give birth to, pursuant to the provisions of this Agreement, and shall freely surrender custody to WILLIAM STERN, Natural Father, immediately upon birth of the child; and terminate all parental rights to said child pursuant to this Agreement.

2. MARY BETH WHITEHEAD, Surrogate, and RICHARD WHITEHEAD, her husband, have been married since 12/2/73, and RICHARD WHITEHEAD is in agreement with the purposes, intents and provisions of this Agreement and acknowledges that his wife, MARY BETH WHITEHEAD, Surrogate, shall be artificially inseminated pursuant to the provisions of this Agreement. RICHARD WHITEHEAD agrees that in the best interest of the child, he will not form or attempt to form a parent–child

relationship with any child or children MARY BETH WHITEHEAD, Surrogate, may conceive by artificial insemination as described herein, and agrees to freely and readily surrender immediate custody of the child to WILLIAM STERN, Natural Father; and terminate his parental rights; RICHARD WHITEHEAD further acknowledges he will do all acts necessary to rebut the presumption of paternity of any offspring conceived and born pursuant to aforementioned agreement as provided by law, including blood testing and/or HLA testing.

3. WILLIAM STERN, Natural Father, does hereby enter into this written contractual Agreement with MARY BETH WHITEHEAD, Surrogate, where MARY BETH WHITEHEAD shall be artificially inseminated with the semen of WILLIAM STERN by a physician. MARY BETH WHITEHEAD, Surrogate, and [illegible words], acknowledges that she will carry said embryo/fetus(s) until delivery. MARY BETH WHITEHEAD, Surrogate, and RICHARD WHITEHEAD, her husband, agree that they will co-operate with any background investigation into the Surrogate's medical, family and personal history and warrants (sic) the information to be accurate to the best of their knowledge. MARY BETH WHITEHEAD, Surrogate, and RICHARD WHITEHEAD, her husband, agree to surrender custody of the child to WILLIAM STERN, Natural Father, immediately upon birth, acknowledging that it is the intent of this Agreement in the best interests of the child to do so; as well as institute and cooperate in proceedings to terminate their respective parental rights to said child, and sign any and all necessary affidavits, documents and the like, in order to further the intent and purposes of this Agreement. It is understood by MARY BETH WHITEHEAD, and RICHARD WHITEHEAD, that the child to be conceived is being done so for the sole purpose of giving said child to WILLIAM STERN, its natural and biological father. MARY BETH WHITEHEAD and RICHARD WHITE-HEAD agree to sign all necessary affidavits prior to and after the birth of the child and voluntarily participate in any paternity proceedings necessary to have WILLIAM STERN's name entered on said child's birth certificate as the natural or biological father.

4. That the consideration for this Agreement, which is compensation for services and expenses, and in no way is to be construed as a fee for termination of parental rights or a payment in exchange for a consent to surrender the child for adoption, in addition to other provisions contained herein, shall be as follows:

(A) $10,000 shall be paid to MARY BETH WHITEHEAD, Surrogate, upon surrender of custody to WILLIAM STERN, the natural and biological father of the child born pursuant to the provisions of this Agreement for surrogate services and expenses in carrying out her obligations under this Agreement;

(B) The consideration to be paid to MARY BETH WHITEHEAD, Surrogate, shall be deposited with the Infertility Center of New York (hereinafter ICNY), the representative of WILLIAM STERN, at the time of the signing of this Agreement, and held in escrow until completion of the duties and obligations of MARY BETH WHITEHEAD, Surrogate, as herein described.

(C) WILLIAM STERN, Natural Father, shall pay the expenses incurred by MARY BETH WHITEHEAD, Surrogate, pursuant to her pregnancy, more specifically defined as follows:

(1) All medical, hospitalization and pharmaceutical, laboratory and therapy expenses incurred as a result of MARY BETH WHITEHEAD'S pregnancy, not covered or allowed by her present health and major medical insurance, including all extraordinary medical expenses and all reasonable expenses for treatment of any emotional or mental conditions or problems related to said pregnancy, but in no case shall any such expenses be paid or reimbursed after a period of six (6) months have elapsed since the date of the termination of the pregnancy, and this Agreement specifically excludes any expenses for lost wages or other non-itemized incidentals related to said pregnancy.

(2) WILLIAM STERN, Natural Father, shall not be responsible for any latent medical expenses occurring six (6) weeks subsequent to the birth of the child, unless the medical problem or abnormality incident thereto was known and treated by a physician prior to the expiration of said six (6) week period and in written notice of the same sent to ICNY, as representative of WILLIAM STERN by certified mail, return receipt requested, advising of this treatment.

(3) WILLIAM STERN, Natural Father, shall be responsible for the total costs of all paternity testing. Such paternity testing [illegible word] at the [illegible word] of WILLIAM STERN, Natural Father, be required prior to release of the surrogate fee from escrow. In the event WILLIAM STERN, Natural Father, is conclusively determined not be the biological father of the child as a result of an HLA test, this Agreement will be deemed breached and MARY BETH WHITEHEAD, Surrogate, shall not be entitled to any fee. WILLIAM STERN, Natural Father, shall be entitled to reimbursement of all medical and related expenses from MARY BETH WHITEHEAD, Surrogate, and RICHARD WHITEHEAD, her husband.

(4) MARY BETH WHITEHEAD'S reasonable travel expenses incurred at the request of WILLIAM STERN, pursuant to this Agreement.

5. MARY BETH WHITEHEAD, Surrogate, and RICHARD WHITEHEAD, her husband, understand and agree to assume all risks, including the risk of death, which are incidental to conception, pregnancy, childbirth, including but not limited to, postpartum complications. A copy of said possible risks and/or complications is attached hereto and made a part hereof.

6. MARY BETH WHITEHEAD, Surrogate, and RICHARD WHITEHEAD, her husband, hereby agree to undergo evaluation by JOAN EINWOHNER, a psychiatrist as designated by WILLIAM STERN or an agent thereof. WILLIAM STERN shall pay for the cost of said psychiatric evaluations, a medical release permitting dissemination of the report prepared as a result of said psychiatric evaluations to ICNY or WILLIAM STERN and his wife.

7. MARY BETH WHITEHEAD, Surrogate, and RICHARD WHITEHEAD, her husband, hereby agree that it is the exclusive and sole right of WILLIAM STERN, Natural Father, to name said child.

8. 'Child' as referred to in this Agreement shall include all children born simultaneously pursuant to the inseminations contemplated herein.

9. In the event of the death of WILLIAM STERN, prior or subsequent to the birth of said child, it is hereby understood and agreed by MARY BETH WHITEHEAD, Surrogate, and RICHARD WHITEHEAD, her husband that the child will be placed in the custody of WILLIAM STERN's wife.

10. In the event that the child is miscarried prior to the fifth (5th) month of pregnancy, no compensation, as enumerated in paragraph 4(A), shall be paid to MARY BETH WHITEHEAD, Surrogate. However, the expenses enumerated in paragraph 4(C) shall be paid or reimbursed to MARY BETH WHITEHEAD, Surrogate. In the event the child is miscarried, dies or is stillborn subsequent to the fourth (4th) month of pregnancy and said child does not survive, the Surrogate shall receive $1,000.00 in lieu of the compensation enumerated in paragraph 4(A). In the event of a miscarriage or stillbirth as described above, this Agreement shall terminate and neither MARY BETH WHITEHEAD, Surrogate, nor WILLIAM STERN, Natural Father, shall be under any further obligation under this Agreement.

11. MARY BETH WHITEHEAD, Surrogate, and WILLIAM STERN, Natural Father, shall have undergone complete physical and genetic evaluation, under the direction and supervision of a licensed physician, to determine whether the physical health and well-being of each is

satisfactory. Said physical examination shall include testing for venereal diseases, specifically including but not limited to, syphilis, herpes and gonorrhea. Said venereal disease testing shall be done prior to, but not limited to, each series of inseminations.

12. In the event that pregnancy has not occurred within a reasonable time, in the opinion of WILLIAM STERN, Natural Father, this Agreement shall terminate by written notice to MARY BETH WHITEHEAD, Surrogate, at the residence provided to the ICNY by the Surrogate, from ICNY, as representative of WILLIAM STERN, Natural Father.

13. MARY BETH WHITEHEAD, Surrogate, agrees that she will not abort the child once conceived except, if in the professional medical opinion of the inseminating physician, such action is necessary for the physical health of MARY BETH WHITEHEAD or the child has been determined by said physician to be physiologically abnormal. MARY BETH WHITEHEAD further agrees, upon the request of said physician to undergo amniocentesis or similar tests to detect genetic and congenital defects. In the event said test reveals that the fetus is genetically or congenitally abnormal, MARY BETH WHITEHEAD, Surrogate, agrees to abort the fetus upon demand of WILLIAM STERN, Natural Father, in which event, the fee paid to the Surrogate will be in accordance to Paragraph 10. If MARY BETH WHITEHEAD refuses to abort the fetus upon demand of WILLIAM STERN, his obligations as staged (sic) in this Agreement shall cease forthwith, except as to obligations of paternity imposed by statute.

14. Despite the provisions of Paragraph 13, WILLIAM STERN, Natural Father, recognizes that some genetic and congenital abnormalities may not be detected by amniocentesis or other tests, and therefore, if proven to be the biological father of the child, assumes the legal responsibility for any child who may possess genetic or congenital abnormalities.

15. MARY BETH WHITEHEAD, Surrogate, further agrees to adhere to all medical instructions given to her by the inseminating physician as well as her independent obstetrician. MARY BETH WHITEHEAD also agrees not to smoke cigarettes, drink alcoholic beverages, use illegal drugs, or take non-prescription medications or prescribed medications without written consent from her physician. MARY BETH WHITEHEAD agrees to follow a prenatal medical examination schedule to consist of no fewer visits than: one visit per month during the first seven (7) months of pregnancy, two visits (each to occur at two-week intervals) during the eighth and ninth months of pregnancy.

16. MARY BETH WHITEHEAD, Surrogate, agrees to cause RICHARD WHITEHEAD, her husband, to execute a refusal of consent form as annexed hereto as Exhibit 'G'.

17. Each party acknowledges that he or she fully understands this Agreement and its legal effect, and that they are signing the same freely and voluntarily and that neither party has any reason to believe that the other(s) did not freely and voluntarily execute said Agreement.

18. In the event any of the provisions of this Agreement are (sic) deemed to be invalid or unenforceable, the same shall be deemed severable from the remainder of this Agreement and shall not cause the invalidity or unenforceability of the remainder of this Agreement. If such provision shall be deemed invalid due to its scope or breadth, then said provision shall be deemed valid to the extent of the scope or breadth permitted by law.

19. The original of this Agreement, upon execution, shall be retained by the Infertility Center of New York, with photocopies being distributed to MARY BETH WHITEHEAD, Surrogate and WILLIAM STERN, Natural Father, having the same legal effect as the original.

WILLIAM STERN Natural Father   DATE   STATE OF NEW YORK(SS.: COUNTY OF NEW YORK) On the 6 day of February, 1985, before me personally came WILLIAM STERN, known to me, and to me known, to be the individual described in the foregoing instrument and he acknowledge to me that he executed the same as his free and voluntary act. NOTARY PUBLIC

AGREEMENT   THIS AGREEMENT is made this Third day of December, 1984, by the (sic) 'between WILLIAM STERN hereinafter referred to as 'Natural Father', and the Primary Research Associates of United States, Inc., d/b/a Infertility Center of New York, (hereinafter referred to as 'ICNY'). WHEREAS, Natural Father is desirous of taking part in the process of surrogate parenting wherein he will attempt to conceive a child by artificial insemination of a surrogate mother; WHEREAS, ICNY is a corporation duly organized and existing under the laws of the State of New York for the purpose inter alia of engaging in research, developmental work and design in the areas of surrogate parenting, ovum transfer and in vitro fertilization with implantation in a surrogate; and additionally providing administrative and supportive services for the above; and WHEREAS, Natural Father is desirous of contracting with ICNY for such services; and

WHEREAS INCY is desirous of contracting with the Natural Father to provide such services;

NOW THEREFORE, in consideration of the mutual promises contained herein, and with the intentions of being legally bound hereby, the parties mutually agree as follows:

(1) Natural Father hereby contracts with ICNY for the services offered by ICNY and ICNY agrees to contract with the Natural Father to use its best efforts to assist the Natural Father in the selection of a 'surrogate mother' as hereinafter defined, it being understood that the final selection of the 'surrogate mother' is solely within the discretion of the Natural Father. In addition to assisting the Natural Father in the selection of a 'surrogate mother', ICNY shall also provide the services set forth in Exhibit 'A' annexed-hereto and made a part hereof and these services shall continue until the completion of the duties and obligations of surrogate or until such time as the Natural Father decides not to utilize ICNY's services, provided that the Natural Father is not in breach of this Agreement.

(2) Natural Father agrees and understands that he must enter into an agreement with the selected surrogate mother whereby Natural Father agrees to the process of artificial insemination with the use of his semen for the purpose of impregnating the surrogate mother. Thereafter, the surrogate mother shall give birth to a child fathered by the Natural Father and voluntarily surrender custody of said child to the Natural Father.

(3) Natural Father hereby agrees to pay ICNY as compensation for the services provided by ICNY the sum of SEVEN THOUSAND FIVE HUNDRED DOLLARS ($7,500.00) incurred by ICNY on behalf of the Natural Father. The Natural Father understands and agrees that said sum is non-refundable. A partial list of costs and expenses is annexed hereto and made a part hereof as Exhibit 'B'. ICNY shall on a periodic basis bill the Natural Father for the costs and expenses incurred on behalf of the Natural Father. The Natural Father agrees that ICNY shall act as escrow agent for the fee to be paid by the Natural Father to the selected surrogate mother.

(4) The following list of definitions shall apply throughout this Agreement:

  (a) 'Child' is defined as all children born simultaneously as a result of the insemination comtemplated by this Agreement.
  (b) 'Natural Father' is defined as the individual over the age of

eighteen (18) who has selected the surrogate mother and whose semen is used in the insemination contemplated herein resulting in the birth of the child.

(c) 'Surrogate mother' is defined as a woman over the age of eighteen (18) selected by the Natural Father to be impregnated by the process of artificial insemination with semen of the Natural Father for the purpose of becoming pregnant and giving birth to a child and surrendering the child to the Natural Father.

(5) ICNY agrees to provide the services detailed in Exhibit 'A'. Said services including the offering, at the option of the Natural Father, of legal representation of the Natural Father in his negotiations and agreement with the surrogate mother. The Natural Father understands and acknowledges that ICNY offers these legal services through the law firm retained by ICNY but, ICNY makes no representations or warranties with respect to matters of law or the legality of surrogate parenting and is not rendering legal services or providing legal advice. However, the Natural Father has the absolute right to seek legal counsel of his own selection in his negotiations and agreement with the selected surrogate mother or her representative. In the event the Natural Father utilizes the legal services of counsel other than the law firm retained by ICNY, all legal fees and cost shall be borne by the Natural Father and such fees and costs shall be in addition to the fees and costs set forth in Paragraph 3 of this Agreement.

(6) Prior to signing this Agreement, each party has been given the opportunity to consult with an attorney of his own choice concerning the terms and legal significance of the Agreement, and the effect which it has upon any and all interests of the parties. Each party acknowledges that he fully understands the Agreement and its legal effect, and that he is signing the same freely and voluntarily and that neither party has any reason to believe that the other did not understand fully the terms and effects of this Agreement, or that he did not freely and voluntarily execute this Agreement.

(7) Natural Father warrants and represents the following to ICNY:

(a) That the Natural Father's semen is of sufficient nature both quantitatively and qualitatively to impregnate the selected surrogate mother.

(b) That the Natural Father is medically free from disease or other hereditary medical problems which could cause injury, defect, or disease to the surrogate mother or child.

(c) That the Natural Father will not make or attempt to make directly or through a representative, a subsequent agreement with the selected surrogate mother or any other surrogates introduced to the Natural Father by ICNY before or at any time after the birth of his child. In the event of a further arrangement with the surrogate for a child is made, the Natural Father agrees to pay to ICNY a second fee in the amount specified in Paragraph 3 of this Agreement.

(8) Natural Father agrees that breach of any of his warranties and representations shall cause this Agreement to immediately terminate but in no way relieve the Natural Father from his obligations under this Agreement. Further, the Natural Father agrees that his warranties and representations shall survive the termination of this Agreement.

(9) Natural Father hereby acknowledges that ICNY makes no representations or warranties with respect to any agreement or understanding which may be reached, or may have been reached, between himself and a prospective 'surrogate mother.' Natural Father further acknowledges that the nature of any such agreement or understanding as well as all ramifications, obligations and enforcement matters relating therein are subjects which he must seek advice from his attorney.

(10) It is expressly understood that ICNY does not guarantee or warrant that the 'surrogate mother' will in fact conceive a child fathered by Natural Father; nor does ICNY guarantee or warrant that if a child is conceived it will be a healthy (sic) child, free from all defects; nor does ICNY guarantee or warrant the 'surrogate mother' (and her husband, if applicable) will comply with the terms and provisions of the separate agreement entered into between herself and Natural Father including but not limited to, the 'surrogate mother's' refusal to surrender custody of the child upon birth.

(11) Natural Father hereby specifically releases ICNY and its officers, employees, agents and representatives from any and all liability and responsibility of any nature whatsoever except willful and gross negligence, which may result from complications, breaches, damages, losses, claims, actions, liabilities, whether actual or asserted of any kind, and all other costs or detriments of any kind, in any way related to or arising from any agreement or understanding between himself and a 'surrogate mother' located through the services of ICNY. Moreover, the Natural Father understands the relationship between ICNY and the relationship of the doctors used in connection with insemination, monitoring and any other medical

or psychiatric procedure or treatment of the surrogate or if the child is that of an independent contractor and that there is no other relationship between the parties.

(12) This Agreement is binding on each party's respective executors, heirs, assigns, and successors.

(13) This Agreement has been drafted, negotiated and executed in New York, and shall be governed by, continued and enforced in accordance with the laws of the State of New York.

(14) In the event any of the provisions of this Agreement are deemed to be invalid or unenforceable, the same shall be deemed severable from the remainder of this Agreement and shall not cause the invalidity or unenforceability of the remainder of this Agreement. If such provision(s) shall be deemed invalid due to its scope or breadth, then said provision(s) shall be deemed to the extent of the scope or breadth permitted by law.

WITNESS   NATURAL   FATHER   WITNESS   BY: PRIMARY RESEARCH ASSOCIATES OF UNITED STATES, INC. d/ b/a INFERTILITY CENTER OF NEW YORK   We have read the foregoing five pages of this Agreement, and it is our collective intention by affixing our signature below, to enter into a binding legal obligation. MARY BETH WHITEHEAD, Surrogate   DATE   RICHARD WHITEHEAD   Surrogate's Husband DATE   STATE OF NEW YORK) SS.:   COUNTY OF NEW YORK) On the 6th day of February, 1985, before me personally came MARY BETH WHITEHEAD, known to me, and to me known to be the individual described in the foregoing instrument and she acknowledged to me that she executed the same as her free and voluntary act.
NOTARY PUBLIC   STATE OF NEW YORK) SS.: COUNTY OF NEW YORK) On the 6th day of February, 1985, before me personally came RICHARD WHITEHEAD, known to me, and to me known to be the individual described in the foregoing instrument and he acknowledged to me that he executed the same as his free and voluntary act.
NOTARY PUBLIC.

Note

1   See *Baby M*, 109 N.J. 396; 5337 A.2d 1227 (1988).

Appendix 3 Model Human Reproductive Technologies and Surrogacy Act[1]

ARTICLE 1: GENERAL PROVISIONS

1–101 Short Title

This [Act] may be cited as the Human Reproductive Technologies and Surrogacy Act.

1–102 Definitions

The following words and phrases, whenever used in this [Act], shall have the following meanings, unless the context otherwise requires:

(1)   'Birth Mother' means a woman who gestates an embryo conceived by insemination, in vitro fertilization, or as a result of a surrogacy arrangement.

(2)   'Donor' means an individual who contributes his or her gametes for the purpose of insemination, in vitro fertilization, or implantation in another, or a woman who contributes a preembryo.

(3)   'Gamete' means the ovum (egg) and the spermatozoa (sperm).

(4)   'Health Care Provider' means a person who is licensed, certified, or otherwise authorized by the law of [this State] to administer health care in the ordinary course of business or practice of a profession.

(5)   'Informed Consent' occurs when a person, while exercising care for his or her own welfare, makes a decision about whether or not to participate in a proposed medical procedure or contractual arrangement that is based on a full awareness of the relevant facts. The relevant facts include: (a) the medical and psychological risks; (b) the legal, financial, and contractual

rights and obligations; and (c) the available alternatives, including the alternative of not participating in any procedure or arrangement and each alternative's attendant risks and obligations.

(6)   'Insemination' means introduction of semen into a woman's vagina, cervical canal, or uterus through noncoital means.

(7)   'Intended Parents,' including 'Intended Father' and 'Intended Mother', means persons who are married to each other and who, complying with the requirements of this [Act], enter into a surrogacy contract with a surrogate by which they are to become the parents of the resulting child.

(8)   'In Vitro Fertilization' means all medical and laboratory procedures that are necessary to effectuate:
    (a) the extracorporeal combining of gametes to allow fertilization to occur, or
    (b) the transfer of a preembryo into the uterine cavity.

(9)   'Licensed Person' means a person licensed or authorized by the [State Department of Health] pursuant to Section 9–101 of this [Act] to engage in the collection, storage, or use of gametes and preembryos.

(10)   'Partner' means an individual specified by an insemination recipient or a preembryo transfer recipient to share equally the rights and responsibilities of parenthood for any resulting child.

(11)   'Person' means individual, corporation, government or governmental subdivision or agency, business trust, estate, trust, partnership or association, or any other legal entity.

(12)   'Preembryo' means the cell mass that results from fertilization of an ovum prior to implantation.

(13)   'Surrogacy' or 'Surrogacy Arrangement' means any arrangement by which a woman agrees to be impregnated by noncoital means, using either the intended father's sperm or the intended mother's egg, or both, with the intent that the intended parents are to become the parents of the resulting child after the child's birth.

(14)   'Surrogate Contract' means an agreement that complies with the requirements of Article 6 of this [Act] providing for a surrogacy arrangement.

(15)   'Surrogate' means a woman who agrees, pursuant to a surrogacy contract, to bear a child for intended parents.

ARTICLE 2: RULES OF PARENTAGE

2–101 Mother–Child Relationship

Except as otherwise provided in this [Act], a woman is the mother of a child to whom she has given birth.

2–102 Father–Child Relationship

(a) A man is presumed to be the father of a child if:

   (1) he and the child's mother are or have been married to each other and the child is born during the marriage, or within 300 days after the marriage is terminated for any reason, or after a decree of separation is entered by a court;

   (2) before the child's birth, he and the child's mother have attempted to marry each other by a marriage solemnized in apparent compliance with law, although the attempted marriage is or could be declared void, voidable, voidable or otherwise invalid; and

   (i)   if the attempted marriage could be declared invalid only by a court, the child is born during the attempted marriage, or within 300 days after its termination for any reason; or

   (ii) if the attempted marriage is invalid without a court order, the child is born within 300 days after the termination of cohabitation;

   (3) after the child's birth, he and the child's mother have married, or attempted to marry, each other by a marriage solemnized in apparent compliance with law, although the attempted marriage is or could be declared void, voidable or otherwise invalid; and

   (i)   he has acknowledged his paternity of the child in a writing filed with the [appropriate court or Vital Statistics Bureau];

   (ii) he is obligated to support the child under a written voluntary promise or by court order;

   (4) while the child is under the age of majority, he receives the child into his home and openly holds out the child as his child; or

   (5) as an unmarried donor of sperm for use in insemination or in vitro fertilization, he and an unmarried woman, who under Section 2–101 would be the mother of the child, follow the procedures in Article 4 or Article 5 and agree in

writing in advance of the procedure that the donor shall be the father.

(b)   A presumption under subsection (a) may be rebutted in an appropriate action only by clear and convincing evidence. The existence of the father and child relationship resumed under paragraphs (1), (2), or (3) of subsection (a) is not, however, rebutted by evidence that the child was conceived by means of insemination or in vitro fertilization so long as the presumptive father complies with the requirements of Section 4–101(c) or Section 5–101(c) of this [Act]. In the absence of such compliance, the presumptive father's consent will be conclusively presumed by his failure to object of (*sic*) paternity [by filing an action to dispute paternity] within 30 days after he knew or should have known of the child's birth. If two or more presumptions of paternity arise which conflict with each other, the presumption which on the facts is founded on the weightier considerations of policy and logic controls. The presumption is rebutted by a court decree establishing paternity of the child by another man.

2–103 Termination and Transfer of Parental Rights to Intended Parents

Parental rights established under this article shall be terminated and transferred to the intended parents or to the surrogate and her husband, if any, only pursuant to Article 6 of this [Act].

2–104 Effect of Noncompliance

Noncompliance with the requirements of this [Act] shall not affect the determination of parenthood under Article 2, nor shall breach of a judicially preauthorized surrogacy contract affect transfer of parentage under Section 6–103(d)(4)

ARTICLE 3: OBLIGATIONS TO AND RIGHTS OF THE CHILD

3–101 Health Care Decisions Concerning the Fetus

(a)   All decisions regarding the health of the birth mother and the fetus are to be made by the birth mother.
(b)   In the case of surrogacy, after birth and prior to:
    (1)   the expiration of the 72-hour period specified in Section 6–103(d)(4), or

(2)   a surrogate's election to keep the child.

Health care decisions regarding the resulting child shall be made by the birth mother, or, in the event of her disability, by the intended parents, unless the surrogacy contract otherwise provides.

3–102 Legitimacy

If, under the provisions of this [Act], a parent–child relationship is created between two persons, the child shall be considered for all purposes of law the legitimate child of the parent.

3–103 Parents' Duty to Support

Any person who is determined to be the parent of a child under the provisions of Article 2 of this [Act] shall support the child.

3–104 Duty of Others for Support

(a)   If the parties who are involved in an insemination, *in vitro* fertilization, or surrogacy arrangement do not substantially comply with the applicable provisions of Article 4, Article 5, or Article 6 of this [Act], then, in addition to the support obligations determined under Section 3–103, the court may impose a support obligation on:
(1)   the sperm donor in the case of insemination;
(2)   the gamete donors in the case of *in vitro* fertilization; or
(3)   the intended parents or surrogate in a surrogacy arrangement.
In imposing this support obligation, the court may consider the seriousness of and the reasons for noncompliance in order to determine which of the parties, if any, should be liable for support.

(b)   If any person wilfully fails to comply with the provisions of this [Act], as determined under Section 8–102(a), and the effect thereof is the authorization of a procedure in violation of this [Act], that person may be liable for support of the resulting child.

3–105 Intestate and Testate Successions

(a)   Subject to the provisions of Section 3–105(b), a child shall be considered a child only of his or her parent or parents as determined under Article 2 of this [Act], and vice versa, for purposes of

(1) intestate succession;

(2) taking against the will of any person;

(3) taking under the will of any person, unless such will otherwise provides; and,

(4) being entitled to any support or similar allowance during the adminstration of a parent's estate.

(b) For purposes of Section 3–105(a), a child born of a surrogate is:

(1) the child of the intended parents from the moment of the child's birth unless within 72 hours of the birth of such child the surrogate gives notice of her intent to keep the child pursuant to Section 6–104(d) of this [Act]; or

(2) the child of the surrogate and her husband, if any, or if none, the person presumed to be the father under Section 2–102(a)(4), from the moment of the child's birth if the surrogate gives notice of her intent to keep the child pursuant to Section 6–104(d) of the [Act].

ARTICLE 4: INSEMINATION

4–101 Eligibility

Insemination shall be performed in accordance with regulations adopted by the [State Department of Health] and shall be available only to a woman:

(a) who is over the age of [18] years;

(b) who, if unmarried, successfully completes the nonmedical evaluation, and who, whether or not married, successfully completes the medical evaluation, receives appropriate counseling, pursuant to Article 7 of this [Act], and provides written certification of the counseling and any evaluation to the licensed person performing the insemination procedure; and

(c) whose husband, if the recipient is married, receives appropriate counseling pursuant to Article 7 of this [Act], and:

(1) successfully completes the medical evaluation, if he is the gamete donor in the insemination procedure,

(2) provides written certification of the counseling and any evaluation to the licensed person peforming the insemination procedure, and

(3) indicates, by a writing, acceptance of the legal rights and responsibilities of parenthood for any resulting child unless

the husband contributes his sperm for the insemination procedure.

(c) whose partner, or husband if the recipient is married, receives appropriate counseling pursuant to Article 7 of this [Act] and:

    (1) successfully completes the medical evaluation, if he is the gamete donor in the insemination procedure and, in the case of a partner, successfully completes the nonmedical evaluation, pursuant to Article 7 of this [Act],

    (2) provides written certification of the counseling and any evaluation to the licensed person performing the insemination procedure; and

    (3) indicates, by a writing, acceptance of the legal rights and responsibilities of parenthood for any resulting child unless the husband contributes his sperm for the insemination procedure.

ARTICLE 5: *IN VITRO* FERTILIZATION

5–101 Eligibility

In vitro fertilization shall be performed in accordance with regulations adopted by the [State Department of Health] and shall be available only to a woman:

(a) who is over the age of [18] years;

(b) who, if unmarried, successfully completes the nonmedical evaluation, and who, whether or not married, successfully completes the medical evaluation and receives counseling, pursuant to Article 7 of this [Act], and provides written certification of the counseling and any evaluation to the licensed person performing the *in vitro* fertilization procedure; and

(c) whose husband, if the recipient is married, receives appropriate counseling, pursuant to Article 7 of this [Act], and:

    (1) successfully completes the medical evaluation, if he is the gamete donor in the *in vitro* fertilization procedure,

    (2) provides written certification of the counseling and any evaluation to the licensed person performing the *in vitro* fertilization procedure, and

    (3) indicates, by a writing, acceptance of the legal rights and responsibilities of parenthood for any resulting child unless the husband contributes his sperm for the *in vitro* fertilization procedure.

(c) whose partner, or husband if the recipient is married, receives appropriate counseling, pursuant to Article 7 of this [Act] and:

(1) successfully completes the medical evaluation, if he is the gamete donor in the *in vitro* fertilization procedure and, in the case of a partner, successfully completes the non-medical evaluation, pursuant to Article 7 of this [Act],

(2) provides written certification of the counseling and any evaluation to the licensed person performing the *in vitro* fertilization procedure, and

(3) indicates, by a writing, acceptance of the legal rights and responsibilities of parenthood for any resulting child unless the husband contributes his sperm for the *in vitro* fertilization procedure.

ARTICLE 6: SURROGACY

6–101 Regulatory Procedures

(a) A surrogate arrangement is lawful only if it conforms to the requirements of this article and if, before the procedure to impregnate the surrogate:

(1) the licensed person performing the procedure receives written certification that the parties successfully completed the medical and nonmedical evaluation and counseling pursuant to Article 7;

(2) the surrogate arrangement has been judicially pre-authorized pursuant to Section 6–103; and

(3) all parties to the surrogacy contract provide the licensed person performing the procedure with written indication of their informed consent to the arrangement.

(b) The procedure to impregnate a surrogate shall be performed only in accordance with regulations issued by the [State Department of Health].

6–102 Eligibility

(a) All parties to a surrogacy contract must be over the age of [18].

(b) The intended mother must be medically determined to be physiologically unable to bear a child without serious risk to her health or to the child's health.

(c) The intended mother or the intended father must provide a complete gamete to be used to impregnate the surrogate.

(d) The intended mother or the surrogate must provide the ovum.

(e) No woman can be a surrogate unless she has a documented medical history of at least one uncomplicated pregnancy and uncomplicated vaginal delivery.

6–103 Judicial Preauthorization

(a) Jurisdiction.

A petition for preauthorization of a surrogacy arrangement must be brought in the [district court] for the [district] in which the surrogate resides at the time the petition is filed.

(b) Petition for Preauthorization Hearing.

(1)   Prior to insemination or *in vitro* fertilization of a surrogate, the parties to a surrogacy contract, as specified in Section 6–104, shall jointly petition the [court] for judicial preauthorization of the surrogacy arrangement.
(2)   the petition shall contain:
    (i)   the full name, age, place, and duration of residence of all petitioners;
    (ii)   the date and place of the intended parents' marriage;
    (iii) the date and place of the marriage, if any, of the surrogate and her husband;
    (iv)   a copy of the duly executed surrogacy contract;
    (v)   all required written consents;
    (vi)   all evaluations and reports required by this [Act]; and
    (vii) the name and address of the licensed person who will perform the procedure.

(c) Time of Hearing; Notice.

(1)   After the filing of a petition for preauthorization, the [court] shall fix a time and place for hearing within [30] days.
(2)   Notice of the filing of the petition and the time and place of hearing shall be given by petitioners at least 10 days prior to hearing to any person who conducted any nonmedical or medical evaluations or counseling pursuant to Article 7 of this [Act].

(d) Hearing and Validation of Surrogacy Arrangement.

(1)   Petitioners must be present at the hearing.
(2)   The parties may offer additional evidence deemed relevant by the [court], and the [court] may require the submission of such

additional information as it deems appropriate under the circumstances.

(3)   An order validating the surrogacy arrangement shall be issued only if, after the hearing, the [court] makes the following findings:

    (i)   All parties to the surrogacy contract have given their informed consent;

    (ii)   The surrogacy contract conforms to all of the requirements of Section 6–104 of this [Act] and contains no prohibited or unconscionable terms; and

(iii)   Evaluations and counseling, pursuant to Article 7, have been completed, and petitioners have been determined by the persons performing the evaluations or counseling to be qualified to enter into the surrogacy arrangement as provided by this [Act].

(4)   The effect of a judicial order validating the surrogacy arrangement shall be the automatic termination of the parental rights of the surrogate and her husband, if any, 72 hours after the birth of a child born as a result of the arrangement and a vesting of those rights solely in the intended parents, unless the surrogate exercises her rights under Section 6–104(d) of this [Act] to keep the child, in which case any parental rights of the intended parents shall be terminated and shall be vested solely in the surrogate and her husband, if any.

(e) Closed Hearings and Record.

(1)   All hearings shall be closed to the public. The only persons admitted shall be essential officers of the [court], parties, witnesses, and counsel.

(2)   All papers and records pertaining to the surrogacy hearing are subject to inspection only upon consent of all petitioners or upon showing of strict necessity supported by a court order.

6–104 Mandatory Terms of Surrogacy Contract

A surrogacy contract must be signed by the intended parents, the surrogates, and, if she is married, the surrogate's husband and shall include the following provisions:

(a)   the consent of the surrogate that she will surrender custody of the child or accept the obligation of parenthood if she gives notice of intent to keep the child as provided in Section 6–104(d) of this [Act];

(b) the consent of the husband of the surrogate, if any, that he will surrender custody of the child or accept the obligation of parenthood if the surrogate gives notice of intent to keep the child as provided in Section 6–104(d) of this [Act];

(c) the consent of the intended parents that they will accept the obligations of parenthood unless the surrogate gives notice of intent to keep the child as provided in Section 6–104(d) of this [Act];

(d) the right of the surrogate to keep the child if, at any time prior to 72 hours after the birth of the child, the surrogate:
  (1) executes a signed writing of her intention to keep the child; and
  (2) delivers the writing to the intended parents or the attending physician.
  This right can only be exercised personally by the surrogate and cannot be exercised by any guardian or other legal representative of the surrogate.

(e) A provision for adequate coverage through insurance or otherwise of health care expenses of the surrogate and the child for the term of the pregnancy and six weeks after the termination thereof for complications caused by the pregnancy or birth;

(f) if the surrogate will receive a fee, a provision that the fee will be deposited into an escrow account at a federally insured institution prior to a conception and held in escrow until:
  (1) relinquishment of parenthood to the intended parents; or
  (2) the contract is terminated before a live birth by means other than a breach by the surrogate. In this case, the surrogate will receive that portion of the fee which the parties to the surrogacy contract shall have provided for in the surrogacy contract.

6–105 No Specific Performance Rule

There shall be no specific performance for a breach by the surrogate of a surrogacy contract term that:
(a) requires her to become impregnated;
(b) requires her to have an abortion; or
(c) forbids her to have an abortion.

6–106 Damages

(a) The intended parents may recover only health care expenses and the fee prescribed in Section 6–104(f) if:

    (1)   the surrogate refuses to become impregnated;

    (2)   the surrogate has an abortion that is not medically necessary without the consent of the intended parents; or

    (3)   the surrogate elects to keep the child as provided in Section 6–104(d).

(b)   If the surrogate fails to become pregnant through no fault of either party within nine months after the surrogacy contract has been judicially approved pursuant to Section 6–103 of this [Act], the contract is voidable at the option of either party.

(c)   If the intended parents breach a material term of the contract, the surrogate may:

    (1)   recover health care expenses that the intended parents were required to pay;

    (2)   collect the fee that is provided for in the contract; and

    (3)   if the breach is refusal to accept the child within 72 hours after birth, the surrogate may file notice pursuant to Section 6–104(d) of this [Act] and the intended parents may be liable for support.

ARTICLE 7: EVALUATION AND COUNSELING

7–101 Nonmedical Evaluation

(a)   A nonmedical evaluation shall be performed by [a person authorized by the State Department of Health] who shall maintain a record of the findings and conclusions and make a copy of them available only to the person evaluated.

(b) The person conducting the nonmedical evaluation shall determine the party's suitability to parent by considering, in accordance with regulations of the [State Department of Health]:

    (1)   the ability and disposition of the person being evaluated to give a child love, affection, and guidance;

    (2)   the ability and disposition of the person being evaluated to provide a child with food, clothing, shelter, medical care, and other basic necessities; and

    (3)   any other factors required by rule of the [State Department of Health].

7–102 Medical Evaluation

(a)   General requirements;

    (1)   Gamete Donors. No gamete shall be used in an insemination procedure, in an *in vitro* fertilization procedure, or in a surrogacy arrangement unless the gamete donor has

been medically evaluated and the results, documented in accordance with regulations promulgated by the [State Department of Health], demonstrate the medical accept-ability of the person as a gamete donor.

(2) Recipients of Insemination or *In Vitro* Fertilization. No woman shall undergo an insemination procedure under Article 4, an *in vitro* fertilization procedure under Article 5, or be a surrogate under Article 6, unless the woman has been medically evaluated and the results, documented in accordance with regulations promulgated by the [state Department of Health), demonstrate the medical accept-ability of the woman to undergo the insemination or *in vitro* fertilization procedure or to be a surrogate.

(b) Until such time as the [State Department of Health] promulgates regulations required by Section 7–102, medical evaluations shall be made in accordance with the relevant sections of the guidelines published by the American Fertility Society.

7–103 Counseling

For any procedure under Articles 4, 5, and 6 of the [Act], the prospective parents of a resulting child and, for a surrogacy arrangement, all parties to the surrogacy contract, shall receive counseling by a [qualified mental health care professional] pursuant to rules promulgated by the [State Department of Health].

ARTICLE 8: LIABILITIES AND IMMUNITIES FOR PARTICIPANTS OF INSEMINATION, *IN VITRO* FERTILIZATION, AND SURROGACY

8–101 Immunities

(a) No person shall be subject to civil or criminal liability for nonnegligent actions taken pursuant to the requirements of this [Act].

(b) A physician or other health care provider, whose actions under this [Act] are in accord with reasonable medical standards, shall not be subject to criminal or civil liability or discipline for unprofessional conduct with respect to those actions.

8–102 Liabilities

(a) A person who acts in wilful noncompliance with this [Act]:
  (1) shall be guilty of [a class misdemeanour];
  (2) shall be liable for resulting damages; and
  (3) may be jointly and severally liable for child support to the resulting child under the laws of [this State].
(b) The sanctions provided in this section are in addition to any other sanctions provided under applicable law.

ARTICLE 9: REGULATORY PROVISIONS

9–101 Licensure and Regulation of Collection and Storage of Human Gametes and/or Preembryos

The [State Department of Health] shall establish standards to be applied by, as well as make rules governing the licensure or authorization of, persons who engage in the collection, storage, or use of gametes and/or preembryos for the uses authorized by this [Act].

9–102 Record Keeping

(a) The [State Department of Health] shall require all licensed persons to keep records in accordance with Section 9–201 of this [Act].
(b) The [State Department of Health] shall periodically review these records for accuracy and completeness to assess the licensed person's compliance with the standards promulgated under Section 9–101 of this [Act].

9–103 Restrictions on Use of Preembryos

(a) No preembryo shall be maintained *ex utero* beyond 14 days postfertilization development.
(b) No preembryo that has been donated for use in research shall be transferred to a uterine cavity.

9–104 Rights in Gametes and Preembryos

Except as provided in Sections 9–105, 9–106, 9–107, and 9–108, no person, other than a donor, can have rights in a donor's gametes or preembryo.

9–105 Transferability of Gametes and Preembryos

(a) Except as provided in Section 9–107, gametes and preembryos may be transferred only to a licensed person.
(b) Gametes and preembryos shall not be transferable by will or intestate succession.

9–106 Rights in Transferred Gametes and Preembryos

(a) Except as provided in Section 9–106(b), a transfer of gametes or preembryos transfers all rights of the transferor with respect to the gametes or preembryos.
(b) A person who tranfers gametes or preembryos may retain such rights with respect to them as are not inconsistent with the provisions of this [Act], by a written agreement with the transferee executed prior to the transfer.
(c) All rights of an individual with respect to gametes or pre-embryos shall terminate at the individual's death.
(d) All rights of any person with respect to a preembryo shall terminate upon implantation.
(e) Unless otherwise provided by written agreement, where two gametes are combined and a preembryo is created, each person who had rights with respect to either gamete shall have the same rights with respect to the preembryo, and conflicting rights with respect to the preembryo shall have priority in the following order:
   (1) First, rights of a sperm donor who had retained rights with respect to his sperm, or the rights of the sperm donor's spouse.
   (2) Second, rights of an ovum donor who had retained rights with respect to her ovum, or the rights of the ovum donor's spouse.
   (3) Third, rights of a licensed person who had rights with respect to the ovum.
   (4) Fourth, rights of a licensed person who had rights with respect to the sperm.
(f) Upon the death or dissolution of the licensed person in possession of gametes or preembryos, such gametes or pre-embryos shall be disposed of in accordance with the provisions of Section 9–108.

9–107 Transfer of Rights with Respect to Gametes and Preembryos

(a) A person may transfer rights with respect to gametes or preembryos by gift or sale, but only by a signed writing, or by a simultaneous transfer of the gametes or preembryos pursuant to Section 9–106(a).
(b) Rights with respect to gametes or preembryos shall not be transferable by will or intestate succession.
(c) A donor may, prior to the donor's death, transfer rights retained by the donor to the spouse of the donor, but only if the donor has no retained rights after the transfer.
(d) Except as provided in Section 9–107(c), a person may transfer rights with respect to gametes or preembryos only to a licensed person.

9–108 Disposition of Gametes and Preembryos Upon the Death or Dissolution of the Person in Possession

(a) Gametes and preembryos in the possession of an individual shall be destroyed at the time of that individual's death.
(b) Gametes and preembryos in the possession of a licensed person who is not an individual shall, at the time of that licensed person's dissolution, be disposed of in the following manner:
    (1) Those gametes and preembryos in which no other person has rights:
        (i) shall be transferred by gift or sale to a licensed person; or
        (ii) shall be destroyed.
    (2) Those gametes and preembryos in which another person has rights:
        (i) shall be transferred by gift or sale to a licensed person, subject to those rights; or
        (ii) shall be destroyed, if, after reasonable efforts to dispose of the gametes and preembryos under Section 9–108(b)(2)(i), no licensed person accepts them.

9–109 Status as Lives in Being: The Rule Against Perpetuities

(a) For purposes of the Rule Against Perpetuities, a person's life ends at the moment of his or her death even though such person may have gametes or preembryos deposited with a licensed or unlicensed person.
(b) For purposes of the Rule Against Perpetuities, a child born as a

result of insemination, *in vitro* fertilization, or a surrogacy arrangement is the child of his of her parents determined under the provisions of Article 2 of this [Act] and is a life in being for the pupose of testing the validity of interests created by such parent, by an ancestor or descendant of such parent, or by any other person, but only if such child was alive at the creation of such interest, or was *in utero* at such time and born within 300 days thereafter.

9–201 Maintenance and Confidentiality of Records

(a)   The [State Department of Health] shall create a Central Registry where all records listed under Section 9–201(b) and any others required by rule shall be kept.

(b)   When a child is born as the result of the procedures governed by Article 4, 5, or 6 of this [Act], the attending physician shall report the following information, if available, to the Central Registry, which shall maintain it in confidence:
   (1)   the identification of the donor, including name, address, and social security number;
   (2)   the identification of the recipient, including name, address, and social security number;
   (3)   the identification of the surrogate and her husband, if any, including name, address, and social security number;
   (4)   the identification of any resulting children born from the donor;
   (5)   the county in which each birth occurred; and
   (6)   such other information as the [State Department of Health] may require by rule.

(c)   Any person who destroys gametes shall notify the Central Registry of that fact, and shall provide such other information as required by rule.

(d)   The [State Department of Health] shall provide by rule who will maintain the records, how long they must be maintained, where they shall be kept, and, subject to Section 9–201(e), the circumstances under which they may be disclosed.

(e)   Access to Records:
   (1)   The identity of gamete or preembryo donors or surrogates shall be available only upon a showing strict necessity supported by court order.
   (2)   The Central Registry shall notify any donor, any surrogate, or the parents of any child born as a result of the procedures governed by Article 4, 5, or 6 of the [Act], if known, of any information it acquires that poses a serious risk to the

        health of the child, the donor, the surrogate, or any other person.

(3)   The records and information maintained in the Central Registry shall be made available for research under such terms and conditions as established by the [State Department of Health].

(f)   Registration fees shall be determined by the [State Department of Health].

Notes

1   From *Iowa Law Review* (1987) **72** p. 943.

Appendix 4 *Baby M*

There is probably no need to rehearse the facts of this well-publicized tug-of-war case except in brief. The Sterns were both professional people, the husband a biochemist and the wife a medical doctor. The latter was told that she might have multiple sclerosis which rendered pregnancy a serious health risk. According to the Supreme Court 537 A. 2d 1227, 1235 (1988),

> . . . [h]er anxiety appears to have exceeded the actual risk which current medical authorities assess as minimal. Nonetheless, that anxiety was evidently quite real, Mrs Stern fearing that pregnancy might precipitate blindless, paraplegia, or other forms of debilitation.

Through a surrogate parenting agency, they were introduced to Mrs Whitehead and they entered into a surrogacy contract in which the latter agreed to surrender the child to Mr Stern, the natural father. After the birth of the child, Mrs Whitehead felt that she could not surrender the child, but kept her word. Finding that she could not live without the child, Mrs Whitehead sought to have the child back for a week from the Sterns who were mindful of Mrs Whitehead's distressed condition and acceded to her request to have the child for a week. The child however was never returned to Mr Stern who then initiated proceedings to obtain custody of the child. An *ex parte* order was made against Mrs Whitehead for the return of the child pending final judgement.

The trial court judge held that the surrogacy contract was valid; he ordered that Mrs Whitehead's parental rights be terminated and that sole custody of the child be granted to Mr Stern and, after hearing testimony from Mrs Stern, an order was made allowing her to adopt the child. The decision of the trial court essentially gave effect to the surrogacy arrangement.

On appeal, the validity of the contract came to be determined by the Supreme Court of New Jersey. Wilentz C.J. delivered the opinion of the court which held that the surrogacy contract was void and unenforceable as it conflicted with the law and public policy of the State of New Jersey. Custody was granted to the father in the best interest of the child, but the court voided both the termination of Mrs Whitehead's parental rights and the adoption of the child by Mrs Stern and remanded the issue of Mrs Whitehead's visitation to the lower court.

Contrary to the view of the trial court,[1] the Supreme Court of New Jersey held the following:

1. *The Contract is Invalid and Unenforceable*
The court took the view that one of the basic purposes of the surrogacy contract is to achieve adoption through private placement. Although private placement is not illegal or prohibited, the surrogacy arrangement violated existing statutes and public policy because of the involvement of money.[2] Further, the termination of Mrs Whitehead's parental rights was not executed in accordance with the statutory provisions governing it.[3] Finally, a contractual arrangement to surrender one's parental rights would not be enforced by the court. In other words, the agreement is not irrevocable.

On the question of public policy, the court took the view that one of the basic principles of family law is that both father and mother have equal rights to the child's custody, the whole purpose of the agreement is to destroy the right of the mother in favour of the father. The agreement also contravenes the general principle in adoption law that the mother's consent to the adoption of the child should be informed consent and that it is generally revocable. The court took a damning view that in this case the surrogate had little or no counselling or independent legal advice. A surrogate mother, under such an agreement is irrevocably committed to surrender the child even before she knows the strength of her bond to the child, and as a result her consent, prior to the birth of the child, is not an informed decision, and after the birth of a child and under the pressure of lawsuit and the inducement of money payment, the act of surrendering the child is less than totally voluntary. The fundamental and predominant interest the contract serves is that of the commissioning parties, and it disregards the best interest of the child; at no stage is the suitability of the commissioning parties examined to determine their fitness to be the custodial parents:

> This is the sale of a child, or, at the very least, the sale of a mother's right to her child, the only mitigating factor being that one of the purchasers is the father. Almost every evil that prompted the prohibition of the payment of money in connection with adoptions exists here. [p. 1248.]

> The surrogacy contract creates, it is based upon, principles that are directly contrary to the objectives of our laws. It guarantees the separation of a child from its mother; it looks to adoption regardless of

suitability; it totally ignores the child; it takes the child from the mother regardless of her wishes and her maternal fitness; and it does all this, it accomplishes all of its goals, through the use of money. [p. 1250.]

The court countered the argument that in this case the surrogate went into this agreement with her eyes wide open. But the court took the view that the evil involved in such a transaction was the same; taking advantage of a woman's circumstances (the unwanted pregnancy or the need for money) in order to take away her child. The spectre of poor women being used exclusively for the rich was in the court's mind and here the evil could not be accepted irrespective of consent:

There are, in a civilized society, some things that money cannot buy. In America, we decided long ago that merely because conduct purchased by money was 'voluntary' did not mean that it was good or beyond regulation and prohibition. [p. 1249.]

Acknowledging that surrogacy may provide satisfaction for many infertile couples and surrogates, the potential degradation of some women cannot be ignored.

In sum, the harmful consequences of this surrogacy arrangement appear to us all too palpable. [p. 1250.]

The court therefore held that the agreement is void as it contravenes the baby-selling statute and is against public policy. A similar conclusion was reached in Michigan in *Doe* v. *Kelly*.

In Kentucky the court in *Surrogate Parenting Assocs.* v. *Commonwealth ex. rel. Armstrong*, 704 S.W. 2d 209 (Ky 1986) distinguished between baby-selling statutes and surrogate arrangements and considered that the former does not apply to an arrangement entered into prior to the conception of the child. The court however took the view, that the surrogate has the right to void the contract if she changes her mind during the pregnancy or immediately after the birth of the child. Just as consent to adoption or to the termination of parental rights five days prior to the birth of the child is invalid, consent of the surrogate before conception must also be caught as unenforceable. [See also in *Matter of Adoption of Baby Girl*, L.J., 132 Misc. 2d 972, 505 N.Y.S. 2d 813 (sur. 1986).]

2. *Restoration of Mrs Whitehead's Parental Rights*
Having considered that invalidity of the surrogate contract, and concluded that parental rights cannot be terminated on the basis of contract, the court restored Mrs Whitehead's parental rights having found that the best interest of the child is not dispositive of the

question, and that constitutional argument does not support the termination of her parental rights.

Both parties put forward constitutional claims; Mr Stern claims the right to procreate, and Mrs Whitehead claims the right to have the companionship of her child. The court held that Mr Stern's right, whether exercised naturally or through artificial means is not affected, but his right does not extend to destroying Mrs Whitehead's right of procreation or her right to custody of the child which is not part of the right to procreate and which involves considerations of different interests.[4]

The court on this point disagreed with the trial court's decision and held that

> there is no constitutional basis whatsoever requiring that Mr. Stern's claim to the custody of Baby M be sustained. [p. 1253.]

> The right to procreate very simply is the right to have natural children, whether through sexual intercourse or artificial insemination. It is no more than that. Mr Stern has not been deprived of that right. Through artificial insemination of Mrs Whitehead, Baby M is his child. [p. 1253.]

The court therefore concluded that the right of parenting, as that asserted by Mr Stern, cannot be enforced without regard to other people's interests, namely, the interests of Baby M. It was argued on behalf of Mr Stern that he was denied equal protection in that a husband who consents to his wife's AID would be regarded as the father of the resulting child. Rightly, the court rejected this argument which seems to draw an analogy between the contribution of a semen donor and a surrogate mother. The court observed that the parallel of this argument should be that of a wife who used a donated ovum for procreation with the consent of the husband. Here the analogy with AID and equal protection would suggest that the wife, as opposed to the ovum donor, should be regarded as the mother of the resulting child.

3. Affirmation of the Trial Court's Decision

On the question of custody, the court concentrated on the best interests of the child. The court found that the trial court's decision should be affirmed.[5] However, the court expressed the view that Mrs Whitehead's conduct had been judged too harshly; namely the way in which she had been characterized for her breach of the contract, violation of the court order, and the portrayal of her as a selfish self-promoting woman. But most important of all, the court passed comment on the initial *ex parte* order of the court and said that, when father and mother are separated and disagree, at birth, on custody, only in an extreme, truly rare, case should the child be taken from its mother *pendente lite* . . . [p. 1261.]

Obviously, this will have substantial practical effects on a father's position in custody disputes of this kind in the future as the mother's bond to the child will effectively render it extremely difficult for the father to argue that it will be in the child's best interests that the child should part with the mother.

Finally, the court said:

the legislature remains free to deal with this most sensitive issue as it sees fits, subject only to constitutional constraints. If the legislature decides to address surrogacy, consideration of this case will highlight many of its potential harms. We do not underestimate the difficulties of legislating on this subject. In addition to the inevitable confrontation with the ethical and moral issues involved, there is the question of the wisdom and effectiveness of regulating a matter so private, yet of such public interest. Legislative consideration of surrogacy may also provide the opportunity to begin to focus on the overall implications of the new reproductive biotechnology – *in vitro* fertilization, preservation of sperm and egg, embryo implantation and the like. The problem is how to enjoy the benefits of the technology – especially for infertile couples – while minimizing the risk of abuse. The problem can be addressed only when society decides what its values and objectives are in this troubling, yet promising, area. [p. 1264.]

Notes

1   The trial court took the view that the various statutes concerning adoption, termination of parental rights and payment of money in connection with adoption did not apply to surrogacy contracts in that the legislature did not have surrogacy contracts in mind when it passed those laws, and therefore they were irrelevant.

2   See N.J.S.A. 9:3–54a:
    No person, firm, partnership, corporation, association or agency shall make, offer to make or assist or participate in any placement for adoption and in connection therewith (1) pay, give or agree to give any money or any valuable consideration, or assume or discharge any financial obligation; or (2) take, receive, accept or agree to accept any money or any valuable consideration.

    9:3–54b says that the above prohibition
    shall not apply to the fees or services of any approved agency in connection with a placement for adoption, nor shall such prohibition apply to the payment for adoption, nor shall such prohibition apply to the payment or reimbursement of medical, hospital or other similar expenses incurred in connection with the birth or any illness of the child, or to the acceptance of such reimbursement by a parent of the child.

3   The court noted that for termination of parental rights under the private placement adoption statute, there must be a finding of intentional abandonment or substantial neglect of parental duties without reasonable expectation of a reversal of that conduct in the future; N.J.S.A. 9:3–48c(1). In relation to adoption through an approved agency, the formal agreement to surrender parental rights occurs only after birth, and then, by regulation, only after the mother has been counselled.

4   [p. 27]:

> The custody, care, companionship, and nurturing that follow birth are not parts of the right to procreation; they are rights that may also be constitutionally protected; but that involve many considerations other than the right of procreation. To assert that Mr Stern's right of procreation gives him the right to the custody of Baby M would be to assert that Mrs Whitehead's right of procreation does not give her the right to the custody of Baby M; it would be to assert that the constitutional right of procreation includes within it a constitutionally protected contractual right to destroy someone else's right of procreation (*sic*).

5   The court agreed with the court's analysis and conclusion. On the analysis side, the court made it clear that contrasting the family life of the Sterns and the Whiteheads, the latter's was less stable financially. On the point of the party's character, personality and home life, the court concluded that

> while love and affection there would be, Baby M's life with the Whiteheads promised to be too closely controlled by Mrs Whitehead. The prospects for a wholesome independent psychological growth and development would be at serious risk.

The Sterns' household and their personalities

> promise a much more likely foundation for Melissa to grow and thrive . . . Their household is stable, and likely to remain so. Their finances are more than adequate, their circle of friends supportive, and their marriage happy. More important, they are loving, giving, nurturing, and open-minded people. They have demonstrated the wish and ability to nurture and protect Melissa, yet at the same time to encourage her independence. . . . All in all, Melissa's future appears solid, happy and promising with them. [p. 33]

List of Reports

Interim Report on Human *In Vitro* Fertilisation and Embryo Replacement and Transfer, *British Medical Journal* (1983) **286**, p. 1594.

Departmental Committee on *Human Artificial Insemination*, London, HMSO, Cmnd. 1105, 1960.

Human Procreation, Ethical Aspects of the New Technique, Report of a Working Party Council for Science and Society, Oxford, Oxford University Press, 1984.

Law Commission *Report on Illegitimacy*, No. 118, London, HMSO, 1982.

Law Commission *Report on Injuries to Unborn Children*, No. 60, London, HMSO, Cmnd. 5709, 1974.

Law Commission *Report on Illegitimacy (Second Report)*, No. 157, London, HMSO, Cmnd. 9913, 1986.

Law Commission's *Working Paper on Illegitimacy*, No. 74, London, HMSO, 1982.

Legislation on Human Infertility Services and Embryo Research – A Consultation Paper, HMSO, London, Cmnd. 46, 1986.

Peel Committee, Report of the Panel on Human Artificial Insemination, **2**, *British Medical Journal* (1973) Suppl., Appendix V, p. 3.

Report of the Commission, Human Artificial Insemination, published in 1948, reprinted in 1952 by S.P.C.K.

Report of the Committee on One Parent Families, London, HMSO, Cmnd. 5629, 1974.

Report of the Committee of Inquiry into Human Fertilisation and Embryology, London, HMSO, Cmnd. 9314, 1984.

Report of the Committee on the Adoption of Children, HMSO, Cmd. 5107, 1972.

Report of the Committee on Homosexual Offences and Prostitution, London, HMSO, Cmnd. 247, 1957.

Report on the Disposition of Embryos produced by IVF, the Committee to Consider the Social, Ethical and Legal Issues Arising from IVF, chaired by Professor Louis Waller, Victoria, Australia, 1984.

Report on Human Artificial Reproduction and Related Matters, 2 Vols., Ministry of the Attorney General, Toronto, 1985.

Report of the Street Offences Committee, London, HMSO, Cmnd. 3231, 1928.

Scottish Law Commission *Consultative Memorandum on Illegitimacy*, No. 53, Edinburgh, HMSO, 1982.

Scottish Law Commission *Report on Liability for Ante-natal Injury*, No. 30, London, HMSO, Cmnd. 5371, 1973.

Scottish Law Commission *Report on Illegitimacy*, No. 82, Edinburgh, HMSO, 1984.

Surrogate Motherhood, Report of the Board of Science and Education, London, BMA, 1987.

Voluntary Licensing Authority for Human In Vitro Fertilisation and Embryology, First Report, London, Medical Research Council/Royal College of Obstetricians and Gynaecologists, 1986.

List of Cases

A. v. *C. Family Law* (1987) **8**, p. 170; *Family Law*, (1984) **14**, p. 241.
A.B. v. *C.B.* 1961 SC 347.
Adoption Application: Surrogacy [1987] 2 All ER 826.
Attorney General (ex rel Kerr) v. *T.* [1983] 1 Qd. R. 404.
Buck v. *Bell* 274 US 200 (1927).
C. v. *S.* [1987] 1 All ER 1230.
C.B. v. *A.B.* (1885) 12 R. (H.L.) 36.
Campbell v. *Croall* (1895) 22 R. 869.
Carey v. *Population Services International*, 431 U.S. 678 (1977).
Clarke v. *Clarke* [1943] P 1.
Corbett v. *Corbett* [1971] P 83
D. v. *A.* (1845) 1 Rob. Ecc. 279.
Dec. Adm. Ap. 6482/74, 10 July, 1975. D & R 7, p. 75(77).
Dec. Adm. Com. Ap. 6482/74, 10 July, 1975. D & R, 7 p. 55(77).
Dec. Adm. Com. Ap. 6564/74, 21 May, 1975. D & R 2, p. 105 (106).
Dec. Adm. Com. Ap. 7229/75, 12 December, 1977. D & R 12, p. 32
    (34–35).
Dennis v. *Dennis* [1955] P 153.
Eisenstadt v. *Baird* 405 US 438 (1972).
Emeh v. *Kensington, Chelsea & Fulham Area Health Authority* [1984] 3
    All ER 1044.
Galison v. *Dist. of Columbia*, 420 A 2d 1263, 1268 (D.C. 1979).
Griswold v. *Connecticut* 281 US 479 (1965).
Harris v. *McRae*, 488 US 297 (1980).
Hope v. *Hope* 8 De G.M. & G. 731.
Humphrey v. *Polak* [1901] 2 K.B. 385.
J. v. *J.* 1978 SLT 128.
K. v. *T.* [1983] 1 Qd. R. 386.
Kerrigan v. *Hall* (1901) 4 F. 10.
MacLennan v. *MacLennan* (1958) S.C. 105.
MacPherson v. *Leisham* (1887) 14 R. 780.
Maher v. *Roe* 432 US 464.
McKay v. *Essex Area Health Authority* [1982] 2 All ER 771.
Op. Com., 1 March, 1979, *Van Oosterwijck Case*, Publ. Court B, Vol.
    36, p. 27.

Op. Com., 12 July, 1977, *Case of Bruggemann and Scheuten*, D & R 10, p. 100.

Paton v. British Pregnancy Advisory Service Trustees [1979] Q.B. 276.

Planned Parenthood Association v. Danforth, 428 US 52 (1976).

Poe et al. v. Gerstein et al. 517 F. 2d, 787 (1975).

Q. v. Q. The Times, 12 May, 1960.

R. v. Ethical Committee of St Mary Hospital, ex parte Harriott, Family Law, 165 (1988).

R. v. Smith 22 L.J. (Q.B.) 116.

R.E.L. (otherwise R.) v. E.L. [1949] p. 211.

Re Andrews (1873) L.R. 8 Q.B. 153.

Re B (a Minor) (Wardship: Sterilisation) [1987] 2 All ER 210.

Re C (a Minor) (Wardship: Surrogacy) [1985] FLR 846.

Re D (a Minor) (Wardship: Sterilisation) [1976] 1 All ER 326.

Re D (a Minor) [1987] 1 FLR 422.

Re Eve (1986) 31 DLR (4th) 1.

Re F (an Infant) [1957], All ER 819.

Roe v. Wade 410 US 113 (1973).

Sciuriaga v. Powell (1980, unreported), CA transcript 597.

Skinner v. Oklahoma 316 US 535 (1942).

Slater v. Slater [1953] P 252.

Surrogacy Twin Babies case, The Daily Telegraph, 13 March, 1987, p. 2.

Sutherland v. Taylor (1887) 15 R. 224.

Syrkowski v. Appleyard 420 Mich. 367 (1985).

T. v. T [1988] 1 All ER 613.

Thake v. Maurice [1984] 2 All ER 513, and [1986] 2 All ER 497.

The Hamer Case, D & R 24, p. 5(14–16).

Udale v. Bloomsbury Area Health Authority [1983] 2 All ER 522.

Vansittart v. Vansittart (1858) 2 De G. & J. 249.

W. v. W. [1952] P 152.

Walrond v. Walrond (1858) Johns 18.

Williams v. States of New York 18 NY 2d. 481 (1966).

Zepeda v. Zepeda 41 Ill App 2d 240.

Table of Statutes

Bibliography

Action, H.B., *The Morals of Markets*, London, Longman, 1971.

Andrews, Lori B., 'Surrogate motherhood: should the adoption model apply?', *Children Legal Rights Journal* (1986) **7**, p. 13.

Annas, George J. and Elias Sherman, '*In Vitro* fertilisation and embryo transfer: Medicolegal aspects of a new technique to create a family', *Family Law Quarterly* (1983) **17**, p. 199.

Annas, George J., 'The baby broker boom', *Hastings Center Report* (1986) **16**, p. 30.

Annas, George J., 'Law and the life sciences: contracts to bear a child; compassion or commercialism?', *Hastings Center Report* (1981) **11**, p. 23.

Annas, George J., 'Making babies without sex: the law and the profits', *American Journal of Public Health*, (1984) **74**, p. 1415.

Appleton, S.F., 'Beyond the limits of reproductive choice: the contributions of the abortion-funding cases to fundamental-rights analysis and to the welfare-rights thesis', *Columbia Law Review* (1981) **81**, p. 718.

Arditti, Rita, Klein, R.D. and Minden, Shelley, *Test-Tube Women, What Future for Motherhood?* London, Pandora Press, 1984.

Atkinson, R.F., *Sexual Morality*, London, Hutchinson, 1965.

Atkinson, Stanley B. 'Life, birth, and live-birth', *Law Quarterly Review* (1904) **20**, p. 134.

Badinter, Elizabeth, *Myth of Motherhood: An Historical View of the Maternal Instinct*, London, Souvenir Press, 1981.

Bartholomew, G.W., 'Legal implications of artificial insemination', *Modern Law Review* (1958) **21**, p. 236.

Bayles, M.D., 'Limits to a right to reproduce', in O'Neil, Onora and Ruddick, William (eds), *Having Children: Philosophical and Legal Reflections on Parenthood*, Oxford, Oxford University Press, 1979, p. 13.

Bentil, J.K., 'Rejection of husband's claim to stop wife's abortion', *Solicitors' Journal* (1984) **128**, p. 288.

Bird, Kathleen, 'Parental rights at issue: Baby M ruling's boldness may invite appellate attack', *New Jersey Law Journal* (1987) **15**, pp. 1, 26.

Blodgett, Nancy, 'Surrogate parent rights: alternative reproduction laws proposed', *American Bar Association Journal* (1986) **72**, p. 33.

Blodgett, Nancy, 'Who is mother? genetic donor, not surrogate', *American Bar Association Journal* (1986) **72**, p. 18.

Blustein, Jeffery, *Parents and Children: The Ethics of the Family*, Oxford, Oxford University Press, 1982.

Bondeson, W.B., *Abortion and the Status of the Fetus*, Boston, D. Reidel Hingham, 1983.

Bowker, W.F., 'Sterilization of the mentally retarded adult: the Eve case', *McGill Law Journal* (1981) **26**, p. 931.

Brahams, Diana, 'Damages for unplanned babies – a trend to be discouraged?' *New Law Journal* (1983) **133**(2), p. 643.

Brahams, Diana, 'The legal and social problems of *in vitro* fertilisation: why Parliament must legislate. 1', *New Law Journal* (1983) **133**(2) p. 869.

Brahams, Diana, 'The hasty British ban on commercial surrogacy', *Hastings Center Report* (1987) **17**, p. 16.

Brahams, Diana, 'Surrogacy: a criminal offence?' *Medico-Legal Journal* (1984) **52**, p. 248.

Brand, Ian, 'Allocation of health care resources', in Brumby, M.N. (ed.), *Proceedings of the Conference on In Vitro Fertilisation: Problems and Possibilities*, Victoria, Monash Centre for Human Bioethics, 1982.

Brody, B.A., *Abortion and the Status of Human Life: A Philosophical View*, London, MIT Press, 1975.

Bromley, P.M., *Family Law* (5th edn.), London, Butterworths, 1976.

Brophy, Katie M., 'A surrogate mother contract to bear a child', *Family Law* (1982) **20**, p. 263.

Campbell, D.T., *The Left and Rights*, London, Routledge and Kegan Paul, 1983.

Campbell, T.D. and McKay, A.J.M., 'Antenatal injury and the rights of the foetus', *Philosophical Quarterly* (1978) **28**, p. 17.

Capron, Alexander M., 'The new reproductive possibilities; seeking a moral basis for concerted action in a pluralistic society', *Law Medicine & Health Care* (1984) **12**, p. 192.

Casler, Lawrence, *Is Marriage Necessary?* New York, Human Science Press, 1974.

Chitty on Contracts, General Principles (24th edn.), London, Sweet & Maxwell, 1977.

Clive, E.M., *The Law of Husband and Wife* (2nd edn.), Edinburgh, W. Green and Son, 1982.

Cohen, Barbara, 'Surrogate mothers: whose baby is it?' *American Journal of Law & Medicine* (1984) **10**, p. 243.

Cohen, Carl, 'Sex, birth control, and human life', in Baker, Robert and Elliston, Frederick (eds), *Philosophy and Sex*, New York, Prometheus Books, 1975, p. 150.

Coleman, Phyllis, 'Surrogate motherhood: analysis of the problems and suggestions for solutions', *Tennessee Law Review* (1982) **50**, p. 71.

Condie, Karen T., 'Surrogacy as a treatment for infertility', *Law Society of Scotland* (1986) **31**, p. 469.

Corea, Gena, *The Mother Machine: Reproductive Technologies from Artificial Insemination to Artificial Wombs*, New York, Harper, 1985.

Cotton, Kim and Winn, Denise, *Baby Cotton: For Love and Money*, London, Kindersley, 1985.

Cowan, M.G., *Children Acts (Scotland)*, Edinburgh, William Hodge, 1933.

Cretney, S.M., *Principles of Family Law* (4th edn.), London, Sweet & Maxwell, 1984.

Current Topic *Australian Law Journal* (1984) **58**, p. 683–5.

Cusine, D.J., 'Artificial insemination', in McLean, S.A.M. (ed.), *Legal Issues in Medicine*, Aldershot, Gower, 1981, p. 163.

Cusine, D.J., *New Reproductive Techniques*, Aldershot, Dartmouth, 1988.

Cusine, D.J., 'Womb-leasing: some legal implications', *New Law Journal* (1978) **128**, p. 824.

Cusine, D.J., 'Artificial insemination with the husband's semen after the husband's death', *Journal of Medical Ethics* (1977) **3**, p. 163.

Cusine, D.J., 'Legal issues relating to AID', in Brudenell, M., *et al.* (eds), *Artificial Insemination, Proceedings of the Fourth Study Group of the Royal College of Obstetricians and Gynaecologists*, RCOG, 1976.

'The Future of Baby M', *The Daily Telegraph*, 3 April, 1987, p. 15.

Davies, Iwan, 'Contracts to bear a child', *Journal of Medical Ethics*, (1985) **11**, p. 61.

Davies, Iwan, 'Fabricated man: the dilemma posed by artificial reproductive techniques', *Northern Ireland Legal Quarterly* (1984) **35**, p. 354.

Davies, Seabourne D., 'Child-killing in English law', *Modern Law Review* (1937) **1**, p. 203.

Davies, Seabourne D., 'The law of abortion and necessity', *Modern Law Review* (1938) **2**, p. 126.

Devlin, P.D.B., *The Enforcement of Morals*, London, Oxford University Press, 1965.

Dickens Bernard, M., *Medico-Legal Aspects of Family Law*, London, Butterworths, 1979.

Dickens, Bernard M., 'The control of living body materials', *University of Toronto Law Journal* (1977) **27**, p. 142.

Digest of Strasbourg Case-law relating to the European Convention on Human Rights, Vol. 3, Carl Heymanns Verlag, Bonn, 1984.

Dodd, Bette J., 'The surrogate mother contract in Indiana', *Indiana Law Review* (1982) **15**, p. 807.

Downie, R.S. and Telfer, Elizabeth, *Respect for Persons*, London, George Allen & Unwin, 1969.

Dunstan, G.R., 'The moral status of the human embryo: a tradition recalled', *Journal of Medical Ethics* (1984) **10**, p. 38.

Dworkin, Gerald, 'Paternalism', in Feinburg, Joel and Cross, Hyman (eds), *Philosophy and Law* (2nd edn.), California, Wadsworth, 1980, p. 230.

Dworkin, Ronald, *Taking Rights Seriously*, London, Duckworth, 1978.

Edwards, R.G., 'Fertilisation of human eggs *in vitro*: morals, ethics and the law', *Quarterly Review of Biology*, (1974) **49**, p. 3.

Edwards, R.G. and Steptoe, P., *A Matter of Life*, London, Hutchinson, 1980.

'Is buying babies bad?', *The Economist*, 12 January, 1985, p. 12.

'The lessons from Baby M', *The Economist*, 21 March, 1987, p. 18.

Eekelaar, John, *Family Law and Social Policy*, London, Weidenfeld & Nicolson, 1978.

Eekelaar, John, 'Second thoughts on illegitimacy reform', *Family Law* (1985) **15**, p. 261–3.

Erickson, Elizabeth A., 'Contracts to bear a child', *California Law Review* (1978) **66**, p. 611.

Fineburg, Joel, *Social Philosophy*, New Jersey, Prentice Hall, 1973.

Fineburg, Joel, 'The nature and value of rights', in Fineburg, Joel (ed.), *Rights, Justice and the Bounds of Liberty*, Guildford, Princeton, 1980, p. 148.

Finegold, Wilfred J., *Artificial Insemination*, Springfield, Illinois, Charles C. Thomas, 1964.

Furrow, Barry, R., 'Surrogate motherhood: a new option for parenting?' *Law, Medicine & Health Care* (1984) **12**, p. 106.

Gary, E. and Clifton, Perry, 'Can claims for "wrongful life" be justified?', *Journal of Medical Ethics* (1983) **9**, p. 162.

Gewirth, Alan, *Human Rights: Essays on Justification and Applications*, University of Chicago Press, Chicago, 1982.

Glover, Jonathan, *Causing Death and Saving Lives*, Harmondsworth, Penguin Books, 1984.

Glover, Jonathan, *What Sort of People Should There Be?*, Harmondsworth, Penguin Books, 1984.

Goldfarb, Carolea, 'Two mothers, one baby, no law', *Human Rights* (1983) **11**, p. 26.

Gordon, G.H., *The Criminal Law of Scotland* (2nd edn.), Edinburgh, W. Green, 1978.

Gordon, Linda, *Woman's Body, Woman's Right*, Harmondsworth, Penguin Books, 1977.

Govier, Trudy, 'What should we do about future people?', *American Philosophical Quarterly* (1976) **16**, p. 105.

Govier, Trudy, 'What's wrong with slippery slope arguments?', *Canadian Journal of Philosophy* (1982) **12**, p. 303.

Hall, Martha, 'Rights and the problem of surrogate parenting', *Philosophical Quarterly* (1985) **35**, p. 414.

Hann, Judith, *The Perfect Baby*, London, George Weidenfeld & Nicolson, 1982.

Hanscombe, Gillian, 'The right to lesbian parenthood', *Journal of Medical Ethics* (1983) **9**, p. 133.

Hardin, Garrett, 'The tragedy of the commons', in Bayles, M.D. (ed.), *Ethics and Population*, Cambridge, Mass., Schenkman, 1976.

Harris, John, '*In vitro* fertilisation: the ethical issues', *Philosophical Quarterly* (1983) **33**, p. 217.

Harris, John, *Value of Life*, London, Routledge & Kegan Paul, 1985.

Hart, H.L.A., 'Bentham on legal rights', in Simpson, A.W.B. (ed.), *Oxford Essays in Jurisprudence*, 2nd Series, Oxford, Clarendon Press, 1973, p. 170.

Hart, H.L.A., *Law, Liberty and Morality*, Oxford, Oxford University Press, 1982.

Herbenick, Raymond M., 'Remarks on abortion, abandonment and adoption opportunities', in O'Neil, Onora and Ruddick, William (eds), *Having Children, Philosophical and Legal Reflections on Parenthood*, New York, Oxford University Press, 1977, p. 52.

Higgs, Roger, 'Lesbian couples: should help extend to AID?', *Journal of Medical Ethics* (1978) **4**, p. 91.

Hilliard, Lexa, ' "Wrongful birth" . . . Some growing pains', *Modern Law Review* (1985) **48**, p. 224.

Hilton, B., *Ethical Issues in Human Genetics*, New York, Plenum, 1973.

Hollinger, J.H.,'From coitus to commerce: legal and social consequences of noncoital reproduction', *University of Michigan Journal of Law Reform* (1985) **18**, p. 865.

Hornblower, Margot, 'Judge awards 'Baby M' to her biological father', *The Washington Post*, 1 April, 1987.

Hubbard, H.A., 'Artificial Insemination: a reply to Dean Tallin', *Canadian Bar Review* (1956) **34** p. 425–51.

Iglesias, Teresa, '*In vitro* fertilisation: the major issue', *Journal of Medical Ethics* (1984) **10**, p. 32.

Ingram, Miranda, 'Adopting the unadoptable', *New Society*, 9 August, 1985, pp. 206–7.

Jacobs, F.G., *The European Convention on Human Rights*, Oxford, Clarendon Press, 1975.

Johnstone, Brian, 'The moral status of the embryo: two viewpoints', in Singer, Peter and Walters, William (eds), *Test-Tube Babies, A Guide to Moral Questions, Present Techniques and Future Possibilities*, Oxford, Oxford University Press, 1984, pp. 49–56.

Joyce, D.N., 'Recruitment, selection and matching of donors', in Brudenell, M. *et al.* (eds), *Artificial Insemination, Proceedings of the Fourth Study Group of the Royal College of Obstetricians and Gynaecologists*, RCOG, 1976, pp. 60–69.

Kant, I., 'Duties to the body and crimes against nature', in Verene,

D.P. (ed.), *Sexual Love and Western Morality: a Philosophical Anthology*, New York, Harper & Row, 1972.

Kass, Leon R., 'Babies by means of *in vitro* fertilization: unethical experiments on the unborn?', *New England Journal of Medicine*, (1971) **285**, p. 1174.

Keane, Noel and Breo, D.L., *The Surrogate Mother*, New York, Everest House, 1981.

Keech, Kristina McDougal and Bruce W., 'Surrogate parenting agreements in Virginia: a proposal for action', *Colonial Law* (1987) **16**, p. 28.

Kennedy, Ian and Edwards, R.G., 'A critique of the Law Commission Report on Injuries to Unborn Children and the Proposed Congenital Disabilities (Civil Liability) Bill', *Journal of Medical Ethics* (1975) **1**, p. 116.

Kerr, M.G. and Rogers, C., 'Donor insemination', *Journal of Medical Ethics* (1975) **1**, p. 30.

Kirby, M.D., 'Bioethics of IVF – state of the debate', *Journal of Medical Ethics*, (1984) **10**, p. 45.

Knoppers, B. and Sloss, E., 'Recent developments: legislative reforms in reproductive technology', *Ottawa Law Review* (1986) **18**, p. 663.

Krause, Harry D., 'Artificial conception: legislative approaches', *Family Law Quarterly* (1985) **19**, p. 185.

Lafollette, Hugh, 'Licensing parents', *Philosophy and Public Affairs* (1980) **9**, p. 182.

Lane, Margaret I., '*In vitro* fertilisation: hope for childless couples breeds legal exposure for physicians', *University of Richmond Law Review* (1983) **17**, p. 311.

Law & Ethics of AID and Embryo Transfer, CIBA Foundation symposium, London, Associated Scientific Publishers, 1973.

Lenow, Jeffrey, 'The fetus as a patient: emerging rights as a person?', *American Journal of Law and Medicine* (1900) **91**.

Levin, Jennifer, 'Reforming the legitimacy laws', *Family Law* (1978) **8**, pp. 35–9.

Liu, A.N.C., 'Wrongful life: some of the problems', *Journal of Medical Ethics* (1987) **13**, p. 69.

Lockwood, M., *Moral Dilemmas in Modern Medicine*, Oxford, Oxford University Press, 1985.

Lynn, S.M., 'Technology and reproductive rights: how advances in technology can be used to limit women's reproductive rights', *Women's Rights Law Reporter* (1982) **7**, p. 223.

MacCormick, D.N., 'Rights in legislation', in Hacker, P.M.S. and Raz, J. (eds), *Law, Morality and Society*, Oxford, Clarendon Press, 1977, p. 139.

MacCormick, D.N., *H.L.A. Hart*, London, Edward Arnold, 1981 Chapter 7, p. 88.

Mady, Theresa M., 'Surrogate mothers: the legal issues', *American Journal of Law & Medicine* (1981) **7**, p. 323.

Maidment, Susan, 'DNA fingerprinting', *New Law Journal* (1986) **136** (1), p. 326.

Mandler, John J., 'Developing a concept of the modern "family": a proposed Uniform Surrogate Parenthood Act', *Georgetown Law Journal* (1985) **73**, p. 1283.

Marietta, Don E., 'On using people', *Ethics* (1971–2) **82**, p. 232.

Mason, J.K. and McCall Smith, R.A., *Law and Medical Ethics* (2nd edn.), London, Butterworths, 1987.

Mason, Stephen, 'Abnormal conception', *Australian Law Journal* (1982) **56**, p. 347.

Matthew, Paul, 'Whose body? People as property', *Current Legal Problems* (1983) **36**, p. 193.

McLean, S.A.M., 'Ante-natal injuries', in McLean, S.A.M. (ed.), *Legal Issues in Medicine*, Aldershot, Gower, 1981, p. 150.

McLean, S.A.M., 'The right to reproduce', in Campbell, T.D., *et al.* (eds), *Human Rights: From Rhetoric to Reality*, Oxford, Basil Blackwell, 1986, p. 80.

McLean, S.A.M. and Campbell, T.D., 'Sterilisation', in McLean, S.A.M. (ed.), *Legal Issues in Medicine*, Aldershot, Gower, 1981, p. 176.

McLean, S.A.M. and Maher, G., *Medicine, Morals and the Law*, Aldershot, Gower, 1985.

McNeill, P.G.B., *Adoption of Children in Scotland*, Edinburgh, W. Green, 1982.

McWhinnie, A.M., *Adopted children: how they grow up: a study of their adjustment as adults*, London, Routledge & Kegan Paul, 1967.

Menning, B.E., 'The infertile couple: a plea for advocacy', *Child Welfare* (1975) **54**, p. 454.

Meyers, D.W., *The Human Body and the Law*, Chicago, Aldine, 1970.

Mill, John Stuart, 'On Liberty', in Feinburg, Joel and Cross, Hyman (eds), *Philosophy and Law* (2nd edn.), California, Wadsworth, 1980, p. 180.

Moggach, Deborah, *To Have and to Hold*, New York, E.P. Dutton, 1987.

Montgomery, J., 'Constructing a family – after a surrogate birth', *Modern Law Reform* (1986) **49**, p. 635.

Morgan, Derek, 'Making motherhood male: surrogacy and the moral economy of women', *Journal of Law & Society* (1985) **12**, p. 219.

Morgan, Derek, 'Who to be or not to be: the surrogacy story', *Modern Law Review* (1986) **49**, p. 358.

Morgan, Derek, 'Legislation', *Modern Law Review* (1986) **49**, p. 358.

Moss, Peter and Lav, Geraldine, 'Mothers without marriages', *New Society*, 9 August, 1985, p. 207.

Nijs, P. and Rouffa, L., 'AID couples: psychological and psychopathological evaluation', *Andrologia* (1975) **7**, p. 187.

Notes, 'Reproductive technology and the procreative rights of the unmarried', *Harvard Law Review* (1985) **98**, p. 669.

'The scars left by Baby M', *The Observer*, 5 April, 1987, p. 11.

O'Donovan, Oliver, *Begotten or Made?*, Oxford, Clarendon Press, 1984.

O'Neil, Onora, 'Begetting, bearing and rearing', in O'Neil, Onora and Ruddick, William (eds), *Having Children: Philosophical and Legal Reflections on Parenthood*, Oxford, Oxford University Press, 1979, p. 25.

Packer, Herbert, *The Limits of Criminal Sanction*, London, Stanford, 1969.

Page, Edgar, 'Book reviews', *Journal of Medical Ethics* (1986) **12**, pp. 45–52.

Parker, Diana, 'Surrogate mothering: an overview', *Family Law* (1984) **14**, p. 143.

Parker, Philip, 'Motivation of surrogate mothers: initial findings', *American Journal of Psychiatry*, (1983) **140**, p. 117.

Parker, Philip J., 'Surrogate motherhood: the interaction of litigation, legislation and psychiatry', 8th International Congress on Law and Psychiatry – June 18–22, 1982, *International Journal of Law & Psychiatry* (1983) **5**, p. 341.

Paton, G.W., *Jurisprudence* (3rd edn.), Oxford, Clarendon Press, 1964.

Pepperill, R.J., Hudson, B. and Wood, C., *The Infertile Couple*, Edinburgh, Churchill Livingstone, 1980.

Petersen, K.A., 'Public funding of abortion services: comparative developments in the United States and Australia', *International Comparative Law Quarterly* (1984) **33**, p. 158.

Plant, Raymond, 'Gift, exchanges and the political economy of health care', *Journal of Medical Ethics* (1977) **3**, p. 166; *Journal of Medical Ethics* (1978) **4**, p. 5.

Pope Paul VI, 'Humane Vitae', in Baker, Robert and Elliston, Frederick (eds), *Philosophy and Sex*, New York, Prometheus Books, 1975, p. 131.

Ramsey, Paul, 'Shall we reproduce?', 'Rejoinder and future forecast', *Journal of American Medical Association* (1972) **220**, pp. 1480, 1481.

Raymond, A. Belliotti, 'Morality and *in vitro* fertilisation', *Bioethics Quarterly* (1980) **2**(1), p. 6.

Reilly, Philip, *Genetics, Law and Social Policy*, London, Harvard University Press, 1977.

Rex, Martin and Nickel, J.W., 'Recent work on the concepts of rights', *American Philosophical Quarterly* (1980) **17**, p. 165.

Richards, David, A., 'Commercial sex and the rights of the person: a moral argument for the decriminalisation of prostitution', *University of Pennsylvania Law Review* (1979) **127**, p. 1195.

Richards, J.R., *The Sceptical Feminist: A Philosophical Enquiry*, London, Routledge and Kegan Paul, 1983.

Robbins, Sara, *Surrogate Parenting: an Annotated Review of the Literature*, Brooklyn, New York, CompuBibs, 1984.

Roberts, Shelley, 'Warnock and surrogate motherhood: sentiment or argument?' in Peter Bryne (ed.), *Rights & Wrongs in Medicine*, King's Fund Publishing Office, London, 1986, p. 80.

Robertson, John A., 'The right to procreate and *in vitro* fetal therapy', *The Journal of Legal Medicine* (1982) **3**, p. 333.

Rushevsky, Cynthia A, 'Legal recognition of surrogate gestation', *Women's Rights Law Reporter* (1982) **7**, p. 101.

Russell, Scott, *The Body as Property*, New York, Viking Press, 1981.

Ruut, Veenhoven, 'Is there an innate need for children?', *European Journal of Social Psychology* (1975) **4**, pp. 495–501.

Samuels, Alec, 'Illegitimacy: The Law Commission's Report', *Family Law* (1983) **13**, pp. 87–90.

Sants, H.J., 'Genealogical bewilderment in children with substitute parents', in *Child Adoption*, the Association of British Adoption and Fostering Agencies, London, p. 69.

Scarlett, B.F., 'The moral status of embryos', *Journal of Medical Ethics* (1984) **10**, p. 79.

Shattuck, J.H.F., *Rights of Privacy*, Illinois, National Textbook, 1977.

Singer, Peter and Kuhse, Helga, 'The moral status of embryo: two viewpoints,' in Singer, Peter and Walters, William (eds), *Test-Tube Babies, A Guide to Moral Questions, Present Techniques and Future Possibilities*, pp. 57–63.

Singer, Peter and Wells, Deane, 'IVF: The major issues', *Journal of Medical Ethics* (1983) **9**, p. 192.

Singer, Peter and Wells, Deane, *The Reproduction Revolution*, Oxford, Oxford University Press, 1984.

Singer, Peter and Wells, Deane, *Making Babies: The New Science and Ethics of Conception*, New York, Scribner, 1985.

Skegg, P.D.G., *Law, Ethics and Medicine*, Oxford, Clarendon Press, 1984.

Sloman, Susan, 'Surrogacy Arrangements Act 1985', *New Law Journal* (1985) **135** (2), p. 978.

Slovenko, Ralph, 'Obstetric science and the developing role of the psychiatrist in surrogate motherhood', *Journal of Psychiatry & Law* (1985) **13**, p. 487.

Smith, J.C. and Hogan, B., *Criminal Law*, London, Butterworths, 1978.

Snowden, R. and Mitchell, G.D., *The Artificial Family*, London, Allen & Unwin, 1981.

Snowden, R. and Mitchell, G.D., *Artificial Reproduction: A Social Investigation*, Allen & Unwin, London, 1983.

St John-Stevas, N., *The Agonising Choice, Birth Control, Religion and the Law*, London, Eyre & Spottiswoode, 1971.

Stevens, Kristy, *Surrogate Mother: One Woman's Story*, London, Century, 1985.

Stumpf, Andrea E., 'Redefining mother: a legal matrix for new reproductive technologies', *Yale Law Journal* (1986) **96**, p. 187.

Sumner, L.W., *Abortion and Moral Theory*, Princeton, Princeton University Press, 1981.

Tallin, G.P.R., 'Artificial insemination', *Canadian Bar Review* (1956) **34**, pp. 1–27, 166–86, 628–31.

Taylor, Ann Spowart, 'Compensation for unwanted children', *Family Law* (1985) **15**, p. 147.

Taylor, Richard, 'Persons and bodies', *American Philosophical Quarterly* (1979) **16**, p. 67.

Teff, Harvey, 'The action for "wrongful life" in England and the United States', *International and Comparative Law Quarterly* (1985) **34**, p. 423.

Teichman, Jenny, *The Meaning of Illegitimacy*, Cambridge, Englehardt Books, 1978.

Teo, Wesley D.H., 'Abortion: the husband's constitutional rights', *Ethics* (1974–5) **85**, p. 337.

Thomson, J.M., *Family Law in Scotland*, London, Butterworths, 1987.

'Judges press for guidelines', *The Times*, 2 April, 1987, p. 8.

Titmuss, Richard, *The Gift Relationship*, George Allen & Unwin, London, 1970.

Treitel, G.H., 'Specific performance and injunction' in *Chitty on Contract, General Principles*, **1** (24th edn.), London, Sweet & Maxwell, 1977, p. 1631.

Tunkel, Victor, 'Modern anti-pregnancy techniques and the criminal law', *Criminal Law Review* (1974) p. 461.

Uniacke, Suzanne, 'IVF and the right to reproduce', *Bioethics* (1978) **1**(3) .

Waldron, Jeremy, *Theories of Rights*, Oxford, Oxford University Press, 1984.

Walker, D.M., *The Law of Contract and Related Obligations in Scotland* (2nd edn.), London, Butterworths, 1985, pp. 540–4.

Walsh, Elizabeth, 'Warnock and after', *Family Law* (1985) **15**, p. 138.

Warnock, Mary, *A Question of Life: the Warnock Report on Human Fertilisation and Embryology*, Oxford, Basil Blackwell, 1985.

Warnock, Mary, 'Legal surrogacy – not for love or money?', *The Listener*, 24 January 1985, p. 2.

Wassertrom, R.A., *Today's Moral Problems*, London, Collier Macmillan, 1979.

Weinberg, S.R., 'A maternal duty to protect fetal health', *Indiana Law Journal* (1983) **58**, p. 531.

Weir, Tony, 'Wrongful life – nipped in the bud', *Cambridge Law Journal* (1982), p. 225.

Wellings, K., 'Sterilisation trends', *British Medical Journal* (1986) **292**, p. 1029.

Williams, Glanville, *Sanctity of Life and the Criminal Law*, London, Faber, 1958.

Winslade, W.J., 'Surrogate mothers – right or wrong?', *Journal of Medical Ethics* (1983) **9**, p. 153.

Wright, Gerald, 'The legal implications of IVF', in *Test-Tube Babies, a Christian View*, London, Unity Press, Becket, 1984, pp. 39–44.

Wright, Moira, 'Surrogacy and adoption: problems and possibilities', *Family Law* (1986) **16**, p. 109.

Index

Note: the following abbreviations are used:

AI(D) = Artificial insemination (by donor)
IVF = *In vitro* fertilization

RIGHTS OF ACCESS TO THE MEDIA

edited by

ANDRÁS SAJÓ

and

MONROE PRICE

KLUWER LAW INTERNATIONAL

THE HAGUE / LONDON / BOSTON

A C.I.P. Catalogue record for this book is available from the Library of Congress.

ISBN 90-411-0166-7

Published by Kluwer Law International,
P.O. Box 85889, 2508 CN The Hague, The Netherlands.

Sold and distributed in the U.S.A. and Canada
by Kluwer Law International,
675 Massachusetts Avenue, Cambridge, MA 02139, U.S.A.

In all other countries, sold and distributed
by Kluwer Law International,
P.O. Box 85889, 2508 CN The Hague, The Netherlands.

Printed on acid-free paper

CONTENTS

INTRODUCTION

by Monroe E. Price

As broadcasting systems transform - both in societies marking a post-communist transition and in the rest of Europe and the United States - opportunities for "access" are frequently put forward and debated. Just as frequently, little is done to analyze what is meant by access and how the concept fits into a theoretical framework. Access issues proliferate, not only for the new statutes concerning broadcasting licenses, but for cable television regimens and for the information infrastructures of the future. Access becomes the hope of social groups, religious organizations, politicians, redemptive in its impact on the democratic process. Given the range of uses, given the consequences imputed to access, in the broadcasting field, more attention to its various meanings is long overdue.

This volume of essays is a partial answer. The book has its origins in a conference held in June 1993 at the Institute for Constitutional and Legislative Policy at the Central European University in Budapest.[1] The purpose of the conference was to gather scholars with a commitment to explore the theoretical and actual implications of various access regimes as they have been or were then being practiced or proposed. The time was a vital one as debates continued throughout the region on the shape of proposed broadcasting legislation.

The conference offered an opportunity to review the political context in which access was being considered at a raw and early moment in the transitions to democracy. Hungary was still deadlocked in its "media wars", a confrontation between the major political parties over the course of society in which the conduct and control of broadcasting was seen as a defining issue. The Czech Republic had just split from its Slovak counterpart and the implications for the role of broadcasting the building of a nation were self-evident. Problems of hate speech and lustration - a negative form of access, namely access by the society for information about the personal past of public figures - compounded the difficulty of policy-making. Access issues yielded concerns about privatization since the ownership of instruments of the press are a key factor in access and that implicated the choice of

---

[1] The conference was part of *The Individual vs. the State* project, funded by the Open Society Institute Budapest, which was developed by *András Sajó, Michel Rosenfeld and Andrew Arato.*

licensees, the conditions under which they should operate, whether and to what extent foreign investment should be allowed. All of these were pending questions.

Overall, there was the inevitable, underlying problem of the role of the state in establishing rules, maintaining a hand in establishing the narratives of continuity and, indeed, in letting go and fostering the processes of change. Here, as through so many concerns, the question was what residual role should the state play as the society emerged from an authoritarian past? What models existed in Western Europe and the United States? How could they be translated, adapted, understood? Should the regulatory distinctions, seemingly fading elsewhere, between the printed press and the electronic media be maintained or abandoned? We have organized the responses in four sections: theories of media access; access to media in Europe and the United States; judicial review of access to the media; and the media and the political arena. The contributions do not neatly fit within these categories and, as a result, some discussion of almost all the issues will be found in each paper.

I.   Theories of Media Access

Two essays on theories of media access begin our exploration. Our first essay, by Monroe E. Price, drawing primarily on the experience of the United States, tries to establish a set of underlying models and approaches for the many uses of the term "access" in American law and practice. Access may be a romantic mode for replicating the circumstances of the village, or something more, namely government assurance that there is fair representation and a sense of inclusion in the dominant narratives of the media. The American experience reveals an unwillingness to be explicit about the role of law in affecting narrative. Often, access rules are used to provide a false sense of fairness rather than fairness itself.

Rules can be established in a taxonomy: one that devolves around ownership access and program access. Ownership access presupposes a relationship between the nature of the owner of the media and the content that the particular ownership will produce. More owners mean more voices. Different kind of owners mean different kind of voices. By regulating or commanding access to ownership, it is presupposed that content diversity will be achieved without program censorship or control. An equivalent in the German and other continental systems is to assure diversity or access to the governing councils with some input in the regulation of the media. This model assumes that, constraints aside, the "market" will not homogenize product, producing a more or less uniform response by owners, regardless of their background. Minorities will speak to their community even if a broader set of messages will enhance market and market share.

Program or producer access regulations provide guaranteed opportunities based on the nature of the program, the social institution or political party presenting it. Often producer access is conditional. The most common example involves rights of reply or personal attack rules. If, for example, a person is maligned, he or she may have some right of access to respond. At other times, access can be absolute, as in provisions, in some countries, furnishing automatic access for political parties.

In general, American access rules reflect an ersatz politics of pluralism: a surface architecture of free speech that combines the trappings of government noninterference with the illusion that narratives - the stories of the good life - are fairly distributed among its tellers. First Amendment "absolutism" embraces a commitment to the right of any group, no matter how spiteful, how antagonistic to the dominant culture, no matter how rooted in the conflicts of the past. Access is assumed, in some part, by a constitutional regime which provides this order of rights. In contrast, talk of assuring unencumbered access may be in transition in societies, still unsure of their very stability. Even in the United States, dissent is sometimes likened to sedition.

Now technological changes have their own compulsion towards means of access, whether the access of multiple channels to be filled or the access of common carrier approaches to the media. In the U.S. context, technology often appears as a kind of access-related *deus ex machina*. More channels mean more access, or at least the idea that more access is possible. If access is to be assured - i.e. the depictions over the air are actually a rich reflection of viewpoints rather than a reflection of capacity to use opportunities - the challenges to governments will increase. This becomes particularly true in terms of control and licensing as governments determine how to intervene in the global environment of new technologies and unimpeded markets.

Our first essay ends with questions about access theory and the public sphere. It is just there that Professor Jean Cohen's submission begins. Professor Cohen finds in the work of Jurgen Habermas - in the concept of the public sphere - a theoretical ground for access provisions. Her essay outlines various critiques on Habermas' essay, particularly those that touch on its relevance for the mass media. For example, to the argument that the public sphere has systematically excluded citizenry on the basis of wealth, race and gender, Cohen counters that the electronic media can open the space to a multiplicity of publics. Cohen also deals with the question whether the mass media is so organized by manufacturers of propaganda that what emerges as the opinion of the public is only an agenda set "from above" and therefore without independent relevance. She reviews and compares Habermas' own changing analyses of barriers to the public sphere in his work of 1962, 1981 and the present. There she traces his sense of countervailing tendencies to the centralizing and homogenizing logic of the mass media.

The concept of the public sphere is important for media theory because it is within that sphere, if at all, that the interaction of groups receive the necessary enlightenment concerning public policy and come to influence policy formation by debating issues of a public concern. Professor Cohen contends that the public sphere - spaces for and processes of open-ended politically relevant yet autonomous societal communication - may have been more effective, stronger and pragmatically potent than what its critics in the West have considered. The public sphere played a critical role in the processes of change in Central and Eastern Europe.

Professor Cohen sees two false directions among those who wish to protect the idea of Habermas' public sphere. One is the call of those who see state control of the media as the appropriate solution. That, for Professor Cohen, is the road to "deadening government controls... with the result that both the cultural and political publics are seriously deformed". Full privatization or marketization does not fare much better: it maximizes the negative phenomena of commercialization. Cohen calls for a strengthening, through both money and law, of those institutions whose logic is neither that of commodification nor of administration. These include foundations and other independent cultural institutions rooted in civil society.

II.   Access to the Media in Europe and in the United States

With some theoretical basis, amplified in the additional essays in the collection, we turn to practices and comparative approaches. In the six essays of this section, specific national regimes to guaranteeing access are delineated.

Professor Michel Rosenfeld employs the example of access by ethnic minority viewpoints - called in the United States as an aspect of "minority preferences" - to plumb access mechanisms in the United States. He argues that neither free competition in the economic marketplace nor state control nor domination of broadcasting assures suitable access for a broad range of diverse viewpoints. He supports American legal initiatives. Indirect procedural, rather than substantive direct government regulation is better suited to promote free speech and democratic self-government.

Rosenfeld's first test is the efficiency of the minority preference measure: is there enough of a nexus between group and access requirements? He answers the question whether ownership or control makes a difference in a market-based system: broadcast content is not exclusively shaped by market forces and "broadcasting programming options consistent with market constraints are generally sufficiently diverse to allow a broadcaster to allocate a certain portion of airtime to the presentation of personally held views without significantly affecting the profitability of his or her station".

Rosenfeld then turns to the relationship between liberty and equality in access considerations. He concludes that there cannot be a genuine liberty in the absence of equality. Furthermore, the broadcast audiences' liberty of political participation depends on the institution of some kind of equality in the electronic marketplace of ideas. Free speech, as does equal liberty, means, that everyone would have the same opportunity for self-expression, though not all kinds of expressions are suited to the broadcast medium. In a world of scarcity, this equal liberty can be resolved by equality of opportunity or the ranking of claims in relative order of importance. Rosenfeld examines the claim that a "significant portion of the broadcasting audience would actually prefer not to be confronted by a large number of views that it regards as personally, morally or politically disturbing, threatening or repugnant" ranking that concern against other competing considerations.

In analyzing the minority preference as an access right, Rosenfeld first determines that viewpoints "seem bound to represent, at least in part, the cultural, social, religious and/or political position of a particular group in society". No neutral scheme leading to genuine equality of opportunity among viewpoints in the context of broadcasting is possible; therefore, the next best result is to minimize government bias and remove barriers to access. Fair equality of opportunity calls for neutralization so that the persuasiveness of arguments, rather than financial ability should be the test of access. Rosenfeld seeks to distinguish between viewpoints that do not receive access because of financial ability, as opposed to viewpoints that do not receive access because of the intrinsic lack of worth of the ideas. There is also the problem of ranking the ideas or viewpoints in terms of their relevance to the audience. Affording a fair opportunity for self-expression to those who have been portrayed as inferiors should rank high, however. Finally, a minority ownership policy does not violate the principle of equality among persons particularly since viewpoint diversity, in the case of minority preference decreased the opportunities for nonminiorities imperceptibly.

Professor Owen Fiss sees a general strategy of privatizing the press, encouraging journalists to see themselves as members of a profession, and creating for the press a constitutionally protected zone of autonomy from state regulation. On the other hand, the state should not be perceived solely as the natural enemy of democracy, though that may be, according to Fiss, a useful starting point in post-authoritarian transition societies. It should be remembered that the market is itself "a structure of constraint" and the constraints placed on the press by the iron laws of capitalist economics might be of special concern from a political point of view. Fiss points particularly to the iron law of minimizing costs, a rule which tends to slight news and public affairs programming. In addition, the reliance on advertizing revenue target audiences based on income or other demographic factors rather than defining the audience in terms of its needs or its cohesion with society. Program decisions, in a privatized market, are made individually (channel by channel), not collectively or by a representative body. All these factors have an impact on the nature of the public discourse.

Fiss points out that while democracy assigns the ultimate responsibility to the public to decide how it wishes to live, it presupposes that the public is fully informed when it makes that judgement. A free press is instrumental in fulfilling this logic. For that reason, "robust public debate" is more important than democratically determined speech. Nation builders should be worried about a broadcasting and press system which does not supply the public with "the information and various opinions it needs in order to exercise its sovereign prerogative." The press should have the responsibility to address large questions of economic and social structure, including the distribution of wealth and the role of workers in the management of their firms - subjects well within the jurisdiction of the demos.

For Fiss, the preoccupation with the means of enforcing constraints, whether it is the state or the private owner who imposes them, misses the point. It is the effect of constraints on public discourse that should be the major concern rather than whether those constraints arise from censorship or from the private dismissal of journalists.

Fiss recognizes that a policy of rapid privatization "is needed to destroy the habits of subservience that the dictatorial practices of the past may have instilled" and that the resulting constraints are more diffuse and less threatening than those emanating from the state. He points out that in the American experience, to temper these private constraints, program regulation, ownership restrictions and funding of public television and radio have been a matter of practice, even if they are under constitutional attack.

According to Fiss, the right to access, unlike most other rights that were articulated in the 1960's in the United States, is not an individual right, not directed at the self-expressive interest of an individual citizen, but rather is intended to further the collective goal of a robust public debate. What is, therefore, important is access to a public, not to a media. The state functions as a "parliamentarian" making certain that all sides are heard from or that arguments are not repetitive. Fiss argues that any procedural approach has a necessary influence on outcomes, so that no intervention can be totally content neutral. To the extent possible, the decision should be taken out of the hands of deeply interested politicians and placed in agencies as independent as possible. Fiss concludes that while access regulations constitute a loss for private owners, "having one's property or wealth used to support activities a citizen detests is but a price of democracy". For Fiss, there is no difference between program and structural regulation and both are constitutionally permissible.

Professor Eric Barendt, in his essay, distinguishes between access rules applicable only to the broadcast media and other kinds of plurality laws (such as competition and merger regulations) which are applicable to the press generally. Drawing generally on the European experience, Barendt points to a variety of examples: an Italian Constitutional Court decision that requires Parliament to provide access opportunities for political, religious and social groups; laws of German Lander that provide access rights to churches and Jewish communities for religious programs; and France, where similar rights exist. Political broadcasting - as opposed to political advertising rights - are also seen as an element of access. In Professor Barendt's experience, these rights are severely limited because they cannot be enforced without complicated administrative regulation and oversight. Furthermore, they are not the most effective means for securing a wide range of balanced programs.

In contrast, Barendt sees more general competition and merger law as a more enduring way of encouraging pluralism. He points to decisions of the French *Conseil Constitutionnel* holding that pluralism of sources of information is a principle of constitutional status, though how this is done is a matter of legislative discretion. In Germany, on the other hand, Barendt finds that the formulation of strict merger controls have been limited out of concern for press freedoms. Furthermore, notwithstanding merger controls, press barons have become ubiquitous, even in the case of broadcasting where restrictions have been more extensive. Barendt points out that the European Union has become more interested in the problem of media competition and that a Commission Green Paper has been issued to suggest the possibility of a need for Community action.

Professor Ulrich Preuss concentrates, in his essay, on the rich experience of German law and German constitutional court decisions. The Constitutional Court has historically emphasized that the right to express one's opinion is "absolutely constitutive of the free democratic order". Preuss provides an overview of the law of communicative freedoms in Germany, tracing the intensity of the German experience, and the development of an institutional understanding of communicative freedoms, to a reaction to the "entire elimination of plurality in all mass media by the Nazi government." In German jurisprudence, "the democratic society itself is essentially interested in the existence and smooth operation of a democratic public sphere...". Because such a sphere will not emerge spontaneously, some intervention by the state is necessary. Freedom has to be organized; the state promotes the realization of individual freedoms by creating the appropriate institutional schemes.

Until the end of 1983, broadcast in Germany was wholly performed by public broadcasting corporations organized along the principles of internal pluralism, in which the governing board was a zone for virtually representative access. There have been problems with this system, primarily the conclusion by the major parties that they are to act as the principal representatives of civil society. Preuss explores the dichotomy between a right of all private entrants to compete in the broadcasting arena and the guarantee of a free communicative process in which the plurality of opinion has to be represented. As a consequence, Preuss explores the dual broadcast system in Germany and the different responsibilities or public and private broadcasters. The unique idea of a basic supply of information, instruction and entertainment gives the public system a constitutional standing that it does not necessarily have elsewhere.

In describing the differences between the German (and continental) systems and the American, Preuss outlines the constitutional reservations on freedoms of expression and communication. These include provisions for the protection of youth and the right to respect personal honour, to avoid illustrations of violence, pornography, crime, racial hatred or glorification of war, and to pursue other public interest if the law is neutral. Preuss compares the German developments to the distinction between "absolutist" and "balancing" approaches in American law. He concludes by examining the application of these principles to hate speech laws and rules concerning lustration - the public exposure of persons compromised by their close relation with the old regime and who then seek the protection of anonymity.

Karol Jakubowicz, the Polish broadcast executive and scholar, explores what is meant by equality, in terms of "both equal access to media channels for everyone, and equal or fair reflection in media content of society in all its diversity of interests, lifestyles and ideologies". To achieve a "full communicative democracy" requires "the creation of some publicly-funded mechanism ensuring exercise of the right to communicate in practice". For democratic communication to exist, society must remove the distinction, "built into many communication patterns" between the sender and the receiver. Direct communicative democracy would have ment that everyone become a "sendceiver".

Given the difficulties of direct communicative democracy, Jakubowicz turns to "representative communicative democracy", which would prevail when "all segments of society could own or control their own media or have adequate access to them for the purposes of communicating to their own members and to society at large".

In Poland, at the time Solidarity first formulated its views, in 1980-1981, social access to the media was a widely expressed goal, meaning, according to Jakubowicz that "the media should be at the disposal of society for the purpose of free, equal and pluralistic communication". It was felt that it is necessary "to abolish all monopolies in this sphere and introduce a system of horizontal, participatory communication ('society talking to itself')". Solidarity is used as a case study of an early model to insure structural guarantees of social feedback, access to, and participation in, media activities and direct media accountability to society. In a "long march" strategy to replace a totalitarian authority, the media would have helped constitute a civil society, supporting alternate institutions independent of and opposed to the sphere of state action.

Jakubowicz captures the moment - the very moment of transition - when social movements, still at their most idealistic stage, sought to fashion innovative ways to make the mass media respond to democratic needs. Among these were creating socially representative governing bodies for public broadcast media. Interestingly, creating a system of "third sector" of non profit private stations representing a wide variety of opinions and beliefs was also a mode for redefining and restructuring the media. Jakubowicz contrasts the treatment of the printed press, where the old systems of controls was generally dismantled, with broadcasting where the process of developing new laws has been "politically contentious and therefore protracted".

Milan Jakobec writes primarily of the experience in the Czech Republic since 1989, establishing stages in the transformation of monopolist broadcasters of the Soviet period. The first step was the establishment of broadcasting Councils, elected according to non-political principles, influenced by Vaclav Havel's original ideas of "apolitical politics". In this mode, there was a direct tie to the Parliament which could dissolve a Council if the Parliament perceived, during a set period, that Czech Radio was not fulfilling its legal mission, namely servicing the citizens of the Czech Republic through the transmission of programs whose subject matter reflects the entire territory and population of the Republic. The statutory responsibility encompasses furthering the development of the cultural identity of the Czech nation and national and ethnic minorities living within the Republic.

The Czech Republic also fostered plurality by developing a systematic approach to the selection of non-state (private) radio and television broadcasters. A framework for licensing and supervision was modeled on the Independent Broadcasting Authority in the United Kingdom and the first private licenses were issued. The first station licensed was subjected to over thirty conditions, including support for domestic television production and conformity with the standards of the Council of Europe. The award of the station was a difficult test of the independence of the Council for Broadcasting given the great interest in the process and disputes over who ought to prevail. Television was more difficult to demonopolize than radio where plurality was furthered by providing access to the FM spectrum to the BBC and Radio Free Europe.

Differences thus emerge between access notions in the United States and in Europe, particularly Central and Eastern Europe. Access in the United States seems a specific, rather narrow set of doctrines, repair mechanisms for a generally unsupervised, unregulated whole. In societies where the social involvement in the rendering of identity is so much greater, access conceptions are more pervasive. They are reflected in the organization of the media, both broadcasting and printed press and the doctrines that emerge from the implementation of media law.

III.   Judicial Review

In each of the societies under review, the courts have played a critical role in determining the meaning and scope of access. This vital task has been played in the United States where the Supreme Court has been an architect of First Amendment values, in Germany where an astonishing set of decisions (reviewed in the earlier section by Professor Preuss) created a jurisprudence of communicative freedom, and in Hungary, where the Constitutional Court was called upon more than once, during the politics-wracked years before 1994, to mediate the struggle between competing parties for control over both the broadcasting system and the process of legislative reform that racked politics there.

Ethan Klingsberg questions whether the criteria used by courts - focusing on the United States Supreme Court - are adequate for ensuring a "rich public debate". The Supreme Court has, from time to time, focused on whether an "individual self-fulfillment"- the "voice" - and whether an idea are being expressed. But, according to Klingsberg, it is more an issue of a "multiplicity of discourses", not just a multiplicity of voices or views. His is an opinion that is stirred by the comment in *Cohen v. California*: "That the air may be filled with verbal cacophony is not a sign of weakness but of strength". Klingsberg proves his point through an analysis of an important strain of American cases that affect access: cases that limit intrusion on "captive audiences". In those cases, individuals cannot avoid the impact of a message by merely averting their eyes or covering their ears. There long has been no absolute freedom for the soundtrack to drown out the natural speech of others. Access doctrines - doctrines that enrich access by assuring or maximizing the possibility of actual, rather than theoretical listeners (or viewers), come close to the problem of captiveness by imposing, or possibly imposing, the speech of others.

While Klingsberg follows a single doctrine, Gábor Halmai emphasizes the comparative and structural aspects of judicial review. He studies and presents the American, Hungarian and German systems. How do judges operate in a period of technological and political transition; where do they find principles, how do they apply them; to what extent do they impose standards on the legislature or Parliament; these are the questions which are answered in Halmai's contribution.

Halmai seeks to locate and specify the function courts have of assuring a mode of access. For him, in doing so they, of necessity, must determine what common feature of laws and constitutional decisions exist where courts "prescribe positive rules in order to ensure the balanced character of television and radio companies and also to ensure their freedom from state intervention". Halmai considers it possibly sufficient, in a new era, one freer of scarcity, to have the government concerned only with the public media, leaving private media to the free market of thoughts and opinion. Halmai may be wishing to retain the now-disappearing distinction between public and private media, and the lost moment of the past where the public media are so immunized that they are not drawn into replicating the private media for competitive reasons. For Halmai, freedom has to be regulated "even though the scarcity of the frequencies ceases to exist". Halmai sees, as a function of the courts, assuring a diversified set of existing opinions conforming with the requirement of a balanced and professional reporting.

Halmai discusses the impact of the 1989 Hungarian Roundtable discussions and the transition in shaping Hungarian regulation of the electronic media. He suggests how the moratorium on making broadcast frequencies accessible to public broadcasters which emerged at the Roundtable talks resulted in limitations on free expression and the launching of new voices impossible. Like the judges of the German Constitutional Court in Karlsruhe, the Hungarian Constitutional Court indicated that it would judge the actions of the legislature by their capacity to guarantee in principle the comprehensive, balanced and objective expressions of all opinions existing in the whole society.

Andrew Arato concentrates on the Hungarian Constitutional Court and its decisions during the deep controversy over control of broadcasting in Hungary. Arato has seized upon a moment of sensitivity: where a new system is emerging from the old, but has not yet done so. The question was whether one could have a system, free of party influence, but subject to parliamentary majoritarian control. Arato traces the story of the dispute over the leadership of the radio and television, the assertion of direct government control and the exercise of budgetary influence. Judicial intervention was frequent and stunningly important: disputes led to a definition of the power of the President, providing him with authority only when his action was taken to avoid "gravely disturbing the democratic organization of the state". The Court was also faced with difficult problems of a transition: how much to honor a decree of the *ancien regime*. The Council of Ministers' control over public broadcasting was based on a clearly unconstitutional 1974 Cabinet resolution. In this situation, the role of the Court is telescoped in its difficulty, in terms of how far it can push against the Parliament and how it, alone, can define the powers of the President. Here was a situation where a discredited and unconstitutional law had to govern pending a revision that could not take place.

IV.   The Media and the Political Arena

We close with several views on media development, access and the political arena. These are snapshots of a phenomenon that is influenced, but not controlled by law, namely the operation of the state, in its cruel splendor, on specific individuals.

Professor Elemér Hankiss, who had been appointed the President of Hungarian Television and served during a turbulent time, called the Hungarian media wars "a sign of relative peace and maturity". Hankiss concludes that there were good and bad reasons to control the media and among the good "let me mention that the extremely difficult process of transition to democracy and market economy calls for common goals of national unity, and broad national support of government plans and policies".

The effort to dismiss Hankiss was labelled by some "the first show trial since the free elections in Hungary in 1990". But Hankiss dismisses this metaphor. Even though "the whole case was prefabricated and the judgment passed before trial", everything else was different. The dispute over his leadership took place in democracy and the stakes were lower: "Instead of the hangman, cheering crowds and sympathizing journalists greeted the condemned".

The essay by Jan Kavan focuses on the political implications of the range of ethical responses by journalists in the transitional Czech Republic. "Many journalists candidly admit that they view themselves primarily as 'citizen journalists', i.e. as reporters who put their civic duty and the health of the republic, as they perceive it, before their journalistic freedom and duty to inform". Therefore, corruption scandals were not covered by those who favored privatization.

Kavan turns to the administration of the then-Czechoslavakian lustration ordinance, and after discussion of the weaknesses in its general administration, discusses its painful application in his own case: "I have been accused of being a former collaborator of the Czechoslovak Secret police". Asked to resign quietly, he refused and was reproached for not "accepting that society has to defend itself against the consequences of the past". His opponents argued not that Kavan was wrong, or that his arguments were false, "but that my defence could discredit government policies". Kavan surveys the coverage of his case in the foreign and domestic press and his efforts to have his name cleared.

Finally, Zsolt Krokovay deals with a number of interrelated issues from a philosophical perspectives. These include the background conditions for the effective practice of political liberty, the problem of government speech and the role of corruption and "political money" in defining freedom of expression.

CHAPTER I

THEORIES OF MEDIA ACCESS

AN ACCESS TAXONOMY

by Monroe E. Price

I.   American Access Talk

When scholars or makers of public policy write about access to the media, they generally intend to initiate a discussion about the means of making more equitable the distribution of opportunities, in a given society, for a citizen or group to address other groups or citizens. The importance of access is almost always assumed to be premised on established notions of democratic theory, the dangers inherent in a non-benign monopoly over the instruments of mass communication and the implications of substantial imbalances in access to pedestals of influence.

The notion of access, even the very word itself, brings forth echoes of easement, of the capacity of one person to go across the property of another. We speak of the right of a land-locked nation to have access to the sea. Access sometimes implies an extraordinary right; a situation in which the property involved is in the control of another, but where circumstances require that the perquisites of ownership be modified for a specific purpose. Ideas of access are vague, but often foundational, a defining or architectural concept, establishing the infrastructure for communications policy. In its most romantic form, access suggests a search to replicate the conditions of the village by the use of high technology: the desire to find a means whereby any person can talk to any other person. Access, in this sense, searches for ways to reconstruct the mass media so it is no longer the few speaking to the many, but, at the least, the many speaking to the many. But access has come to mean something more, namely government assurance that there is fair representation, a sense of inclusion, a mode of altering monopolies of narrative. "Providing access", as a political agenda, may mean locating those who have, for a variety of reasons, been excluded from the community's dialogue and provide them with the opportunity to speak to the whole. Access can also mean providing

1

A. Sajó (ed.), Rights of Access to the Media, 1-28.

the kind of internal communications network to inchoate or disabled minorities that permits the majority effectively to function. And, finally, providing access can mean creating gateways to sources of information for those who have been deprived of such sources in the past or conversely, providing access by such speakers to an audience from which they have been precluded. More cynically, concepts of access may mean constructing a set of artificial decorations, a *mosaic faux*, a means of legitimating the dominant voices by showing a toleration of difference and dissent. "Access" has the ring of neutrality to it; but its invocation implies specific structures of state and society.

In this essay, I seek to outline a kind of taxonomy of access, at least as the term has developed in the United States. Some contextual qualifiers are fairly obvious. The distinction between the printed press and broadcasters, central to so much of American thinking about the power of government to regulate, seems less in evidence in Europe. In general, outside the United States, if governmental authority to introduce or establish access is available to government, there is not so sharp an inherent or historical reason to distinguish among modes of information distribution as there is in the United States. The United States debate differs from the European in another way: American legal doctrine is obsessed with factual determinations of "scarcity" and bottlenecks in the distribution of information. The existence of scarcity is thought by some to be a sine qua non for anchoring the power of government to regulate. Not only has the American doctrinal basis for access been rather narrow, but even where access approaches have been congressionally authorized and judicially approved, the usual forms of obtaining access have proved quite ineffective at achieving stated goals.

Even at a time when the federal regulatory agencies and courts were sympathetic to notions of access, implementation or enforcement was cumbersome and unsatisfactory. The European and American context differ, perhaps most profoundly in the institutional, legal recognition of pluralism, in the forms of encouraging or masking, suppressing or rendering explicit the status of historic ethnic or other minorities. The history of access regulation in the United States is very much a history of a public inability or unwillingness to be explicit about the relationship of narrative to social context and of ownership structures to the nature of the narrative. The entire project of explicitly providing guaranteed forms of access to specified groups seems antithetical to an American legal tradition of non-differentiation based on race or class or gender or political perspective. But a mass media perceived as exclusionary by large segments of the population could have a destabilizing impact and concern with "access" is a means of forestalling perceptions of political injustice.

In fact, while there has been much access talk in the United States, and much concern with access by Congress and the Federal Communications Commission, the different modes of American regulation have not been analytically organized and tied to different models of democratic theory. This article is an effort at initiating that process, though there are lots of pitfalls. Like all categories, the categories I propose are somewhat arbitrary and the examples cited are thrown, perhaps too casually, in one categorical box rather than another. Also, the introduction of cable and other new technologies has altered the nature of the discussion of access; access becomes a different subject in each technological and social transformation of the media. The relationship between access and these transformations needs systematic exploration. The flip side of granting access is controlling it. Some forms of television regulation assume that citizenship is enhanced by limiting access from outside a nation's borders; here a notion of national identity comes into play. This is a kind of negative access. Another kind of negative access arises when conditions are placed upon the kinds of speakers who, under a general rule, should have the opportunity to speak. The American rule that obscenity is not protected by the First Amendment and that "indecent" speech may also be unprotected in some circumstances, has been used to circumscribe the class of producers who have access.[1] In a recently adopted charter for independent media in the former Soviet Union, for example, a provision that guaranteed access for political parties was amended to exclude those parties and speakers whose views were inimical to democratic values.

Out of the American experience, I suggest four broad categories of law-imposed access (ownership access, producer access, common carrier access and Hyde Park corner "public access") and one broad category of semi-coerced access,

---

[1]   This notion was affirmed by the U.S. Supreme Court in *Roth v. United States*, 354 U.S. 476 (1957), in which Justice Brennan noted history has rejected obscenity for being "utterly without redeeming social importance." The lack of constitutional protection was fine-tuned and narrowed in *Miller v. California*, 413 U.S. 15. Here the court introduced the criteria that enable states to regulated obscenity:

> a) whether "the average person, applying contemporary community standards," would find that the work, taken as a whole, appears to the prurient interest; b) whether the work depicts or describes in a patently offensive way, sexual conduct specifically defined by the applicable state law; and c) whether the work, taken as a whole, lacks serious literary, artistic, political, or scientific value (citations omitted). Id. at 24.

namely political and pressure group access. Each of these forms is discussed, together with something of their history and justification and something of their shortcomings.

II.1.   Ownership access

What I am calling "ownership access" has been the technique used most broadly by the Congress and the Federal Communications Commission to cope with the perception of needed access while avoiding direct responsibility for altering narrative or content. Rules concerning control of broadcasting licenses are based on the assumption that diversifying ownership is a method of achieving the substantive goal of achieving a richer more diversified source of information. Rules that provide privileged opportunities for certain groups to have access to broadcast licenses are based on similar assumptions. Early in its concern over concentration in control of broadcasting, the FCC limited an owner to one station in a radio and television market[2] and, in the 1960's, barred the cross-ownership of newspaper and television stations in the same market.[3] The most marked recent example of ownership access - and the example that most dramatically makes assumptions about the relationship of ownership to narrative - is the policy of the FCC toward encouraging minority -

---

[2]   That rule was changed for radio stations in 1992. A single owner can now have as many as three AM and three FM stations in a single city. That owner may also control as many as 30 AM and 30 FM stations nationwide, up from 12 of each. 7 F.C.C.R. 2755 (1992). Those who favor deregulation would not view this as an assault on access. Rather, it could reflect a stark economic reality, namely that a majority of radio stations nationwide were losing money when the ownership order was issued. In fact, 153 stations went dark in 1991. See Edmund Andrews, *F.C.C. Loosens Restrictions On Owning Radio Stations*, N.Y. Times, March 12, 1993, at D1.

Still, the ruling may have the effect of preventing small entrepeneurs or minority owners from entering the larger markets where minority populations are based if larger companies with more cash can more easily snap up stations that might come up for sale. Id.

[3]   For example, when Rupert Murdoch bought the Metromedia television stations, including WNEW-TV (now WNYW) in New York, he was forced in 1988 to divest the New York Post. Murdoch regained control of the newspaper in March 1993 as it teetered on the brink of extinction under the stewardship of previous owners. He applied to the FCC for a waiver of the cross-ownership ban. By a 2-1 vote, the FCC approved the waiver. Commissioner Barrett dissented, fearing other financially troubled media outlets would want the same treatment. David Henry and Elizabeth Sanger, *FCC Says Murdoch Can Buy NY Post*, N.Y. Newsday, June 30, 1993.

including black, Hispanic, Native American and Asian - ownership of radio and television stations.[4] In the 1970's, the FCC adopted a policy that provided tax incentives and advantages in comparative hearings[5] that would result in the transfer of some existing radio and television licenses to minority owners or businesses controlled by members of minority groups.[6] When the FCC announced its ownership policies, it made it clear that the goal had to be altering the social narrative. At the same time, the Commission constantly adverted to constitutional limitations precluding government from affecting the stories told, the figures on the screen in a way that would entail establishing categories of content. Affecting ownership was the solution. And in the Supreme Court decision upholding the constitutionality of the minority preference, the majority of the Justices accepted the assumption, adopted by the FCC, that minority ownership would likely produce more diversified speech.[7]

---

[4] As of 1991, there were 182 radio stations and 15 television stations that were minority owned, up from 30 radio stations and one television station in 1976. Joe Flint, *Minorities see an indifferent F.C.C.*, Broadcasting & Cable, Aug. 24, 1992, at 25. The FCC conceded the minority ownership numbers are at a "disturbingly low level." 7 F.C.C.R. 2755, 2769 (1992). Indeed, FCC Commissioner Andrew Barrett noted in a partial dissent to the 30/30 rule that just 1.64 percent of all radio stations were black-owned in 1991, compared to 1.57 percent in 1980. Barrett, who is black, said, "Clearly, more progress is needed." Id. at 2814, n.12.

[5] Minority Ownership Policy Statement, 68 F.C.C. 2d 979, 983. The purpose of such a hearing was to determine "whether there is a substantial likelihood that diversity of programming will be increased." The presumption running through many of the FCC's rulings on ownership is that diversity is equated with access, a comparison that may in some instances be adequate if a little too convenient. The majority in the 30/30 decision felt relaxation of the caps would "actually enhance viewpoint diversity." It cited a 1984 report which concluded that commonly owned stations offer more public service programming and that stations in a group make editorial decisions autonomously. 7 F.C.C.R. 2755, 2765 (1992).

[6] 68 F.C.C. 2d 979, 983. The FCC established a tax certificate policy, whereby the seller of a broadcast outlet could defer the gains on a sale if it sells to a minority-controlled interest. The FCC also has a policy that allows a broadcast licensee whose license has been designated for revocation to sell to a minority at a below-market rate before the hearing commences. Minority owners, prior to the 30/30 rule, were also able to have up to 14 AM and 14 FM stations, compared to 12 of each service for non-minorities. Id. at 2769.

[7] *Metro Broadcasting Inc. v. FCC.*, 497 U.S. 547 (1990). For an exhaustive and cogent discussion of the case, see Michel Rosenfeld, *Metro Broadcasting, Inc. v. FCC: Affirmative Action at the Crossroads of Constitutional Liberty and Equality*, 38 U.C.L.A. L. Rev. 583 (1991).

6

The evidence to support this vital assumption is fragile, as Justice O'Connor, in her dissent, sought to demonstrate.[8] Most licensees seek an affiliation with one of the national networks, if available, and adopt or "clear" most of the network's program offerings. Even if the programming that the local licensee selects is from non-network offerings, there are patterns of great similarity, based on what will maximize audience or advertising revenues. Seldom does ownership diversity - except in specific market circumstances - lead to the kind of program diversity that has overtones important in furthering pluralist goals. At the very margin, stations owned by minority groups are somewhat more sensitive to minority issues; perhaps they have better affirmative action records. But there has not been a convincing showing that, where the owner is interested in maximizing profit, the nature of the operation varies with the nature of the owner.

The ownership access policy, - not with respect to minorities, - but in terms of the cross-ownership rule and the one-to-a-market rule, seems to have a mechanical truth to it. More owners are said to be better than fewer from the point of view of diversified speech. It would be wrong to have a single owner, in a major city, of all newspapers or of the daily newspaper, the television station and the radio station (the way in which markets were once constructed). The FCC has never been tolerant of the argument, made so long by the BBC, that a single manager of frequencies would maximize audience by purposely and rationally diversifying, playing to small segments, in only the way that a monopolist can do.

Technology has its odd tricks, however. Cable television, which is considered a harbinger of diversity, comes close to playing the role of benificent monopolist. While there are now many more channels available to each household - 50 or 150[9] or 500[10] - the cable operator now more or less controls the entire

[8]   "[B]oth the FCC and Congress have determined that a relationship does exist between expanded minority ownership and greater broadcast diversity." 497 U.S. at 569. Justice O'Connor further noted: "Evidence suggests that an owner's minority status influences the selection of topics for news coverage and the presentation of editorial viewpoint, especially on matters of particular concern to minorities." Id. at 580-81. The majority also accepted the conclusion from several studies, cited by the FCC, that "a minority owner is more likely to employ minorities in managerial and other important roles where they can have an impact on station policies." Id. at 591.

[9]   Time Warner began in 1992 a test of a 150-channel system in the New York City borough of Queens, which included fifty-seven pay-per-view channels, or what the company called "virtual video on demand." *Virtual Movies-on-Demand Service Starts in Queens*, Comm. Daily, Dec. 30, 1991, at 2.

system. Diversity becomes a strategy to expand the number of subscribers subscribing to the system. While neither the FCC nor Congress has limited the scale of ownership of cable, the 1992 Cable Television Consumer Protection and Competition Act[11] was designed to encourage competition by ensuring program sources for new multi-channel video distributors;[12] and FCC regulations extend the tax incentives for sale to minority purchasers of cable systems that exist for minority purchasers of broadcast licenses.

II.2. Producer access

Another technique for addressing access is to focus not on the owner, but on the producer of programming. "Producer access" is government regulation that requires that a carrier of programming (a television station or a cable operator, for example) take certain categories of programs or certain packagers of programs. In some ways this is an awkward term and I have included a wide variety of mechanisms under its umbrella. The United States does not have one of the most familiar European forms of producer access provisions, namely national or regional producer quotas. In the age of deregulation, the FCC has virtually foresworn producer quotas, even for news and public affairs. Producer access provisions are imposed not only to affect content, but because of some bottleneck in the distribution of programming or control of vehicles for distribution in monopoly or near-monopoly hands. The medium, as

---

[10]   As outlandish as 500 channels may seem, it is fast becoming part of the video landscape. Tele-Communications Inc., the largest cable company in the United States, was slated to begin installing in 1994 cable boxes to offer at least 500 channels, offering everything from movies on demand to interactive video games. *See generally* Richard Ernsberger Jr., *The Patron Saint of Channel Surfing*, Newsweek, May 31, 1993, at 46; Kevin Maney, *A New Media World-Interactive Technology Fades Borders*, USA Today, May 18, 1993, at 1B.

[11]   47 U.S.C. §§ 521-558 (1993) (hereinafter "1992 Cable Act").

[12]   One could also characterize the preference for a local owner a form of ownership access. The preference for local ownership and for integration of ownership and management would imply a kind of access, especially given the philosophy of the FCC during its first twenty-five years, that localism was to be valued and local ownership was more likely to produce a station that was the "mouthpiece" of the community.

gatekeeper, is required to provide opportunities for given entities, at given times, to air their programs and views. Producer access, in this sense, takes many forms.[13]

II.2.a. *Access by Political Parties or Candidates*

The most familiar and accepted form of producer access rules involve those specifically related to the political process. These rules, in conjunction with many other campaign structuring provisions, usually ensure that recognized or qualified political candidates are entitled to time at a regulated price or a rate that is nondiscriminatory among political candidates. Federal law assures that candidates can have access to television and radio stations at the lowest available rates[14] and gives one candidate equal time when another candidate receives time, under prescribed circumstances.[15] Rules that set aside time for political parties at no

---

[13]   Access by the general public, so-called "public access" provides a special case of producer access and is treated separately, infra.

[14]   47 U.S.C. § 315 (b), which reads:

> The charges made for the use of any broadcasting station by any person who is a legally qualified candidate for any public office in connnection with his campaign for nomination for election, or election, to such office shall not exceed:

> (1) during the forty-five days preceding the date of a primary or primary runoff election and during the sixty days preceding the date of a general or special elction in which such persons a candidate, the *lowest unit charge* of the station for the same class and amount of time for the same period; and

> (2) at any other time, the charges made for comparable use of such station by other users thereof (emphasis added).

[15]   47 U.S.C. § 315(a). It reads in relevant part:

> If any licensee shall permit any person who is a legally qualified candidate for any public office to use a broadcasting station, he shall afford equal opportunities to all other such candidates for that office in the use of such broadcasting station: *Provided*, that such licensee shall have no power over censorship over the material broadcast under the provisions of this section.

The principal exceptions for the equal time rule include a bona fide newscast, interview or documentary and on-the-spot coverage of news events, including, but not limited to, political conventions. However, this does not mean broadcasters can simply relieve themselves from the potential headaches of the equal time rule by not

charge and rules that require televised debates fit within this category, though these rules do not exist under American law. There are no political access rules that apply to newspapers or magazines in the United States.[16]

Access rules that relate to political parties can serve pluralistic ends. They can encourage smaller parties; they can be so described as to encourage or discourage parties that represent particular historically defined ethnic groups to have privileged access. In the United States, political access rules do not serve very well the reflection of pluralist tendencies. Indeed, some think that the rules are designed to favor the major parties, the two-party system and incumbency.

The 1992 campaign demonstrated an unusual, perhaps unique, aspect of access rules, namely the capacity of personal wealth to capture access. What might be called Perotist access in the United States is a newly-important manifestation, namely, the opportunity of a person or group with a message to purchase large amounts of time on a major network - not "advertising" - as a way of reaching a national audience. In the pre-Perot period, the major broadcast television networks were reluctant to lease out their time for the presentation of controversial views, or for the views of any group except for specific candidates for office or the recognized

---

covering news and public affairs. This section also reminds broadcasters that they still have an obligation, under the conditions of their license, to "operate in the public interest to afford reasonable opportunity for the discussion of conflicting views on issues of public importance".

[16] The landmark case that affirmed this notion was *Miami Herald v. Tornillo*, 418 U.S. 241 (1968). The Supreme Court invalidated a "right to reply" statute in Florida that granted political candidates newspaper space equal to the amount of space used by the newspaper to criticize the candidate or attack his record. The Court found the statute restrained expression, intruded on the editorial function and thus violated the First and Fourteenth amendments.

Tornillo is a celebrated case as much for its message as for its frequent misreading by courts and commentators who have applied the case to resolve access issues in other media, particularly cable television. Jerome Barron, who wrote the Supreme Court brief supporting Tornillo, notes how some courts perceived Tornillo as foreclosing on First Amendment grounds any media regulation based on economic scarcity when the court left that issue unresolved. Jerome Barron, *On Understanding the First Amendment Status of Cable: Some Obstacles in the Way*, 57 G.W. L. Rev. 1495, 1499-1500 (1989).

Barron notes this misreading has influenced cases where cable operators were found to have First Amendment rights analogous to newspapers and thus could not be regulated by governments like other natural monopolies such as utilities. *See Preferred Communicatons, Inc. v. City of Los Angeles*, 754 F.2d 1396 (9th Cir. 1985), *aff'd* and *remanded*, 476 U.S. 488 (1986).

political parties.[17] Indeed, as recently as March, 1993, Perot's offer to purchase an hour's prime time was refused by ABC. NBC rationalized the sale of time to Perot on the basis of an in-house process of determining what kinds of applicants had national appeal and warranted the time.[18]

II.2.b. *Conditional Access*

Conditional access involves a regulatory pattern which provides a given speaker or producer the right of access if certain circumstances occur. The best example of this in the United States is the personal attack rule or the reply to editorial rule.[19] If a broadcaster airs a personal attack, the person attacked has the right to respond. Similarly, an editorial is aired, parties with competing views have some right to respond. This fairness doctrine has been a self-administered conditional access rule. If a broadcaster, in certain settings, airs material that is one side of a controversial

---

[17]   This designation extended beyond the mainstream Democratic and Republican candidates. For example, radical Lyndon LaRouche, nominally a Democratic candidate, bought time on CBS in September 1992, spending $240,000 to give a speech from prison. Sharon D. Moshavi, *CNN just says no to Bush ad*, Broadcasting & Cable, Sept. 14, 1992. Another unusual candidate was John Hagelin of the Natural Law Party, who plunked down $225,000 on NBC to espouse such views as using meditation to help solve the problems of the nation. Ben Smith III, *Natural Law candidate to plug meditation as cure for nation's ills*, Atl. Jour. and Const., Oct. 23, 1992, at A6

[18]   Ed Bark, *Television critics question Perot about Sunday's 'town meeting'*, The Dallas Morning News, March 20, 1993, at 8A.

[19]   47 C.F.R. § 73.1920. It reads in relevant part:

When, during the presentation of views on a controversial issue of public importance, an attack is made upon the honesty, character, integrity . . . of an identified person or group, the licensee shall, within a reasonable time, and in no event later than one week after the attack, transmit to the persons or group attacked:

1) Notification of the date, time and identification of the broadcast;

2) A script or tape (or an accurate summary if a script or tape is not available) of the attack; and

3) An offer of a reasonable opportunity to respond over the licensee's facilities.

This is actually one aspect of the fairness doctrine.

question of public importance, there has been, at times, some obligation to air other sides of the issue.[20] Strictly speaking, the fairness doctrine is not an access mode, because groups do not have the right to use time themselves to respond. As a consequence of recent congressional action relating to the Corporation for Public Broadcasting and the legislated requirement of objectivity, the CPB announced a policy under which the Corporation would seek out and provide financing for producers with points of view different from those already aired if the productions presented were controversial and, in some determined way, not "objective".[21]

---

[20]   The fairness doctrine imposed on broadcasters an affirmative duty to devote a reasonable amount of their air time to covering public issues and providing a chance for opposing viewpoints to be aired. The doctrine hovers on being antithetical to First Amendment values when taken to its extremes. Nevertheless it withstood its greatest constitutional challenge in *Red Lion v. FCC*, 395 U.S. 367 (1969) (Holding that the government's role in frequency allocations properly meshed with the legitimate claims of those unable, without the government's help, to gain access to those frequencies in order to express their views).

The debate over *Red Lion* has raged long and hard over the years. A bibliography of commentary related to the fairness doctrine can be found in William Van Alstyne, *The Mobius Strip of the First Amendment: Perspectives on Red Lion*, 29 S.C. L. Rev. 539, 547-48, n.49 (1978). All of this commentary may have had a role in influencing the FCC to gradually shy away from aggressively enforcing the doctrine. *See* Monroe E. Price, Taming Red Lion: The First Amendment and Structural Approaches to Media Regulation, 31 FED. COMM. L.J. 215, 216 (1979). A full-scale retreat began in the 1970's. The FCC stated "we no longer believe that the fairness doctrine, as a matter of policy, serves the public interest." Notice of Inquiry Concerning General Fairness Doctrine Obligations of Broadcast Licensees (1985 Fairness Report), 102 F.C.C. 2d. 143, 147 (1985).

> Two years later, the FCC finally repudiated the doctrine as unconstitutional and has not enforced it since. "The First Amendment was adopted to protect the people *not from journalists, but from government* . . . We therefore believe that full First Amendment protections against content regulation should apply equally to the electronic and printed press." In re Complaint of Syracuse Peace Council against WTVH, 2 F.C.C.R. 5043, 5057. The decision was upheld by a federal appeals court. *Syracuse Peace Council v. FCC*, 867 F.2d 654 (D.C. Cir. 1987). Subsequent Congressional attempts to definitively codify the fairness doctrine have failed. The latest version was attached to campaign reform legislation, which passed the Senate in June 1993, and was being considered by the House. See Comm. Daily, June 21, 1993, at 11 (available in Lexis/Nexis Library).

[21]   See Jane Hall, *Public Broadcasting Board OK's Objectivity Measures*, L.A. Times, Jan. 27, 1993, at F1.

II.2.c. *"Must Carry Channels"*

The 1992 Cable Act requires that cable operators carry local commercial broadcast stations[22] and public broadcasting stations,[23] reflecting a long history in which, for economic and social reasons, the FCC had provided guaranteed access, through cable, for much of the existing broadcast structure.[24] These rules could be called an exercise in ordered transition; but the cable operators have been bitterly opposed to them and have hit upon a way of providing an emotional challenge, namely by characterizing themselves as speakers[25] and then arguing that these rules force them to utter the expressions of others, in violation of the first amendment (and human) rights.[26] From an access perspective, the problem of definition is an important one.

---

[22]   47 U.S.C.A. § 534 (1993).

[23]   47 U.S.C.A. § 535 (1993).

[24]   Must-carry cases were thrown into limbo by two cases which found that FCC rules requiring carriage were unconstitutional. *Century Communications Corp. v. FCC*, 835 F.2d 292 (D.C.Cir. 1987), *clarified*, 837 F.2d 292 (D.C.Cir. 1987), *cert. denied*, 476 U.S. 1169; *Quincy Cable TV, Inc. v. FCC*, 768 F.2d 1434 (D.C. Cir. 1985), *cert. denied*, 476 U.S. 1169.

Understandably, cable operators may have believed overturning the must-carry rules in the 1992 Cable Act, 476 U.S.C. §§ 534-535, should not have been difficult. A panel of district court judges felt otherwise in *Turner Broadcasting System, Inc. v. FCC*, 819 F. Supp. 32 (D.D.C. 1993). In a 2-1 decision, the judges noted that Century and Quincy never determined that must-carry rules are *per se* unconstitutional, only that the FCC had failed to "demonstrate that the means it had chosen to employ to its putative end were necessary at all." Id. at 41. This time around, however, the court agreed that the must-carry rules were necessary to preserve broadcasters from the growing dominance of cable. "The Court does not find improbable Congress' conclusion that this market power provides cable operators with both incentive and present ability to block non-cable programmers' access to the bulk of any prospective viewing audience; unconstrained cable hold the future of local broadcasting at its mercy." Id. at 46.

[25]   See Stuart Robinowitz, *Cable Television: Proposals for Reregulation and the First Amendment*, 8 Cardozo Arts Ent. L.J. 309 (1990). Robinowitz, who represents cable operators, including Time Warner Cable, is among many who argue that cable operators are speakers in the same way as newspapers or any other protected medium, and that to regulate them infringes on their First Amendment rights. It should be noted that the Supreme Court has yet to decide this matter, thus far going only so far as to say that cable operators engage in speech protected by the First Amendment without specifying the precise mode of speech. *Los Angeles v. Preferred Communications, Inc.*, 476 U.S. 488 (1986).

[26]   See *Turner Broadcasting System, Inc. v. FCC*, 114 S. Ct. 2445 (1994).

If cable is characterized as a conduit or highway, then such access rules are less difficult to justify than if cable operators are, themselves, considered social communicators.

One reading of the legislation is that it was designed to preserve a certain stock of programming (like sports) in a mode of delivery that was "free", i.e. advertiser supported, not requiring additional payment by citizen viewers.

In part, this was programming that included local news, programming that carried important elements of the political debate and federally funded public cultural and instructional presentations. The must-carry rules have reoriented the way in which commercial broadcasters perceive their public responsibilities. In some way, it is only if they provide a kind of access, serve the goals that are behind access rules, that the requirement that they be carried on cable is justified.[27] Furthermore, to the extent that the public broadcasting system sees as a goal the inclusion of minority cultures, the "must carry" rules could be understood as mandating access for them.[28]

II.2.d. Mandated Government and Education Channels

When the FCC established its Table of Allocations for the distribution of television broadcast licenses in the early 1950's, it reserved channels for educational purposes. This was access to spectrum, not access across the broadcast license reserved by

---

[27]   Keeping this criterion in mind, it is all but unfathomable how the FCC determined that home shopping channels should be lumped in to the must-carry strictures. By a 2-1 vote on July 2, 1993, the commissioners somehow determined that such channels, of which about 100 exist carrying the signals of the Home Shopping Network, met the public-service standard the must-carry rules mandate. Between the frenzied pitches for cubic zirconia rings and overpriced baseball cards, this stations stick in five minutes of "community programming" each hour, along with several hours of public affairs shows early each Sunday. But if this is the standard to meet, is there any meaningful standard left? In re-regulating the cable industry in 1992, it is highly doubtful Congress intended to open the window for such video hucksters to climb inside. See Edmund Andrews, *F.C.C. Lets TV-Shopping Stations Demand Access to Slots on Cable*, N.Y. Times, July 3, 1993, at 1, 40.

[28]   This is of particular concern in the New York area, where two public stations, WNYE-TV and WNYC-TV, provide an extensive amount of programming not normally seen on other PBS channels. Much of it is foreign-language programming that would otherwise be without a television home.

14

others. It was out of that reservation that the public broadcasting system emerged.[29] The reservation can be seen as a wholesale act of providing access, first for colleges and municipalities that wished the opportunity to use the new medium to accomplish their public responsibilities to instruct and then for a far broader range of cultural institutions.

Twenty years later, many local governments, as part of a highly competitive system for awarding local cable franchises, required that cable operators set aside a certain amount of channel time for governmental, educational and public uses. The franchising process for cable television franchise, reserved channels for education and government purposes. Mostly, these latter reservations lie unused.[30]

II.2.e. Prime Time Access

An arcane genre of access regulation provides preferred opportunities for "independent" producers (those not linked to the major networks) to gain access to broadcast time in the periods of maximum audience viewing. This form of access is a reflection of concerns about competition among producers of programming and the power of the television networks. While the goal of the prime time access rule[31]

---

[29]   The current regulations governing the table of allotments and the criteria for noncommercial educational television stations can be found in 47 C.F.R. § 73.606 (1992) and 47 C.F.R. § 73.621 (1992), respectively.

[30]   One notable exception is New York City, where the dominant cable operator is Time Warner Cable. As part of its franchise renewal in 1990, the city received five governmental channels, including one for the City University of New York and another for an institutional network that would be employed mostly for training sessions for city employees. Time Warner also agreed to pay a minimum of $9 million for equipment for the channels (mostly for the institutional network), which are collectively known as the Crosswalks network. The network began operation in 1992, and all channels were to be on-line by 1994. Cable Television Franchise Agreement for the Borough of Manhattan between the City of New York and Manhattan Cable Television Inc., (Appendix E) (1990) (on file in the New York City Department of Telecommunications and Energy).

[31]   The FCC passed this rule in 1971, limiting network affiliates in the top 50 markets to no more than three hours of prime-time programming (8-11 p.m.) from Monday-Saturday. Prime-Time Access Rule, 47 C.F.R. §73.658 (1992). There are some notable exceptions to the rule. They include: programs for children, public affairs programs and documentaries, fast-breaking news events, runovers of live sports events, but not to post-game shows and broadcasts of international sports events such as the Olympics. Id.

was to make more broadly available a wider set of perspectives, the rule has been exploited most by such shows as "Jeopardy" and "Wheel of Fortune". Access has led, perhaps, to debasement of taste, not a broadening of it. Prime time access rules have merely served as another effort to bring to broadcasting general views about anticompetitive behavior and vertical integration. For example, if the distributors of information are also producers of information, there is a danger that the distributor will discriminate against other producers who are competitors. The 1992 Cable Act had, as a principal thrust, producer access provisions of this sort. The new law prohibits cable operators from insisting that they gain equity ownership in cable network services as a condition for carrying them, especially if these cable operators have affiliated network services themselves.[32] Similarly, there are restrictions on the capacity of the new cable networks to deny their product in such a way as to limit competition at the consumer distribution level.[33] In other words, distributors, in this example, have access to the work of producers.

II.2.f. Access by Specific Minority Groups

I have mentioned the historical antipathy for the FCC or Congress forcibly to alter social narratives by compelling networks, stations and cable operators from carrying works solely on the ground that they were produced by representatives of particular racial or ethnic groups. In the 1992 Cable Act, however, Congress provided that a cable operator can dedicate channel capacity otherwise designated for leased access for a "qualified minority programming source", defined as a programming source which "devotes substantially all of its programming to coverage of minority viewpoints, or to programming directed at members of minority groups" and which

---

[32]   47 U.S.C. 548

[33]   Direct broadcast satellite systems and other non-cable services had long complained that cable companies had blocked access to premium services or charged high prices for services they owned or controlled (e.g. Time Warner owns Time Warner Cable and Home Box Office). The largest cable operators and programmers were sued by forty states seeking more parity in pricing. After five years, the companies, without admitting guilt, agreed in 1993 to make their programming available at more uniform prices. However, bulk discounts would still be allowed to large cable systems, which could undercut any cost savings for upstart wireless systems. *Cable TV Programmers Settle Antitrust Suit With Noncable Services*, Satellite Week, June 14, 1993; Edmund Andrews, *Cable Pact is Reached by States*, N.Y. Times, June 9, 1993, at D1.

is over fifty percent minority-owned.[34] This is an extremely interesting access rule because it has both an ownership and a content feature.

III.3. Common carrier and leased access

Common carrier approaches to access are, in some ways, the antonym to ownership access. Ideas of access are intrinsic in the very aesthetic of the common carrier model. The common carrier is the invention of custom to establish the fair and nondiscriminatory use of an essential instrument for the conduct of the society. A common carrier for transportation allows, within predetermined limits, assurance concerning travel. Common carriers, providing transit at a set rate and without preference, was the model for ferrying across rivers since time out of mind. And in the twentieth century, the telephone has been the common carrier first for voice, and now for data and hope of video.

Some think of the common carrier model as the perfect mechanism for a free market society dedicated to unencumbered speech and access to modes of distribution of that speech. Multi-channel common carrier systems, the *deus ex machina* of the new technology, avoids the need for intrusive government intervention. But common carriers provide equal opportunity, not equal access. The social narratives may change as a result of the introduction of a common carrier system, but not necessarily toward a more pluralistic set of stories, and one that reflects historically excluded racial and ethnic groups. Of course, a general common carrier model can be combined with features that seek to assure access: subsidies to preferred groups, specific mandated reductions in fees for such groups and similar methods.

The common carrier model for the media - for video and press applications - represents, at its full embodiment, an architectural decision that some distribution modes, such as cable or optical fiber, or at least some part of it, should be like the telephone, with published non-discriminatory rates and ownership separated from control of content. Access would be much eased. One might say that there would be no gatekeeper. Common carrier access is appealing because it has the aura of eliminating government intervention to choose among speakers.

---

[34]   47 U.S.C.A. § 532 (i)(1), (2) (1993).

The 1934 Communications Act[35] precluded the FCC from treating broadcasters as common carriers, and the 1984[36] and 1992 Cable Acts place substantial restrictions on local governments and the FCC in terms of its regulation of cable. There is a limited treatment of the cable operator as a common carrier, at least imposing an obligation to carry existing broadcast stations and certain specialized carriers which the local franchising authority requires. There is intense current American debate about whether to allow telephone companies to preempt or absorb cable television companies and about the nature of the next generation of broadband video distribution.[37] This debate concerns, in significant ways, these access questions.[38] Broadening the number of channels should, in theory, bring down the cost of access (though there may always be preferable platform channels and though the access cost may be low relative to the cost of production). An additional step, permitting full switching and digital compression, may mean that the concept of channels themselves will be obsolete, replaced by new marketing, storage and pricing strategies that will allow each person to have access to whatever message or program he or she wants (though not necessarily the right of each producer of a message to have automatic access to the desired homes).

---

[35] 47 U.S.C.A. §§ 151-609 (1991).

[36] Cable Communications Policy Act of 1984, 47 U.S.C.A. §§ 531-532 (1991), *amended by* 47 U.S.C.A. §§ 531-532 (1993).

[37] It should be noted that both sides are seeking to ensure that the debate concludes before it seriously got started. In May 1993, Time Warner, the second-largest cable operator, announced that US West, a major telephone company, would invest $2.5 billion to build advanced cable networks. Geraldine Fabrikant, *US West to Work with Time Warner*, N.Y. Times, May 17, 1993, at A1. AT&T & Viacom soon followed with a joint venture to deliver movies on demand and shopping services over cable. Edmund Andrews, *Market Test of New Video Technology*, N.Y. Times, June 2, 1993, at D1.

[38] Beyond alliances with telephone companies, cable system operators are taking bold steps to exploit the capacity of the fiber optic cable they are now using to upgrade its cable service and expand it for other users. The nation's three-largest operators, TCI, Time Warner and Continental Cablevision, have all announced plans to build their own information superhighways, which will put the operators in direct competition with the Baby Bells and AT&T in the years to come. Peter Lambert, *TCI's $1.9B Pledge for Superhighway*, Multichannel News, Apr. 19, 1993, at 1; Carl Weinschenk, *Time Warner's Message*, Cable World, Feb. 1, 1993, at 1; Carl Weinschenk, *Continental Joining 'Superhighway' Parade*, Cable World, Apr. 19, 1993.

One of the provisions of the 1984 cable legislation[39] was to require that most cable television operators set aside channel capacity for unaffiliated companies seeking access to subscribers. The statutory provisions were enacted to provide a way for producers who would not otherwise be selected by the cable operator to gain channel space at a reasonable fee. The "leased" channel is something less than a common carrier, and the operator has extensive control of rates and sufficient control of the situation that the leasing provision has not been much used. The fact of its existence as a possible way of breaking the monopoly power of the cable operator was sufficient, however, for a judge, dissenting in the "must carry" cases, to hold that any other effort by Congress to impose programming access on cable operators was unconstitutional.[40]

II.4.   The Hyde Park corner or "public access" model

Perhaps this is, quintessentially, the access channel of populist dreams. For almost twenty years now, some cable systems in the United States have had a form of access that is derivative of the model of the aggressive personal or individual speech typified by the romanticized soapbox in a corner of Hyde Park.[41] These are the so-called public access channels, available to anyone, with no guarantee of audience, but with the notion that there ought to be a space for anyone to release passion, show talent, articulate a point of view.[42] The channels are designed to be used for

---

[39]   47 U.S.C.A. § 532(b)(1) (1991).

[40]   *Turner Broadcasting System, Inc. v. FCC*, 819 F. Supp. 32 (D.D.C. 1993) (Williams, J. dissenting) "In requiring cable systems to carry a special group of competing speakers, Congress directly, not incidentally, restricts the cable operators' exercise of editorial discretion. None of the interests advanced by Congress supports such a burden." Id. at 67.

[41]   For the uninitiated, this is the famed London park where an area is reserved for literally anyone to launch into a speech, tirade or polemic about anything on their mind. It is the ultimate in street theater.

[42]   But see, Andrew A. Bernstein, *Access to Cable, Natural Monopoly, and the First Amendment*, 86 Colum. L. Rev. 1663 (1986) (Access rules are unconstitutional because they abridge the rights of cable operators to make editorial decisions and because there are less intrusive means of serving the public). Courts have for years frowned on mandating public access channels. See, e.g., *Midwest Video Corp. v. FCC*, 571 F.2d 1025 (8th Cir. 1978), *aff'd on other grounds*, 440 U.S. 689 (1979).

individuals or community groups. They are often first-come, first-served. In many communities, low-tech facilities are provided to allow these groups or individuals to make the videos. The public access channels incorporate into television a kind of public pathway, an echo of the use of the streets, from time immemorial, to hector, implore and change the nature of the debate. Of course, a soapbox in a small village is different from a soapbox in a global village, the equivalent of shouting into the void. And without the necessary care, this is often what the public access channel has become.[43] In practice, public access channels have been an unkempt corner, a place of disarray and margin, but not a significant contributor to public debate. A number of issues of interest have arisen with respect to these public access channels. Cable operators have argued that it is a violation of their speech rights to be forced to carry the programming of this grab-bag of producers. When marginal and unpopular views have been propounded, cities and others have gone to court to try to censor them, as occurred with a Ku Klux Klan use of public access channels in California.[44] Congress, in the 1992 legislation, reduced the broad freedom of public

---

Nevertheless, however tenuously, they remain a part of the cable firmament.

The 1992 Cable Act codified this ambivalence by allowing a cable operator to prohibit the use of any public, educational, or governmental access channel for any "obscene" programming. 47 U.S.C.A. § 532 (h) (1993). No definition of obscene is provided, which has led to a lawsuit by producers fearful of capricious operators who are skittish of controversy and lawsuits. The latter situation could arise because the Act also imposes liability on those operators for carrying the obscene programming. 47 U.S.C.A. § 558 (1993). See *Allience for Community Media v. FCC*, 15 F.3d 186 (1994) (vacated and hearing granted en banc).

[43]   More often than not, public access shows are desiccated affairs; talk shows or call-in programs that interest no one but the host and guest. But then there are shows like "Morbid Underground" in Tampa, which aired a video tape of a punk rock singer defecating and urinating on stage. The appropriately named "Worst Show" in San Antonio sparked an uproar when it broadcast a skit about teen suicide. Politicians are also part of the mix, particularly in election years. They were apparently crowding the access channel in Houston to the point where cable officials considered of hours allowed to any one group or individual. Bill Duryea, *Cable TV obscenity issue flares*, St. Petersburg Times, March 21, 1993 at 1B; David McLemore, *Trying to pull the plug; San Antonio cable TV suicide guide angers many*, Dall. Morn. News, Nov. 14, 1992, at 1A; Julie Mason, *Access Houston may limit political rivals' air time*, Hous. Chron., Jan. 3, 1993, at C1.

[44]   Invariably, these communities find the uproar is muted by the reality that these programs cannot be censored unless they are obscene. Even obscenity, in this instance, is narrowly defined. So that means suburban New York residents will be startled by a self-proclaimed high priest of the Black Israelites saying, "We're going to be beating the hell out of you white people." Joseph Berger, *Forum for Bigotry?*

access users by establishing new guidelines for what constitutes unacceptable obscene or indecent programming.

II.5.   Consumer access or pressure group access

The first four categories of access arise as a consequence of specific statutory or regulatory initiatives. They are forms of access that are the consequence of law. But there is another form of access that is not purely "voluntary", namely a kind of access that exists because of the political or economic pressure of interest groups. Describing and circumscribing this category is difficult. One could say that most specific items in the media are there for reasons externally determined (by a need to appeal to a substantial audience, by a need to appeal to advertisers, by a need to appeal to those who grant government licenses, by a need to appeal to other funding sources, such as foundations).

What is meant here is something more specific: namely a rising form of access which involves the efforts of pressure groups, who consider themselves to be excluded, to influence the decisions of producers of news programs, situation comedies, dramas and other television offerings to include them in the everyday narratives of television life. This is, perhaps, an unusual use of the term access. The more common term to describe these activities is threatened boycott, bringing of undue pressure, and censorship. Rather than formal access or primary access - the opportunity of the group itself to broadcast a message - the group seeks to modify what they deem to be the negative messages of others or to insert what they consider a more favorable mix of images and narratives.

These groups include, most famously, religious groups arrayed against what they deem to be indecent sexual imagery or undue violence.[45] But they also include

---

Fringe Groups on TV, N.Y. Times, May 23, 1992, at 29. A neo-Nazi based in Florida, through a local sponsor, was able to get air time in Manhattan for his anti-Semitic ramblings.

[45]   Perhaps the most famous - or, for the networks, notorious - of these morality police is the Rev. Donald Wildmon, a former Mississippi preacher who founded the Coalition for Better Television (read no sex or violence, just "traditional" American values). The typical modus operandi of Wildmon, whose bailiwick is now called the American Family Association, is to threaten to wage economic war with advertisers and networks if they do not disassociate themselves from a particular program. For a revealing look at Wildmon, see Kathryn C. Montgomery, *Target: Prime Time*

gay and lesbian organizations seeking a more positive depiction of plural sexual orientations;[46] minority groups concerned with enhanced depiction of black and Hispanic subjects; the Anti-Defamation League, a group with Jewish roots, and others. One can consider Hollywood a vast field where these groups or their representatives are camped out, seeking to influence the imagery that affects millions of people in the United States and throughout the world.

What is interesting about this form of access is that it moves the process of decisionmaking from the formal political system to a different kind of market. The leverage that is used, often, is the leverage of the consumer. Rather than seeking the intervention of the government to influence programming, the interest group works with the advertiser, or the threat of the advertiser.[47] At times, the group seeks leverage, also, through appeal to the shareholders either in the media corporation or in the businesses which buy advertising on the medium. In essence, the power of the consumer is the voting strength, silent and in temporary abeyance, that will be used to influence the outcome.[48] This is not to say that these pressure groups do not seek

---

154-73 (1989). See also Marvin Kitman, *Best PR Money Can't Buy*, N.Y. Newsday, July 15, 1993, at 89, for a denunciation of Wildmon's crusade against "NYPD Blue", an ABC-TV program purportedly containing saucy language and some nudity. The program had not even been shown yet, and already Wildmon was trying to shut it down.

[46] The highest-profile group working in this area is the Gay and Lesbian Alliance Against Defamation (GLAAD). The group gained national attention in 1992 during its protest against the movie "Basic Instinct," which featured a homicidal lesbian. See Andrea Heiman, *Gay, Lesbian Alliance Honors Image Makers*, L.A. Times, Apr. 13, 1992, at F4; *GLAAD seeks Fox's apology for off-'Color' skit*, Daily Variety, Dec. 22, 1992, at 8.

[47] Donald Wildmon inspired some imitators. A dentist in Fort Worth, Texas, carried out a one-man, but nontheless highly visible, campaign to try to get the "Donahue" talk show moved from the morning to a late-night time slot and get advertisers to stay away from the show because of its provacative program topics. The dentist, Richard Neill, claimed more than 130 advertisers stopped sponsoring the program. Geraldo Rivera's saucy talk show was the target of a similar campaign in Fort Worth by a housewife who claimed 70 advertisers bailed out of that program after she wrote to them. The shows' 9 a.m. time slots were not changed, and the advertiser claims cannot be verified. See Ed Bark, *Phil follows path trod by Geraldo*, The Dallas Morning News, Apr. 14, 1993, at 1C.

[48] The actual effect of these boycotts, threats and protests is unclear. Time has shown it depends on the timidity of the broadcaster, how much money is at stake and how much publicity is garnered. Wildmon, for example, targeted NBC shows for a boycott in 1982, at a time when NBC was running a distant third in the ratings and could ill afford to lose revenue. But still, NBC's profits doubled that year from $48.1 million to $107.9 million. Montgomery, supra note 56, at 171-73.

government involvement as well. Political interest groups certainly seek to create an environment which, to the extent feasible, encourages producers "voluntarily" to accede to their wishes. In the United States, hearings in Congress, speeches by senators and Congressional members all were used to encourage producers and networks to reduce depictions of violence or improve representations of those underrepresented.[49] But these have been the backdrop for consumer actions. It might be recalled that the most effective aspect of McCarthyism, in the 1950's, leading to the blacklisting of a large number of writers and actors, was marshalling of advertisers to bring pressure on radio and television stations and the networks. Once individuals were identified in the newsletter *Red Channels*[50] as risky, a station or network or producer would not take the risk of employing them.

III.   Access and the Public Sphere

This has been a rough taxonomy of historical access alternatives. But there is something tinny about access talk. Access claims in the United States are neither sufficiently grounded in theory nor adequately justified empirically. They reflect a search for an ersatz politics of pluralism; a surface architecture of free speech that combines the trappings of government noninterference with the illusion that narratives - the stories of the good life - are fairly distributed among its tellers. There is a kind of hubris in the fashioning of access doctrine, the shaping and taming and channeling of the massive and unruly forces of opinion and difference in society. Talk of assuring unencumbered access may be a luxury of societies, like the United States, where dissent, for the moment, is not perceived as sedition; not

---

[49]   The four television networks announced in 1993 they would voluntarily post short warning announcements on violent television programs, following intense pressure from Congress, where legislation to regulate violence had repeatedly been threatened. Edmund Andrews, *Mild Slap at TV Violence*, N.Y. Times, July 1, 1993, at A1. But not every lawmaker was pleased, leaving open the continuing specter of legislation, or at the very least, a public relations nightmare for the networks. Rep. John Bryant of Texas called the violence warning "laughable and contemptible." The actual warning reads: "Due to some violent content, parental discretion advised." Robert Jackson, *House Gives TV Plan Mixed Review*, L.A. Times, July 2, 1993, at F1.

[50]   Red Channels championed the 1950's version of "outing," namely unmasking Communists who the magazine believed were masquerading as television and movie stars in Hollywood. See John Cogley, *Report on Blacklisting; Movies* (1956).

in states where the very existence and composition of sovereignty is in a kind of armed equipoise. It is interesting that broadcasting statutes of the transition societies, mirroring the European model, tend to exclude material, from permitted speech, that would stir up racial and national hatreds.

In the United States, as I have suggested, the efforts to produce diversity of ownership or ownership access did not, during the broadcast era, produce meaningful diversity of content. Great store, at least rhetorically, was placed in ownership access, though special steps to create ownership by minority licensees might have been accepted as a way to avoid harsher pressures for programming changes among the industry at large.[51] To the extent there is somewhat greater program diversity, greater breadth of narratives now on American television, one has to look elsewhere. These changes are a result of some combination of the following: a) subtle pressures of the licensing process on television broadcasters; b) what I have called consumer or group access, including the consequences of social and cultural changes over the last decades; and, finally, the marketing changes and programming possibilities occasioned by the combined satellite-cable revolution of the last fifteen years.

The satellite enabled the efficient delivery of competing programming sources to land-based, multi-channel ground distribution sources. The marketing potential of increased channels produced increased diversity for a simple reason: after mainstream subscribers were enrolled, cable entrepreneurs and some broadcasters dependent on cable had an incentive to present programming at the margin that would attract additional subscribers and additional viewers. In the New York cable market, one now can receive not only Black Entertainment Television and several Spanish-language channels but the news from Russia and Poland and programming from Italy, Taiwan, India, Korea and elsewhere.[52] Splintered direct programming, virtually private networks, begin to be introduced as they make economic sense within the present regulatory framework. The new potential of pay-per-view may permit previously ignored audiences to demonstrate the intensity of their desire for special interest programming through collective bidding for time. As

---

[51]   See supra notes 6-11.

[52]   See Susan Spillman, *Warner Cable Breaks Language Barrier*, Electronic Media, June 13, 1988, at 32.

an example, a local system in Manhattan recently offered a cricket Test match for $19.95.[53]

Because most elements of access regulation have been halting, half-way and under-theorized, the yield, as I have suggested, has been relatively unproductive in terms of contribution to democratic dialogue. What we have gotten in the United States is a failing fairness doctrine, clumsy must-carry legislation, a badly conceived and damaging set of rules concerning the political process (with many built in irrationalities). It is important to determine, anew, how the structure of television relates to democratic values and citizenship as a grounding for considering public intervention.

One can argue that modern television - not as an instrument of news and information, but as a blanket aspect of culture and education - is antithetical to citizenship and democratic values. The approach to reform with the most integrity might be the abolition of television, as we know it; but resurrecting print as the dominant mode of communication is probably fantasy.[54] The behemoth of television, in its massive impact, can be construed as belittling treasured differences, mauling history, subverting belief patterns. Provision of access by minorities to their constituencies, or to a larger whole, may merely be a counterfeit counterweight to such an overarching tendency. In a sense, modern television does not pay its own way, one could argue. It eats away at qualities of citizenship, at the capacity to read and analyze, without having those who consume it pay for the costs to society.

More affirmatively, there is the view of television and broadcasting as creating or reinforcing a public sphere. Public discourse is reinvented as media discourse. We are required to ask how access regulation can serve to adapt the medium to increase its function as an auxiliary to the democratic process. Perhaps it is possible to think of the categories of access as a way of groping toward a public sphere: searching not for ethnic and minority representation, but for assurances that

---

[53]   The match was also shown in San Francisco, Los Angeles and other major markets. Peter D. Lambert, *Viewers Choice, Request Find Room for Triplecast,* Broadcasting, May 18, 1992, at 27.

[54]   On the one hand, it is estimated that 62 percent of American adults, or 115 million people, read a newspaper on an average weekday. However, the number of newspapers has fallen 10 percent since World War II. Moreover, between 1970 and 1990, newspaper readership fell 18 percent among women, and 12.5 percent among men. See *Newspapers, Research Alert,* Jan. 1, 1993 (Available in Lexis/Nexis library); James Cox, *Bottom line puts women in focus,* USA Today, Nov. 24, 1992, at 8B.

there exist the conditions of supervision, involvement and discourse necessary for a modern democracy. If elements of the principal agenda of access are to find building blocks of the public sphere, then mechanisms beyond traditional modes of political access must be reviewed. The American 1992 Presidential campaign, for example, suggested some change in terms of the public sphere and the role of the citizen in shaping the public agenda. A combination of telephony, communications technologies such as the fax machine, forms of participatory broadcasting, such as the radio phone-in, new ventures taken together, seemed to be part of a new electronic public sphere.

Modern access doctrines might be adopted, interpreted or evaluated as successors to historical developments in the eighteenth century. This was the period, as Michael Warner has written, of the Republic of Letters,[55] novel ways of using print to provide intercommunication among citizens and the growth of a public sphere. It was not exactly free speech that made modern democracy possible; nor was it exactly the existence of the technology of print. Some magical combination of changed industrial practice and technology were attributes of the new democratic possibilities. Studying the organization of television against the backdrop of the organization of print in the eighteenth century allows us a different way of asking about the relationship of technology to culture. We can harken back to the literature relating the history of print (and its technology and organization) to democracy and transfer that learning to the study, as it were, of television capitalism.

We can hardly reinvent the eighteenth century, and we certainly cannot transplant it into the twentieth. The question is rather what elements of emerging processes with respect to television create a kind of public sphere, a Republic of Letters. To situate radio and television in this discussion of the public sphere is somewhat problematic since these instruments of communication are late developments of democratic societies. Radio was not necessarily the descendant of the newspaper, as opposed to vaudeville and the music hall, though it claims the mantle of succession today. Indeed, there is something about the emergence and history or radio (and later television) that is almost antithetical to the idealized notions of the public sphere. Almost from the beginning, radio was a vehicle of entertainment, a toy, a soother or organizer of the masses rather than a locus for interpersonal rational discourse among individuals dedicated to the public welfare.

---

[55]   Michael Warner, *The Letters of the Republic: Publication and the Public Sphere in Eighteenth Century America* (1990).

And in too many places, in the 1930's, radio, and television after it, became instruments to rearrange loyalties rather than more perfect tools for debating the public good. The new technologies have been a too useful weapon for the sale of goods (or of ideas) for it to be conceptualized as a neutral forum for public discourse.

The public sphere in the twentieth century cannot be described without thinking about the role of radio and television. Over time the electronic media have become so pervasive, so linked to political institutions, so seized with importance that the public sphere cannot be imagined outside of broadcasting. Yet, how vital and how configured is dependent on the overall framework of discourse in a society. Our immediate impulse is to think that broadcasting is actually at the core of a healthy public sphere in modern society. But to determine that is to avoid the process of analysis that may shed light on how debate is conducted. We have yet to see whether broadcasting, at least with respect to the public sphere, is a cheap technological illusion.

IV.   Conclusion: From Micro to Macro Access

I have focused on a taxonomy of internal access issues, what might be called micro access, particularly within the United States. But I should close with some words about access through a more global perspective. One could look at the history of radio and television through the lens of transnational access, but that would be another article. Transnational access has been designed either to expand markets for goods or markets for ideologies and influence. Radio started as a mechanism to get from ship to shore; and among the earliest legal questions was whether and how Great Britain could end transmissions to its people emanating from the Eiffel Tower. International conventions were, in part, mechanisms to limit trans-border terrestrial transmissions. In the 1970's, various bodies connected with the United Nations began debate over access issues against the background of the introduction of the direct broadcast satellite.[56] The principal question was whether external

---

[56]   One approach was advanced in 1973 by the Soviet Union, who espoused the need for a concrete international treaty on the matter. The Soviets also argued that broadcasts to foreign states could only happen with the consent of the receiving country. Nowhere did the Soviets talk about the free flow, or access to, information. At the other end of the spectrum was a more *laissez-faire* plan Canada

programmers of any sort should have access to domestic audiences without the consent of the state.[57]

Transborder access questions are more than domestic access issues writ large. Practical, legal regimes for channeling and limiting access seem increasingly doubtful. Ostankino[58] is transforming itself from the powerful voice of the Soviet Empire to a transnational service serving former Republics and a suddenly dispersed Russian audience. Turkey faces satellite-delivered signals that can threaten constitutional secularism, a more modern equivalent of the Ayatollah Khomeini's audio and video tapes. The United States has decided to merge the Voice of America with its European rivals, Radio Liberty and Radio Free Europe.[59] The BBC has

---

and Sweden collectively released a year earlier. Predictably, an impasse developed between these viewpoints, and efforts toward forging a compromise stalled until 1982, when the United Nations General Assembly adopted *Principles Governing The Use By States of Artificial Earth Satellites for International Direct Television Broadcasting*, G.A. Res. 37/92, U.N. Doc. A./37/646 (1982). However, the DBS principles are in actuality rather weak, as they are only contained in a resolution that fails to satisfactorily resolve the conflict between prior consent (in the name of state sovereignty) and freedom of information. The United States was among thirteen nations voting against the resolution. Since then, the United Nations has failed to bridge what could invariably become a troubling issue. Rita Lauria White and Harold M. White, Jr., *The Law and Regulation of International Space Communication* 246-51 (1988); David I. Fisher, *Prior Consent to International Direct Satellite Broadcasting*, 45-7 (1990). See also Sharon L. Fjordbak, *The International Direct Broadcast Satellite Controversy*, 55 J. Air L. & Com. 903 (1990).

[57]   The European Community has put a different twist on this question through the passage of the Television Without Frontiers Directive, 32 O.J. Eur. Comm. No. L 298/23 (1989). See Laurence G. Kaplan *The European Community's "Television without Frontiers" Directive: Stimulating Europe to Regulate Culture*, Emory Int'l L. Rev. 255 (1994).

[58]   The Russian state broadcasting service.

[59]   Radio Free Europe broadcast to the former Eastern Bloc countries and Baltic states, while Radio Liberty aired in the former Soviet Union. Based in Munich, Germany, both were created in the early 1950's by the Central Intelligence Agency. The fall of Communism and the end of the cold war made these agencies expendable. David Binder, *U.S. to Merge Its International Radio Operations*, N.Y. Times, June 14, 1993, at A16. The latest cutbacks ended RFE broadcasts in all languages except Bulgarian and Romanian. Radio Liberty will continue. *Radio Free Europe Will Drop 7 Languages*, N.Y. Times, June 22, 1993, at A13. Washington-based Voice of America, broadcasts throughout the world to an estimated 100 million listeners in 49 languages, offering news, music and a healthy dose of English lessons. RFE/RL were intended more to be of an alternative to the Soviet propaganda for the countries where the two stations broadcast. Lynne Marek and Marianna Kozintseva, *End of Cold War puts pressure on government broadcasters to justify their existence*, Chi. Trib., May 25, 1993, at 1. See also Malcolm Forbes Jr., *With*

launched a new world television service to compete with CNN.[60] Hungary's new satellite service reaches Hungarian populations outside its borders in a manner that could be perceived to have political overtones. In Britain, the MBC[61] delivers, via satellite and cable, Middle Eastern news and entertainment programming to an intensely loyal audience.

These initiatives present the great, global access questions of the future: Will satellite footprints replace national borders as relevant boundaries of the mind? Will global patterns of access unite ethnics across national borders in ways that challenge existing patterns of sovereignty? Will patterns emerge that allow the unrepresented and the powerless to speak to the whole, or to each other? Will global interconnection be primarily a force for enlarging commercial markets? And finally, can there be a regulated public sphere, a world community of discourse, a fulfillment of the right to information?

all thy getting get understanding, Forbes, June 7, 1993.

[60]   Brian Donlon, *CNN, BBC fight for shares of global news audience*, USA Today, Jan. 12, 1993, at 3D.

[61]   The Middle East Broadcasting Centre, which is London-based and owned by Saudi investors.

THE PUBLIC SPHERE, THE MEDIA AND CIVIL SOCIETY

by Jean L. Cohen

I. Introduction

The concept of the public sphere has been one of the most important focal points around which democratic theory has been renewed in our time.[1] As is well known, it refers to spaces for and processes of open-ended, politically relevant yet autonomous societal communication. Oddly enough, this concept has also been crucial for democratic politics, especially (but not exclusively) in Eastern Europe. What was initially a primarily theoretical revival in the West, stimulated by the impasses of neo-Marxist critical theory and Hannah Arendt's republicanism, took place on the level of the politics of democratic oppositions in East-Central Europe.[2]

Here a crucial paradox manifests itself. In the path of Habermas' theory, the most influential single source of the revival in the West,[3] normative and more importantly, historical reservations about the liberal concept of the public dominated the discussions. In East-Central Europe, however, it was precisely this version of the concept that was revived in the self-understanding of the "alternative" (Poland) or the "second" (Hungary) public spheres, as well as in post-1989 struggles around the media.

There are two ways of addressing this paradox. First, one may wish to argue that because of historical difference of phases, the East European struggles

---

[1]   See Craig Calhoun, ed., *Habermas and the Public Sphere* (MIT Press 1992); Jean L. Cohen and Andrew Arato, *Civil Society and Political Theory* (MIT Press 1992); John Druzek, *Discursive Democracy* (Cambridge University Press 1990); James Fishkin *Deliberative Democracy* (Duke University Press, 1991); Anne Phillips, *Engendering Democracy* (Pennsylvania State University Press, 1991).

[2]   For a discussion of the debates in democratic theory in the West see Cohen and Arato, *Civil Society and Political Theory*, supra note 1, at 4-8.

[3]   J. Habermas, *Strukturwandel der Öffentlichkeit ("The Structural Transformation of the Public Sphere")* (Neuwied: Luchterhand, 1962). This was true even in Hungary where a translation was published in 1971. Here the democratic opposition has understood its central activity in the 1980's as that of building a "second" public sphere. From the late 80's, the Publicity Club has been the most forceful advocate of press and media freedom. The recent translation of the book into English, in 1989, has been an important stimulus to discussions in articles in many journals in the U.S. on democratic theory.

A. Sajó (ed.), Rights of Access to the Media, 29-50.
© 1996 *Kluwer Law International. Printed in the Netherlands.*

against their own version of the authoritarian state merely repeat the experience of anti-absolutist movements of earlier Western history. This argument would imply that we would have to declare the Eastern struggles to be normatively backward and imitative. We would also have to predict the decline of the newly constructed public spheres in line with Western experience. Such seemed to have been the direction in which Habermas himself was initially headed after the transformations of 1989.[4]

Alternately, one may wish to argue a more complex thesis with two parts: first, that the liberal concept is normatively stronger than Habermas himself initially supposed, or rather, that it is capable of being reconstructed in a normatively and institutionally compelling way; and second that the thesis of the unambiguous decline of the public sphere cannot be sustained, even in the West, and thus need not have deterministic consequences for the developments in the East. In this argument both parts are essential: the reaffirmation of the (reconstructed) norm, and the case for its historical possibility.

It is the complex thesis that I wish to argue here. I am not the right person either to evaluate the applicability of the analogy of older Western political experience to the new democracies of East-Central Europe, or to analyze the alternative outcomes of contemporary "media wars" - the struggles around the autonomy of some of the central institutions of the public sphere. What I would like to show, however, through a series of normative and social theoretical considerations, is that the objective of an autonomous public sphere is worthwhile, and that it is not historically (or theoretically) obsolete.

I shall do so in the following steps. After a brief restatement of the normative concept of public space, I shall turn to four key types of criticisms of this conception (normative and empirical) and present my replies to these criticisms. I shall focus primarily on the claims regarding the mass media - in particular I shall try to counter prevalent skepticism as to the possible autonomy and/or critical function that such media can play in post-liberal societies. I will try finally, to sketch a normatively attractive framework which I believe should guide institutional design in this area of public space.

---

[4]   Habermas, *Die nachholende Revolution* (1990).

II. Decline of the Public Sphere?

The concept of the public sphere, of *Öffentlichkeit* refers to a juridically private space where individuals without official status seek to persuade one another through rational argumentation and criticism about matters of general concern.[5] While rational critical discussion is in itself the ideal type of communication of the civil public, however, it has the important additional purpose of controlling and influencing the formation of policy in the juridically public institutions of the state. Moreover, in terms of its (inevitably counter-factual) ideal, the public sphere is universally accessible, inclusive, and freed from deformations due to economic or political power, and social status. The normative conception of rational critical discussion, which Habermas distilled from his analysis of the forms of "social intercourse" and the institutional self-understanding typical of the public sphere as it emerged in 18th century Europe, thus included the principles of individual autonomy, equality of status, parity of discussants,[6] the free and open problematization of previously unquestioned issues that become of common concern, and rational critique.[7]

The historically new type of public analyzed by Habermas is normatively speaking liberal, in that the sets of rights deemed necessary to secure the autonomy of this sphere (freedoms of speech, press, assembly, and communication), together with those dimensions of individual autonomy it presupposes ("privacy rights"),

---

[5]   See Habermas, *The Structural Transformation*, supra note 3, at 1-26.

[6]   Whose "common humanity" formed the basis on which the authority of the better argument could assert itself. Id. at 36 and 85.

[7]   Despite his gloomy assessment of the fate of the bourgeois model of public space, Habermas never altered his allegiance to its underlying normative principles. Indeed, his theory of discourse ethics can be seen as an attempt to construct a philosophically coherent conception of the moral core of the principle of public discourse, in procedural terms. He has reconstructed this core in terms of a moral theory and a theory of democratic legitimacy.

In brief, he argues that a norm of action can be considered legitimate (justified) only if all those possibly affected by it would, as participants in a practical discourse, arrive at an agreement that such a norm should come into or remain in force. The procedural principles underlying the possibility of arriving at such a consensus on the validity of a norm are symmetry, reciprocity, and reflexivity. For a statement of his discourse ethics see J. Habermas, *Discourse Ethics: Notes on a Program of Philosophical Justification in Moral Consciousness and Communicative Action*, 43-115 (MIT Press, 1990).

simultaneously constitute the public and private domains of modern civil society and serve as limits to the reach of state power.[8] Legally separated from the state, this sphere and its members have a polemical, critical, argumentative relation to the polity rather than a directly participatory one. From the point of view of a discursive theory of democratic legitimacy, the public sphere (and all the rights of communication and association)[9] provides the only possible setting in which all concerned can equally participate in the discussion of contested norms and policies. From this normative perspective, collective will formation occurs through the medium of rational unconstrained communication, *with the civil public itself becoming the critical authority vis a vis the genesis of power and the legitimacy of norms.*

Additionally, with this theory of (a democratic) civil society, the public sphere represents the level where the legally framed interaction of groups, associations and movements can both receive its necessary enlightenment concerning public policy, and come to influence policy-formation by thematizing and debating issues of general concern. Finally, from the point of view of parliamentary democracy, the openness of representative bodies to and their continuity with the civil public sphere represents the only source of democratic control over them, and hence a key element of their democratic legitimacy. The representative political public sphere is supposed to be open to the influence of civil society - the themes, issues, debates and public opinion contested and developed in the latter ought in principle to be among those that are taken up by the former. Indeed, the emergence of a new form of unified, depersonalized, bureaucratic public authority, the modern state, is to be checked, supervised, responsive to and controlled by not only the rule of law but also by the emergence of a second politically relevant public sphere

---

[8] See Cohen and Arato, *Civil Society and Political Theory*, supra note 1, at 210-254 for a full discussion of Habermas' theory of the public sphere.

[9] See generally Cohen and Arato, *Civil Society and Political Theory*, supra note 1, for a discussion of the double character of "civil rights"- many of which preserve both individual autonomy and privacy as well as publicity.

I am thinking for example of freedom of association - crucial to the formation of parties, interest groups, or unions, all of which face and seek to participate in power, political or economic. But freedom of association is also crucial to private individuals who wish to form clubs, voluntary associations, intimate associations etc. Here what is protected is private and civil as distinct from political forms of group life. A similar point can be made regarding the doubleness of other rights such as freedom of conscience and speech.

(within society and penetrating the state in the form of parliaments) that challenges *raison d'etat* as well as *arcana imperii*. Thus, the civil politically-oriented public, a dimension of the public sphere rooted in the communication processes of civil society which penetrate the state through the legislature, is the most important mediation between the citizenry and its elected officials in a constitutional democracy.[10]

There are four lines of criticism that are directed at this conceptual model. First, beyond Habermas' concession of the actual historical limits of access to the public sphere,[11] it has been argued that the very concept of the *liberal* public, including the emphasis on rational speech, deliberation and discourse, along with the separation of the public and the private implies exclusion, hierarchy and inequality.[12] Second, following Carl Schmitt and even extending his argument, it has been maintained that liberal democratic parliaments do not now, or never did, even minimally satisfy the conditions of rational deliberation and attempted persuasion. Instead, liberal parliaments are dominated by party discipline as well as backroom, non-public negotiation that reduces public deliberation to mere show. Thus, with the rise of modern party systems, parliaments are not extensions of a societal public, rather they involve political processes entirely discontinuous with societal discussion and debate. Third, both Schmitt, Habermas and their followers have all claimed that with state interventionism into all spheres of society, and assumption of public functions by corporate, private bodies whose internal processes and interactions are not exposed to public scrutiny, the autonomous space *between* the state and private life is eliminated. Accordingly, far from influencing or indirectly controlling the political public sphere of the state, developments outside

---

[10]   Of course, one ought not forget that there is also the bourgeois dimension of the new public sphere. The new public analyzed by Habermas in *Structural Transformation* is bourgeois because in it independent owners of property, divided in their competitive, egoistic economic activities that have grown vastly beyond the limits of the household, deem themselves capable of generating, at least in principle, a collective will through the medium of rational, unconstrained communication. The original limitation of access to the newly emerging public sphere to the propertied and the educated, attest to its bourgeois character.

[11]   Habermas, *Structural transformation*, supra note 3, at 37.

[12]   See Nancy Fraser, *Rethinking the Public Sphere: A Contribution to the Critique of Actually Existing Democracy*, and Sheyla Benhabib, *Models of Public Space: Hannah Arendt, the Liberal Tradition and Jürgen Habermas, in Habermas and the Public Sphere*, supra note 1. See also Iris Young, *Justice and the Politics of Difference*, Ch. 4 and 6 (Princeton University Press, 1990).

the civil public sphere have allegedly led to its disappearance. Fourth, in the path of the older Frankfurt school, it has been repeatedly argued that the massification, commodification, and industrialization of culture, especially dominant in the electronic media, transforms the medium of social communication in such a way that individual response becomes distracted, passive and uncritical, easily manipulable through advertising techniques and political propaganda. Thus, the space for a critical, autonomous, and influential civil public sphere is also destroyed from within. I would like to briefly deal with each of these arguments.

1. The fact that historical exclusion from the public sphere has operated not only through differences in wealth and education (i.e. class differences) but also through gender, ethnic, racial and regional differences does not alter the normative context or core principle of publicity analyzed by Habermas. The legitimacy of the public sphere is tied up with its potential for inclusion, and the existence of the public sphere as the central context of democratic access calls for programs of inclusion.

> "[T]he public sphere of civil society stood or fell with the principle of universal access. A public sphere from which specific groups would be eo ipso excluded was less than merely incomplete; it was not a public sphere at all. Accordingly the public that might be considered the subject of the bourgeois constitutional state... anticipated in principle that all human beings belong to it."[13]

Thus, formal legal guarantees (equal rights) together with mechanisms for the facilitation of equality of access to the public sphere such as public education, civil and social rights, affirmative action, provisions for child care, policies supporting alternative cultural forms of expression etc., become all the more important in relationship to a functioning public sphere.

As for the essentialistic objection that the very processes of rational, critical public discussion and deliberation favor one particular class, race, ethnic group or gender, I would argue that this claim defames just those whom the argument wishes to protect. To be sure, by enshrining a particular form of discourse, a particular style of argumentation, a particular understanding of what is appropriate rhetoric, or a particular body-language as the only acceptable form of public speech, dominant groups can indeed silence those who are no longer de jure or even de facto excluded from the public sphere, yet who differ in important ways from those who have

---

[13]   Habermas, *Structural Transformation*, supra note 3, at 85.

previously had privileged access to it. But such would clearly be a deformation of the normative principle of public discourse rather than its expression.

The related objection, that the stress on the public sphere privileges intellectuals or experts, is itself based on the fallacious assumption that intellectuals are themselves a class. In reality, in modernity, all classes, ethnic groups, regions, races and sexes always had and will have their intellectuals. Indeed, the general civil public is not *per se* specialized in esoteric language games (typical of specialized publics such as the public of science, high art, or academia). Rather, it operates through levels of communicative interaction for which mastery of a natural language suffices, because it is tailored to the general comprehensibility of everyday communicative practice. To be sure, the civil public, especially if one has the mass media in mind, involves the virtual rather than the actual presence of readers, listeners, and viewers. This virtual presence entails context generalization and growing anonymity. On the one side, this is what allows for greater inclusion, on the other, it also has an intellectualizing effect. Nevertheless, the latter need not entail the esoteric use of specialized codes or technical vocabularies. Instead, the orientation of the civil public sphere to lay persons implies the redifferentiation or rather the retranslation of special technical vocabularies back into ordinary language and the general elevation of the intellectual level of comprehension of all concerned.

While it is true that access to centralized *electronic* media in complex societies requires accumulated resources of money, power and influence, this is not the case for other forms of the civil public nor even for the print media. I shall return to the issue of access to electronic media below. For the present, let me make the more general point that the issue of access/exclusion can be defused if one abandons a unitary conception of the public sphere in favor of a pluralistic model. In other words, I would build on an early proposal of Habermas, and argue that the very norms of publicity in a modern society imply the pluralization of public fora, in the sense of cultural, civil and political publics.[14] *Indeed, the most effective way to parry the charge of constitutive exclusiveness is to argue that the normative principle of publicity has an elective affinity (Wahlverwandtschaft) with a multiplicity of public spaces and a plurality of types of publics.*

---

[14]   In his most recent work on the subject Habermas has begun to stress the multiplicity and plurality of types of publics, having accepted the general outlines of our theory of civil society. See *Facticity and Validity*, Ch. 8, 60 (in particular) and 50-60 generally (MIT). (page citations refer to the previously unpublished English manuscript).

Only a unitary and monistic conception of public space would perforce have to involve exclusion. Let me explain. That there was always a multiplicity of publics in modern civil society is hardly a new idea.[15] But few have stressed the plurality of types of publics. I have in mind two types of pluralization: functional and segmental. Functionally distinct publics are necessarily specialized and tend to be esoteric. The publics of science, politics, religion, art, the various academic disciplines, etc. are of this sort.

But this is not true of segmental pluralization, which can be conceived of in two complementary forms. The first refers to the multiplicity of publics that develop in the milieu of social movements, voluntary associations, interest groups, clubs, etc. which are not functionally differentiated yet are limited in purpose and scope. On this level, there can be as many civil publics as there are groups that generate issues of common concern to their members. The second aspect involves what I would like to call a non-specialized, civil "public of publics" that allows for the communicative interaction of members of different functional spheres or social groups. It is crucial to see that alongside the myriad publics of a differentiated and pluralist society there is a general civil public - and here I have in mind the disincorporated society-wide forms of public communication which, though incapable of decisional power, can influence political publics specialized in decision-making as well as the more specialized civil publics.

The history of social movements has shown that the influence of the open-ended processes of communication in a civil public of this amorphous type (itself in turn influenced by the discourses of specific publics) can be far reaching both for collective learning and indirectly for the generation of policy. As Habermas has recently pointed out,[16] all partial publics constituted by ordinary language remain porous for each other, as does the abstract public sphere of readers, listeners, and viewers scattered around the national society and brought together through the mass media. I shall return to the relation of the mass media to this general society wide public of publics in a moment. My point here is to show that when interpreted in terms of multiplicity and plurality of forms and locii, the liberal concept of the public need not be associated with exclusion or silencing of particular groups. If it

---

[15] Here Habermas' critics are simply wrong when they argue that he assumed there was only one unitary public sphere in *Structural Transformation of the Public Sphere*. See Nancy Fraser, and Iris Young, supra note 12.

[16] Habermas, *Facticity and Validity*, supra note 14 at 60-61.

took this form in the past, this was due to the bourgeois, not the liberal character of the public sphere examined by Habermas.

2. In my view, Habermas' early work did not go far enough in distinguishing political from civil/cultural publics because it remained under the influence of republican conceptions of public space.[17] While cultural and civil communication processes remain open-ended and in principle unconstrained if fundamental freedoms are not violated, evidently the political public sphere of parliament, even before the origin of modern political parties, always involved temporal, formal and substantive limitations of free and open ended discussion. The existence of powerful, non-public processes of the executive administration that always penetrated law making bodies implied further limitations on what the deliberative process could directly accomplish. Admittedly, the coming of modern parties, parliamentary discipline, and the structure of committee negotiations further limited the opportunities for free discussion, and the possibility of its direct influence on policy making. But understanding that the parliamentary public sphere could not fulfill the same norms of openness and unconstrained communication, even ideally, as the civil, cultural, reasoning public, saves us from overreacting to these changes brought on by the party system.

The danger of overreaction is that it could lead to a fundamentalist rejection of party politics as *per se* inimical to democracy. We should note instead that parliamentary publicity did not disappear as modern parties came to dominate the

---

[17] Hence, his own ambiguities concerning the problem whether the public of civil society exercises power, or only controls and influences the holders of power. In his most recent text on the topic, however, Habermas has adopted mine and Arato's position contained in *Civil Society and Political Theory*, which stresses the role of the civil public in influencing and indirectly (through its effect on political society) controlling the holders of power, but not in exercising power. Following our lead, Habermas has come to recognize the importance of the category of influence to democratic theory. He has seen that it is not just through the general debate and discussion of norms and policies that an abstracted public of communication "controls" political society and generates democratic legitimacy.

In addition, it is through the mobilization of concerned groups into movements and collective actions, including acts of civil disobedience, that influence can be exercised by civil on political actors. "Strong publics" or actors exercising political decision-making and power can of course proliferate throughout society through the decentralization and the division of "sovereignty" along various lines. These decentered political publics can exercise counter-powers vis a vis the centralized holders of state power, as well as exercising influence in their own right. But they differ in kind from the civil publics I have been discussing. Unfortunately, I cannot go into this further here. But see Cohen and Arato, *Civil Society and Political Theory*, supra note 1, at Ch. 8, and Habermas, *Facticity and Validity*, supra note 14, at Ch. 8.

scene, and in a sense became even more important than before. When party discipline very much reduces the likelihood of rational persuasion in debates within parliament, the same debates undergo a change of function. Their role is now to address the extra-parliamentary public first and foremost, informing it and asking for the approval of rationally defended policies or of opposition to them. Thus, in contemporary contexts, parliamentary argument operates through the wider circuit of societal communication and attempted persuasion. The constraint of the better argument has a chance to be effective through persuading the electoral public, whose control function becomes more important at a time when persuasive discourse by no means automatically carries the day in parliament itself. Without additional arguments, it remains unpersuasive to claim, as did Schmitt, that the appeal in parliamentary debates to extra-parliamentary publics is merely a call for plebiscitary approval.

3. The undeniable trends toward state interventionism and corporatism have certainly reduced the political importance of terrains of consequential public communication. The point is not so much that the private and the public are so fused that any space between them actually disappears.[18] Rather, as economic, cultural, family, and welfare policy become provinces of the state administration and of large private associations dealing with one another in specifically non-public forms of interaction, the significance of public discussions decline. Thus, the control function retained with respect to the open processes of legislation, loses its meaning in relation to bureaucratic and corporatist processes that are closed to open scrutiny. Nevertheless, the survival of the norms of publicity create legitimation problems for both state interventionism and corporatist interest representation.

Unlike the apparently spontaneous results of the market, state action that produces differential outcomes calls for more and more explicit justification of the actions of the executive. Intervention has been thus coupled with the growth of social demands on the state. Even the return to neo-liberal economic policies has not reduced the increasing social scrutiny of the internal dealings, arrangements and decisional processes of the executive. And while neo-corporatist arrangements do reduce some of the excess demand on the state, and are acceptable to the members of influential groups, they remain illegitimate from the point of view of all those

---

[18]   Hence the mechanical and spatial dimensions of the fusion argument are certainly untenable. See Cohen and Arato, *Civil Society and Political Theory*, supra note 1, at 247, 308-309.

who are inevitably excluded. Demands for the democratization and publicization of bargaining processes, as well as the self-organization of civic initiatives and movements thrive precisely where neo-corporatism has been the strongest.

4. Finally, the acceptance of the Frankfurt thesis on the culture industry, according to which the democratization of culture and communication is merely pseudo-democratization of something that is no longer either culture or real communication, would mean that the classical literary public splits into "a minority of reasoning no longer-public experts, and the great mass of public consumers".[19] Even more important, it would also mean that in such a context political communication can remain effective and competitive only if it imitates the techniques of advertising and "public relations". Propaganda - the advertising and selling of political leaders, parties, and policies - presupposes, and is required by, already formed, passive, uncritical, privatized yet mobilizable audiences.

Under these circumstances, what goes under the heading of public opinion would not really be public opinion in the normative sense. For what makes opinion public, what makes its influence legitimate is, *au fond*, the way it comes about and the broad agreement it expresses.[20] But once propaganda techniques predominate in the media of communication, once issues are chosen and agendas are set "from above" by small circles of the powerful and/or the rich, once public debate and critical discussion disappear from the generalized media of communication, the public opinion that is measured by opinion polls or "expressed" on talk shows cannot be considered autonomous or of any normative weight. It is simply a statistical aggregate of singly solicited and privately expressed individual opinions, normatively indistinguishable from survey results. Such "opinion" is, in short, no longer the product of a public debate in which peers can have an influence on one another's way of seeing things through rational argument, arrive at an agreement on key principles and therefore *legitimately* exercise influence on the powers that be.

---

[19]   Habermas, *Structural Transformation*, supra note 3, at 175.

[20]   The formal criteria (procedural principles) governing how a qualified public opinion comes about is articulated on the most abstract level by Habermas in his theory of discourse ethics. But more concretely one might argue that the rules of a shared practice of communication which is egalitarian and symmetric in principle, are what allow for agreement on topics and norms - agreement which develops as the result of an exhaustive public debate in which proposals, information, and reasons can be more or less rationally worked through.

This argument is especially serious, because if it were fully compelling, it would remove the ground from my replies to arguments 2 and 3 above. Even if the existence of an open, unconstrained public sphere outside of parliament linked to the more restricted deliberative forms of the legislature could rehabilitate the liberal and democratic claims on behalf of political publicity, the elimination of a reasoning, critical public by the modern media would effectively end this possibility. This is because the normative thrust of the public media, and of the general civil public, would be completely undermined. If the general public of publics neither can nor will reason critically because its "organs"- the mass media - have been structurally transformed in the epoch of organized capitalism such that their critical thrust is blunted, then neither the increased range and effectiveness of the media nor even the multiplication of chances to have access to them (the future promises 500 tv stations) would make much difference.[21] Accordingly, if elections were now organized in such a way as to reward only those who replace the rational presentation of programs most effectively by advertising techniques, a crucial sanctioning link between parliamentary and public discussions would disappear. If, in other words, one could sell a candidate to the voters on the basis of the right advertising techniques, irrespective of the positions he and his party argued for in parliament, it would be senseless to claim that parliamentary debates still have a rational function. Similarly, neither the public scrutiny of the executive, nor the discourse of new movements and civic initiatives could rehabilitate public life, if the very media of public information and communication were deformed by an all pervasive logic of commodification. There would be no possibility for the self-enlightenment of the public through the general airing of views in the media if issues, approaches, attitudes and concerns are pre-packaged and determined on the basis of non-neutral

---

[21]   This is the thesis succinctly stated in page 188 of Habermas's *Structural Transformation*. Beyond the stage of commodification, the mass media in late capitalism are penetrated by societal, yet private interests (individual or collective) such that the very debates, topics, and forms of discussion shaped by these rather than generated by an autonomous public of private persons:
"[A]ccording to the liberal model of the public sphere, the institutions of the public engaged in rational-critical debate were protected from interference by public authority by virtue of their being in the hands of private people. To the extent that they were commercialized and underwent economic, technological and organizational concentration, however, they have turned during the last hundred years into complexes of societal power, so that precisely their remaining in private hands in many ways threatened the critical functions of publicist institutions". Id.

extrinsic considerations such as the maximization of profit, or of the power of political parties.

III.   Public, State and Market(s)

Thus, our overall argument converges on the problem of the media of communication. If the interpretation along the lines of the Frankfurt School were correct, it would throw a great deal of doubt on any effort seeking to reconstruct the liberal public sphere today (irrespective of the normative rationale for doing so). Habermas stood in that tradition when he wrote his seminal work on the topic. He was thus was unable to go beyond a species of *Verfallsgeschichte*, to which the term *Strukturwandel* in the end reduces. It is otherwise with Habermas as the author of *The Theory of Communicative Action* ("TCA"),[22] as well as with my collaborative work with Andrew Arato, *Civil Society and Political Theory*, which builds on Habermas's methodological foundations. Indeed, in *TCA*, Habermas became skeptical of his own thesis on the liquidation of the essence of the public sphere in postliberal societies, insisting instead on the "ambivalent potential" of the mass media.[23] It is on the basis of this new framework that I wish to respond to the

---

[22]   In his most recent book, *Facticity and Validity*, Habermas develops the analysis of the media begun in *Theory of Communicative Action* on the basis of a synthesis of the theoretical framework developed in that book, with the analysis of myself and Andrew Arato of civil society. See *Theory of Communicative Action*, Vol. 2, chapter 8 (1989).

[23]   He revises his assessment because of two key theoretical developments in his work: the differentiated analysis of communicative interaction itself, and a more sophisticated analysis of the two-sided character of the institutional framework of modern societies. With respect to the first, the new argument is based on the insight that unlike the "steering media" of money and power, which uncouple the coordination of action from building consensus in language altogether and which substitute for discursive interaction, the generalized forms of communication do not replace reaching an agreement in language but merely condense it and thus remain tied to lifeworld contexts.

The mass media belong to these generalized forms of communication. They free communication processes from the provinciality of spatiotemporally restricted contexts and permit public spheres to emerge, through establishing the abstract simultaneity of a virtually present network of communication contents far removed in space and time and through keeping messages available for manifold contexts. Their ambivalent potential lies in the fact that they both hierarchize (and select) contents while removing restrictions on the horizon of possible communication. Habermas, *Theory of Communicative Action*, supra note 22. The key point here is

fourth argument (whose successful refutation as we have seen is a precondition of the validity also of the answers given to the previous two arguments).

Let me first indicate where the public sphere fits into our own framework. Like Habermas, we operate with a three part conception of lifeworld, and two media steered subsystems, the political and the economic systems. We understand civil society as the institutional dimension of the lifeworld, composed of family, associations and the public sphere (the lifeworld conversely is the socio-cultural substratum of the reproduction of civil society). Unlike Habermas, we postulate political and economic society between civil society and each of the subsystems, representing institutional frameworks where ordinary language communication processes coexist with forms of interaction steered by money or power.

The public dimension of parliamentary bodies for example is a part of political society that is necessarily constrained by the logic of administration, but which preserves to an important extent the communication structures (patterns of argumentation, criteria of validity, standards of respect and civility etc.) of the public of civil society which remains its cultural presupposition. If the civil public remains the reason why argument and debate are both possible and necessary in the political public, the latter (the political public) is still the precondition of the political influence of the former (and of civil society as a whole).

In this framework one can speak neither of a fusion between civil society (lifeworld) and the state, nor of the total commodification of civil society. Such a conception, aside form the weaknesses of the metaphor itself, presupposes a much too passive lifeworld, without important resources of its own. But forms of communication, solidarity, and personality in everyday life are just such resources. While administration and economic rationality can *colonize* the lifeworld and take over or replace some of its processes of reproduction by the logic of money or power, they cannot completely do so without provoking the cultural and social psychological dysfunction of society, and/or organized forms of resistance. At the limit such a reduction would imply dedifferentiation, and the end of the affectivity of the economy and the state as modern frameworks of interaction. Thus, a genuinely modern state establishes forms of self-limitation, such as rights, also for

---

that they are no longer seen by Habermas as by definition reified tools of the culture industry. For a discussion of the doubleness of modern institutions, see id. at Ch. 8.

its own sake.[24] It is important to note finally that colonization of the lifeworld by state and market can be seen as two competing processes. However, opposing one with the other leads only to a different form of colonization, not its abolition.

This last point should be made more precise, because state interventionism into the lifeworld, when direct, has a different logic than any type of commercialization or commodification. The motivational bases of direct state control of culture (societal communication) is always in part a negative sanction, linked to fear. In the context of governmental control of the media or under censorship and especially under the conditions of a police state, the creators and disseminators of culture face direct or implicit orders whose violation leads to specific punishments (ranging from demotion to imprisonment). Such power is inescapable, and the individual cannot turn to a competitor for better treatment.

Interestingly, the addressees of propaganda, unlike those of advertisement are also more manipulable in terms of their fears than their hopes. Direct state intervention into the media, both its creation and reception, has always the friend-enemy logic of authoritarian politics. And yet the ability of such intervention to streamline society and culture is limited; only by terroristic means can this form of intervention fully eliminate older or newly emerging competitive cultural forms. The potential of administration to produce new cultural meanings is notoriously weak. The affectivity of such cultural creation depends in fact of the ability of a state-party to mobilize existing, autonomous forms for its own purposes, a project more successful under nationalist than under communist dictatorships for obvious reasons.

Commodification of the lifeworld, of cultural life, operates through positive rather than negative sanctions. Having a homogenous medium at its disposal, namely money, economic markets require only one outcome of creators and disseminators of culture: monetary success. Having diverse markets to address, such outcome permits alternative solutions. While one cannot be an artist fully obeying a censor who punishes precisely autonomy, the market can reward both the genuine creator and the hack under given conditions, even those who work for great cultural *apparati*, can potentially offer their services to competitors or try their hands at small entrepreneurship. To be sure, the big *apparati* that greatly reduce competition among the producers of culture do industrialize rather than merely commodify

---

[24]   This assessment of the limits to reification is what distinguishes Habermas' conceptual framework as well as his evaluation of the mass media, among other institutions, from his early work on the public sphere.

culture. This means not merely that the market success is a precondition of cultural success, which would entail only the supplementation of cultural production by a sales or advertising effort, but that marketability becomes from the outset the principle of production.

Here, as elsewhere, the big firms do not only respond to market signals, but are able to structure the markets themselves. Nevertheless, as the existence of thriving counter-cultures show, the industrial producers of culture never have the field fully to themselves. All analogous options would tend to transgress the line to illegality under consistent state control of culture. Illegality and repression cut off culture at the roots, while lack of economic success punishes only deviant results with sanctions that members of counter cultures and *avant-gardes*, always far more numerous than political dissidents under stable authoritarian regimes, are willing to pay. Finally, while authoritarian rule is notoriously unable to base its cultural production on contemporary autonomous creation, the cultural industry has always relied on the integration of the most advanced forms and techniques.

At the same time, commodification of culture, by permitting some autonomy and working through positive sanctions, penetrates deeper into human motivation than colonization by the state. Whereas the rigid following of orders in a hierarchical structure of command is daily proven absurd under conditions of a modern industrial society (hence success always involves a precarious, and secret violation of rules), market-oriented strategic action is functional and leads to success. Possessive individualism and civil privatism provide for a space of independence where the individual can cultivate his or her specific interests, inclinations and forms of personality.

Cultural autonomy within the limits of economic success does not exclude creativity. But, and this is the point that remains valid in the challenge of the older Frankfurt school, such creativity takes place at the margins, while the cultural life of large majorities remains apparently centralized, homogeneous, coordinated, and open to strategic manipulation. For most people, privatism means to be receivers of prepackaged information, rather than the to have the chance to be creative in niches of autonomy. Under such conditions we need not be surprised, that so many elements of Habermas' 1962 depiction of electoral politics as a sales, advertising, and public relations effort rings as true as ever 30 years later.

And yet new media research has forced an abandonment of some of the crucial elements of the diagnosis. In 1981 Habermas presented the following catalog of factors not taken into account in the original Frankfurt thesis:

1.   the difficulty of integrating competing interests (political, economic, aesthetic) in broadcast networks;

2.   the conflicting imperatives of journalistic ethics and network interests;

3.   the penetration of competing messages through the appropriation of autonomous and popular culture;

4.   the reinterpretation of ideological messages in the context of specific subcultures;

5.   the hostile response of everyday communication to attempts at direct manipulation; and

6.   the development of new media technologies opens up possibilities for both decentralized, as well as centralized forms of communication. [25]

Habermas, rightly, does not consider these factors sufficient reason to entirely disregard the original Frankfurt diagnosis, but only to reintegrate it in an two-sided analysis pointing to contradictions and ambiguities. The large scale, industrial production of culture retains its centralizing and homogenizing logic, but as the list above reveals, there are important countervailing tendencies. This is also the case with political colonization of the media. To be sure, it remains true that in a society with a market economy that has deeply penetrated cultural communication, political entrepreneurs do learn to use commercialized patterns of expectation for the sake of delivering their message, selling their parties and policies. Indeed, with Germany in mind, Habermas argues that it depends entirely on the legal organizational form and the institutional establishment whether television companies are more open to the influence of parties and associations or to private firms with large advertising outlays.

It would nevertheless be intriguing to repeat Habermas' list in this context as well: political sales efforts could have many of the same limits as the propagation

---

[25]   Habermas, *Theory of Communicative Action*, supra note 22, at 390-391.

of ideology by the cultural industry. But there is one crucial difference in this context. While the forms of resistance to cultural manipulation do yield some measure of autonomy, resistance to political manipulation may not yield an alternative politics but only a turn away from this sphere altogether in terms of privatism, apathy, and anti-political forms of protest. Political sales efforts do not have to completely succeed in order to be successful in general: the votes of the non-voters are not counted, and the political entrepreneurs can generally mete out the votes of the rest.

Much depends in fact on the strength, the institutional supports, and the strategies behind the countervailing tendencies. But a lot also depends on which normative model of the media one operates with when one devises such strategies. Recall that despite the tendency of political and economic colonization of the media to foster the depoliticizaiton of public communication, the effects of the media remain uncertain. The wealth of empirical investigations does not permit a definitive answer to the question of how autonomous the position-taking of the public is as a result of these distortions of the electronic media. Habermas thus suggests that insofar as we engage in empirical studies, we direct our attention to the "strategies of interpretation" employed by viewers. For, "[e]ven if we know something about the importance and operation of the mass media and about the distribution of roles among public and various actors, and even if we can make some reasonable conjectures about who has power in the media, it is by no means clear how the mass media intervene in the unsurveyable circle of communication in the political public sphere."[26]

But such empirical studies would have to be at least implicitly guided by a normative preunderstanding of how the media and the civil public should interrelate. Thus, it remains worthwhile to develop a normative conception of how the media

---

[26]   Habermas, *Facticity and Validity*, supra note 14, at 71-72. Habermas points out that many of the great themes of the last decade - ranging from issues of ecology, nuclear energy, large-scale technological projects, genetic engineering, feminist concerns, problems of immigration, etc. - were initially brought up not by exponents of the state apparatus, large organizations, or socio-functional sub-systems, but rather by actors in the civil public. Thus, at least in perceived crisis situations, the civil public is able to get the media to listen and to place its concerns on the "public agenda". That this may require spectacular collective actions on the part of the civil public, including incessant campaigns, pass protests and even civil disobedience does not obviate the basic point. The influence of the civil on the media public is in principle possible, according to Habermas, because the principle that the players in the arena owe their influence to the assent of those in the gallery, is built into the internal structure of every public sphere (in a democratic society) including the normative self-understanding of the mass media.

ought to work. Accordingly, in his latest text, Habermas provides us with another list, this time enumerating the tasks that the media ought to fulfill in constitutional political systems:

1. surveillance of the socio-political environment, reporting developments likely to impinge, positively or negatively on the welfare of citizens;

2. meaningful agenda-setting;

3. platforms for an illuminating advocacy by politicians and spokespersons of other causes and interest groups;

4. dialogue across a diverse range of views, as well as between power-holders and mass publics;

5. mechanisms for holding officials accountable for how they exercised power;

6. incentives for citizens to learn, choose, and become involved;

7. a principled resistance to the efforts of forces outside the media to subvert their independence; and

8. a sense of respect for the audience.[27]

These principles ought to orient both the professional code of journalism and the laws governing mass communication. The regulative idea that they express, which complements the concept of democratic politics is simple:

> "[T]he mass media ought to understand themselves as the agent of an enlightened public whose willingness to learn and capacity for criticism the media simultaneously presuppose, demand, and reinforce; like the judiciary, they ought

---

[27] Habermas, *Facticity and Validity*, supra note 14, at 66 I have abridged this list slightly. Habermas has taken the list from M. Gurevitch and G. Blumler, *Political Communication Systems and Democratic Values in Democracy and the Mass Media* 270 (J. Lichtenberg, ed. 1990).

to preserve their independence from political and social actors . . . to look after the public's concerns and proposals in an impartial manner and, in light of these topics and contributions, submit the political process to a course of legitimation and intensified critique."[28]

The power of the media would thus be neutralized in that the conversion of administrative or social power into political-publicist influence would be blocked.

It is this normative understanding that undergirds our approach to the problem of bringing the power of the media under control and avoiding both political and economic colonization. Our theory points to two false roads which those seeking to oppose the colonization of the public sphere and its media of communication might be tempted to take. Some of the most strident critics of the tendencies toward commodification, manipulation through advertisement, and replacement of artistic with market values typical of a commercialized culture, call for state control of the media, as the appropriate solution. This was the implication of cultural criticism as practiced by the socialists historically, and today's nationalist - radicals rarely hide their corresponding intentions.

As we have seen through ample historical experience, however, this road leads to deadening governmental controls in the form of censorship or other types of softer pressure, with the result that both the cultural and political publics are seriously deformed. Evidently, the political process can be damaged even under a democratic government when ruling parties or coalitions control information about themselves and their competitors. But the solution proposed above to commodification would inevitably lead in this direction.

Because of the different consequences of "commodification" and "governmentalization" the second false road that attacks authoritarian controls over culture and publicity in the name of full privatization or marketization seems initially preferable. But its advocates are wrong (and, in face of the statist critics, imprudent) to close their eyes to all the negative phenomena of commercialization. In fact the advocates of both roads are similar to the extent that their uncompromising criticism of each other leads them to absolutize their own option. Such a posture in turn leads to the mistaken identification of alternatives that are neither statist nor purely market-oriented as "collectivist" by the liberals, and as "liberal" by the statists.

And there are such options, both in our theory of civil society and in empirical experience. Beginning with the recognition that in a complex, modern

---

[28]   Habermas, *Facticity and Validity*, supra note 14, at 67.

society cultural life cannot do without both economic resources and outputs of the political system (money and legal regulation) we nevertheless need to focus on institutions of large scale communication whose logic is neither that of commodification nor of administration. Both money and law can be used to allow institutions to become relatively independent of the economic and political systems. Our best models for such independence are cultural foundations, universities and public service forms of broadcasting.

While there are plenty of examples of institutions of this type being themselves penetrated by political and commercial criteria, we generally consider such forms of penetration to be pathological and inconsistent with the mission of the institutions. On the level of remedies, it is evident that methods of funding and legal regulation can be devised that would simultaneously maintain the political and economic independence of cultural institutions along with their openness to the variety of interests, associations, cultural and life forms of civil society. The media that were funded by such institutions would thus be able to serve the normative role outlined above, that is, to foster and help develop a critical civil public able, hopefully to influence political publics.

Of course, it would be utopian to imagine that under present conditions, media and cultural institutions rooted in civil society could largely displace commercially or government based forms. Indeed, even if it became more prevalent, I do not believe that it would be normatively desirable for the public service option to entirely displace privately-owned or state-controlled media. There is no better reason to absolutize this form of media any more than either of the other two. Instead, I would argue for the importance of all three ways of structuring the media for the simple reason that a plurality of forms ensures a healthy competition among the various types such that stultification is less likely. On its own, each form tends to be deformed and to succumb to special interests. The presence of other forms would not only increase the chances for technological innovation, it would also tend to make each type of media more responsive to the other and to society at large.[29]

---

[29]   This is obvious in the case of the presence of privately-owned media where the impetus to innovation is strongest. But even in the case of state-run media, it is hard to find a convincing argument against the mere existence of a state-run channel on television or radio. While the dangers are obvious, the claim that the state too needs its voice, to ensure an airing of its own assessment and justification of important policy decisions is certainly not to be rejected out of hand.

Nevertheless, in all likelihood, in most countries, civil society-based cultural institutions are going to remain in a minority. But their significance should not thereby be underestimated. In the context of civic initiatives and movements these institutions (as it happened in the case of ecology, feminism, etc.) give a national voice to particular constituencies that allows them to become effective if the needs addressed are universal enough. Moreover as we have seen both in the case of state-controlled and heavily commercialized publics, the emergence, and even temporary stabilization of alternative publics or forms of cultural transmission present the dominant public with competition to which it must respond by in part altering its own substance (e.g., C-Span in the U.S.; alternative publics in Hungary and Poland).

It is impossible to tell *a priori* whether such competition would lead to disappearance of the alternative form and things going back to "normal", or to the longer term alteration of the dominant form along with the coexistence of its alternative. Again, much would depend on the forms of legal regulation, available economic resources, and social pressures supporting the older forms. Only adequate, many levelled support for cultural institutions rooted in civil society, would in the long term justify Adorno's secret hope that, in spite of his own culture industry thesis, the rate of the growth of intelligence of people may very well be rising at a faster rate than the attempts to reduce them to stupidity.[30]

---

[30]   Adorno & Horkheimer, *Dialectic of Enlightenment* 145 (1975).

CHAPTER II

ACCESS TO THE MEDIA IN EUROPE AND IN THE UNITED STATES

FREE SPEECH, EQUALITY AND MINORITY
ACCESS TO THE MEDIA IN THE UNITED STATES

by Michel Rosenfeld

I.   Introduction

A broad range of diverse viewpoints must find access to the electronic media as a precondition to the realization of democratic self-government in a contemporary society. Such access, however, is not easily achieved, even in societies where the state does not control or dominate broadcasting. For example, in the United States, where an overwhelming majority of broadcasting outlets are in private hands, minority - and in particular African-American - viewpoints have been historically grossly underrepresented over the electronic airwaves. Moreover, not only have minority viewpoints been largely absent in American broadcasting, but portrayals of minorities on American radio and television have tended to be negative and stereotypical.[1] Accordingly, free competition in the economic marketplace by no means assures suitable access to the electronic marketplace of ideas for a broad range of diverse viewpoints. As neither state control nor unrestrained market competition are likely to yield a genuinely free marketplace of ideas in broadcasting, this calls for an alternative scheme of regulation which is better suited to generate the requisite viewpoint diversity. One such alternative scheme of regulation, based on a blending of government regulation with reliance on economic market mechanisms has been developed in the United States. In this article, I assess the American experience with broadcast regulation predicated on a mixed public and private market-oriented approach, in terms of the vexing quest for adequate means

---

[1]   See *Metro Broadcasting, Inc.* v. *FCC*, 110 S. Ct. 2997, 3004 and 3021 (1990).

A. Sajó (ed.), *Rights of Access to the Media*, 51-85.

to improve access in broadcasting for minority viewpoints consistent with free speech and equal protection rights.

Based on my evaluation of the American experience, I will argue that a mixed public and private scheme of media regulation, while far from entirely satisfactory, is preferable to state control or unrestrained market competition. Moreover, I will also argue that, among different models of mixed public and private regulation, those that place greater emphasis on indirect procedural, rather than direct substantive, governmental regulation are better suited to promote free speech and democratic self-government. Furthermore, while these conclusions are supported by exclusive reference to the situation in the United States, they may be of some relevance in other contexts, provided that proper account is taken of significant political, social and cultural differences between the American context and the particular context in relation to which one may wish to test these conclusions. To facilitate this latter task, Part II of the article is devoted to a brief discussion of the relevant constitutional, institutional, social and political context in which the American regulation of the media is embedded. Part III presents three different models of regulation that rely on the interplay between government action and private enterprise, and discusses them in terms of their suitability for promoting viewpoint diversity in the media. Part IV focuses on salient aspects of United States regulation of broadcasting in the pursuit of a free electronic market place of ideas. And, finally, Part V zeroes in on the problem of minority access to the media, and assesses it in terms of the models of regulation presented in Part III.

II.   Free Speech, Equality, the Marketplace of Ideas and the Institutional and Regulatory Structure of Broadcasting in the United States.

Free speech is not only a fundamental constitutional right in the United States, but also one of America's most revered cultural symbols.[2] Furthermore, prominent in the American conception of free speech is the notion of a "free marketplace of ideas"[3] encompassing a wide range of diverse ideas and viewpoints in the context

---

[2]   See Lee C. Bollinger, *The Tolerant Society: Freedom of Speech and Extremist Speech In America* 7 (1986).

[3]   The original judicial formulation of the "marketplace of ideas" metaphor was Justice Holmes' famous dissent in *Abrams* v. *United States*, 250 U.S. 616 (1919).

of a "profound national commitment to the principle that debate on public issues should be uninhibited, robust and wide open".[4] Open debate of a wide range of diverse viewpoints is particularly valued, moreover, on account of two strong convictions broadly shared by Americans: First, a pragmatic conception of truth as gradually and incrementally discoverable through examination and discussion of all available ideas, theories and hypotheses;[5] and, second, a belief that legitimate democratic self-government requires affording every member of the polity the opportunity to have an input in the formulation, deliberation, choice and implementation of programs and policies to be pursued for the common good of society.[6]

Open public debate of all issues relevant to democratic self-government requires the availability of a public forum to which all those who wish to participate should have access. Traditionally, the paradigm for such public forum was the town meeting where all citizens gather to discuss the issues confronting their community.[7] Access to the town meeting, moreover, could be secured though negative liberty,[8] thus making it possible for every citizen to have an input in the public debate, provided only that no one prevented him or her from coming to, and speaking at, the public gathering place where the town meeting was scheduled to take place.

Consistent with the town meeting paradigm, only active state interference or purposeful interference carried out by some citizens against others could mar the integrity of the public debate over political issues. But as the town meeting paradigm becomes largely obsolete, and as the electronic media come to assume, at least in part, some of the essential functions of the town meeting, mere negative freedom is

---

[4]   *New York Times* v. *Sullivan*, 376 U.S. 254, 270 (1964).

[5]   For the intellectual origins of this philosophical position see John Stuart Mill, *On Liberty* in *Utilitarianism; On Liberty; Essays on Bentham* 180-81 (Mary Warnock ed. 1970).

[6]   See Alexander Meiklejohn, *Free Speech And Its Relation to Self-Government* (1948).

[7]   See id.

[8]   Negative liberty requires that a person be left alone by others to do as he or she chooses. Positive liberty, on the other hand, "involves an affirmative course of assistance designed to put a person in a position meaningfully to pursue a particular good." Michel Rosenfeld, *Substantive Equality and Equal Opportunity: A Jurisprudential Appraisal*, 74 California L. Rev. 1687, 1692 (1986).

no longer sufficient to secure access to public debate. Accordingly, preventing purposeful interference against citizen participation in the public debate cannot, standing alone, legitimate such debate. Moreover, to the extent that broadcast outlets suitable for public debate remain scarce, and that it is impossible for every citizen who wishes to present views personally to participate in the public debate, the issue of *equal* access (or of equal opportunity to have access) to the forum of public debate becomes critical. In short, in a society like the United States, where broadcasting plays a key role in shaping public debate, the integrity of the public forum for political issues depends on allocation of positive freedoms in a way that does not contravene each citizen's equal claim to access to that public forum.

At the same time that freedom of speech in America has evolved from a purely negative to a partially positive liberty, perception of the principal threat to free speech has shifted. Three different stages of free speech in America can be distinguished according to the principal perceived threat against uninhibited wide open debate of public issues.[9] In stage one, the principal threat to free speech comes from government;[10] in stage two, from the tyranny of the majority;[11] and in stage three, from apathy resulting from widespread consensus on essential values, which promotes a tendency to refuse to listen to novel or unorthodox ideas.[12] Consistent with these respective threats, in a stage one society the most important function of free speech is to prevent government from censoring citizens; in a stage two society, to protect speakers who hold views shared only by a minority of their fellow citizens from attempts by the majority to silence them; and, in a stage three society, to shift the focus from *speakers* to *listeners* in order to expose the latter to politically relevant views which they would prefer to avoid. Although government and majority threats to free speech by no means disappear in a stage three society like the United States, they appear to recede in importance as compared with audience hostility or

---

[9]   See Lee C. Bollinger, supra note 2, at 143-45.

[10]   Id.

[11]   Id.

[12]   Id.

indifference which results in marginalization of dissonant viewpoints.[13] Accordingly, a stage three society must promote free speech both through the protection of speakers and through the opening and preservation of channels of communication between speakers and listeners.

Broadcasting in the United States was from the outset virtually exclusively in private hands. Moreover, it was not until it became plain that the scarcity of available airwaves made it impracticable to leave entry into broadcasting exclusively to market forces, that government instituted a scheme of regulation requiring broadcasters to operate in the public interest.[14] In devising a regulatory scheme for broadcasting, the United States Congress rejected both the imposition of direct state controls over the operations of broadcasters and obligating broadcasters to provide general access over the airwaves in the manner of common carriers. Instead, Congress specifically prohibited state censorship of broadcast programming, and cast broadcasters in the dual roles of journalist and of trustee responsible for serving the broadcast audience's public interest. As journalists, broadcasters are supposed to enjoy the same freedom from state intrusion as their printed press counterparts. As trustees, however, broadcasters are supposed to be answerable for their programming in order to insure the use of their airwaves in furtherance of the public interest.

Since it is impossible neatly to disentangle a broadcaster's acts as journalist from those as trustee, state regulation of broadcasting confronts the vexing task of successfully reconciling two apparently conflicting distinct objectives. Indeed, to the extent that private broadcasters bent on making a profit tend to shy away from their public interest obligations, active state regulation looms as particularly desirable. On the other hand, any governmental regulation relating to broadcast programming seems likely to have some inhibiting effects on broadcasters' journalistic zeal. Mindful of the twofold danger of underregulation and overregulation, and consistent with its obligations to respect constitutional rights to freedom of speech and of the

---

[13]   It is of course quite conceivable that government and the majority would not simply stay on the sidelines in a stage three society, but that instead they would play an active role in promoting audience indifference and the marginalization of dissonant viewpoints.

[14]   See Federal Communications Act of 1934, 48 Stat. 1064 codified at 17 U.S.C. §§ 151, et seq. For a description of the advent of the current scheme of governmental regulation of broadcasting in the United States, see Michel Rosenfeld, *The Jurisprudence of Fairness: Freedom through Regulation in the Marketplace of Ideas*, 44 Fordham L. Rev. 877, 887-890 (1976).

press, the Congress opted for a scheme of broadcast regulation that revolves around government licensing of private broadcasters for a term of five years, with options for license renewals based on satisfactory fulfillment of the broadcast licensee's public interest obligations.[15]

Before looking into how this regulatory scheme deals with viewpoint diversity and with minority access, it is necessary to examine briefly different ways in which a scheme of regulation might promote the right mix of state regulation and private enterprise.

III.   Three Models of Regulation

In a society like the United States, where the bulk of income producing property is in private hands, one can generally distinguish three distinct models of regulation according to the relative roles reserved respectively for the state and for private economic actors. The first of these models, which is usually associated with a laissez faire economy, can be called the "purely procedural" model of government regulation. Under this model, the state's only legitimate role is to provide the requisite support to a free market economy exclusively animated by the endeavors of private economic actors. Under the purely procedural model, legitimate state regulation is essentially limited to the protection of life and property and to the enforcement of private contracts. Accordingly, the purely procedural model emphasizes negative liberties and precludes the state from tampering, directly or through regulation, with market mechanisms in order to promote any particular conception of the common good.

The second model, which may be characterized as the "substantive" model of government regulation, is associated with active government intervention, the promotion of positive liberties, and concerted private and public action designed to further some articulated conception of the common good. This substantive model is characteristic of the welfare state with its proliferation of regulation in the public interest. Consistent with this model, moreover, the state may intervene directly, as when it takes over and runs certain industries, such as banks, airlines or railroads. Or the state may impose a regulatory scheme on private actors in order to achieve some articulated socio-political objective, as when it sets in place an administrative

---

[15]   47 U.S.C. § 307 (c).

bureaucracy responsible for implementing a particular policy, such as fair labor standards or adequate protection of the environment.

The third model of governmental regulation is characterized by a combination of state pursuit of articulated substantive objectives with procedural devices designed to pave the way towards realization of such objectives. This model, which relies on a mix of positive and negative liberties can be referred to as the "mixed substantive and procedural" model. Unlike the purely procedural model, the mixed substantive and procedural model is not indifferent to outcomes, thus confining procedural devices or reliance on market forces to a relatively narrower range of activities.[16] On the other hand, unlike the substantive model, the mixed substantive and procedural model does not contemplate direct state implementation of adopted substantive objectives. Instead, this third model envisages that for reasons of efficiency or legitimacy it is preferable to pursue a particular substantive objective through indirect and largely procedural means than through direct state intervention or prescription. For example, it may be more efficient to pursue every citizen's basic welfare needs through economic competition within the constraints imposed by minimum wage and maximum hour laws than through the dispensation of direct state subsidies.

Ideally, broadcast regulation should be patterned on the purely procedural model. Scarcity, however, precludes achieving equal access and viewpoint diversity through purely procedural means. Moreover, even if the proliferation of cable television outlets has, strictly speaking, done away with broadcasting scarcity in the United States, other factors, such as the economic structure of the broadcasting industry, still appear to rule out achieving a satisfactory regulatory scheme through

---

[16]   It should be emphasized that the purely procedural model is indifferent to outcomes only in a very special sense. Indeed, in theory at least, in a pure laissez faire economy, the state would have no preference among private competitors and would remain indifferent as to how the market apportions winners and losers among competitors much as the referee in a football match is presumably indifferent as to which, of the two teams involved in the match, turns out to be the winner. By choosing a market economy over other alternatives, however, the state evinces a preference for certain kinds of likely outcomes over others, and for certain kinds of economic actors over others. So long as it remains clear that the market is indifferent or neutral only in the limited sense indicated above, it may be convenient to refer to the market as a neutral baseline and to view departures from the laissez faire paradigm as requiring the embrace of substantive values and objectives.

58

the purely procedural model.[17] The substantive model, on the other hand, is also unsuitable for broadcast regulation because it would put the state in the position of controlling access to, and exclusion from, the electronic marketplace of ideas, thus facilitating state censorship of critical ideas and viewpoints. Because of legitimacy concerns, therefore, the mixed substantive and procedural model seems to be the most appropriate for broadcast regulation in the United States. As we shall now see, this model has been implemented - although not without misgivings or controversy - in the United States.

IV.   Broadcast Regulation to Promote Viewpoint Diversity:
        The Case of the Fairness Doctrine

The Fairness Doctrine,[18] which was an integral part of American broadcasting regulation until 1987[19] was supposed to promote viewpoint diversity - including increased access for minority viewpoints - in broadcasting in a way that protected broadcasters against both government censorship and common carrier status. Mindful

---

[17]   For an argument that the present economic structure of the American broadcast industry justifies the same kind of regulation originally justified on the basis of scarcity, see C. Edwin Baker, *Human Liberty and Freedom of Speech* 262 (1989). Another factor worth mentioning is that access alone appears insufficient in the age of cable television, particularly, if one focuses on the problem of reaching a significant audience. Indeed, as "broadcasting" gives way to "narrowcasting", every person wishing to express a point of view over the airwaves might well get an opportunity to get on television. But as the number of outlets increases, the audience for each new voice heard on television is bound to diminish. Ultimately, in an age of virtually unlimited cable outlets, the important issue is not merely access to television but rather access to those channels which command a sufficiently large audience to constitute a veritable forum for public debate. Accordingly, particularly in a stage three society, so long as access to the latter channels remains highly restricted, the technical elimination of broadcast outlet scarcity may be of little consequence in terms of genuine access and viewpoint diversity.

[18]   See generally Applicability of the Fairness Doctrine in the Handling of Controversial Issues of Public Importance, 29 *Fed. Reg.* 10,415 (1964) (hereinafter "Fairness Primer").

[19]   The Fairness Doctrine requirements were abrogated by the Federal Communications Commission ("FCC") in 1987 during the Reagan Administration. See *Syracuse Peace Council* v. *Television Station WTVH*, 63 *Rad. Reg.* 2d (P & F) 541, 543 (FCC 1987); 52 *Fed. Reg.* 51,768 (1987). See also, Edward J. Markey, *Congress to Administrative Agencies: Creator, Overseer, and Partner* (1990) Duke Law Journal 967.

that the United States Congress had intended "that the air waves be used as a vital means of communication, capable of making a major contribution to the development of an informed public opinion",[20] the FCC imposed on broadcasters the obligation to address issues of public importance.[21] To avoid government interference with broadcasters' programming decisions, however, the FCC embraced the Fairness Doctrine, which qualifies as a mixed substantive and procedural means of regulation, provided both its requirements and its modes of implementation are properly taken into account.

The Fairness Doctrine imposes two distinct affirmative duties on broadcasters. First, broadcasters have the duty "to provide a reasonable amount of time for the presentation over their facilities of programs devoted to the discussion and consideration of public issues".[22] Second, the implementation of this obligation carries the further affirmative duty to encourage and afford reasonable opportunity for the presentation of contrasting views on all issues of importance.[23]

These two affirmative duties restrict the freedom of a broadcaster in two significant respects: First, the broadcaster cannot avoid devoting some programming to the discussion of issues of public importance; and second, with respect to such programming, the broadcaster is not free to present one among a series of contrasting views on a controversial issue while ignoring all the others. These two affirmative duties, moreover, constrain broadcast journalism in a way that has been adjudged impermissible when it comes to print journalism.[24]

Although the Fairness Doctrine restricts the freedom of broadcasters, its implementation and enforcement by the FCC was deliberately designed to minimize government intrusion upon the day to day operations of broadcasters. Accordingly, the FCC made it clear that the broadcaster was to remain the sole judge concerning

---

[20]   Fairness Primer, supra note 18, at 10,425.

[21]   13 F.C.C. 1246, 1247-48 (1949).

[22]   Id. at 1249.

[23]   Id. at 1250-51.

[24]   The Fairness Doctrine was upheld as constitutional against a challenge of the grounds that it violated the broadcaster's freedom of speech in *Red Lion Broadcasting Co.* v. *FCC*, 395 U.S. 367 (1969). Similar regulation imposed by a state on the printed press, however, was held unconstitutional in *Miami Herald Publishing Co.* v. *Tornillo*, 418 U.S. 241 (1974).

the determination of the subjects to be considered, the different shades of opinion to be aired, and the spokespersons for each point of view.[25] Moreover, to dispel concerns that government regulators would be called upon to take stands on the merits of particular issues, the FCC made it clear that its role in this area would be limited to a consideration of the broadcast licensee's overall program service, provided that the licensee act in good faith and make reasonable determinations as to particular issues. In the FCC's own words: "The question is necessarily one of the reasonableness of the station's actions, not whether any absolute standard of fairness has been achieved".[26]

Under the Fairness Doctrine, the broadcast licensee enjoyed great latitude in the selection of issues, viewpoints and spokespersons, but failures in compliance could lead to drastic consequences, such as revocation of a license or denial of a license renewal application.[27] In addition to overall periodic reviews of broadcaster compliance with the Fairness Doctrine (primarily in connection with license renewal applications), a licensee could be confronted by a "fairness complaint" filed with the FCC by a private individual, group or organization alleging that the licensee had failed to present contrasting views in programming devoted to a controversial public issue. For example, if a broadcaster presented a series of programs on abortion where only pro-abortion views were heard, some anti-abortion organizations would in all likelihood file a fairness complaint with the FCC.

Because of the standards employed by the FCC in dealing with fairness complaints, these had very little chance of success, thus placing virtually no added direct burden on broadcasters.[28] Indeed, all that FCC required was that the licensee's contention be a "reasonable one".[29] Thus, for instance, if a licensee were to dispute the contention made in a fairness complaint that a given program

---

[25]   13 F.C.C. at 1251.

[26]   Id. at 1255.

[27]   47 U.S.C. § 312(a) (1970).

[28]   For example, out of 5,000 fairness complaints filed with the FCC in 1986, only 6 were forwarded to broadcasters for response. H.R. Rep. No. 108, 97th Cong., 1st Sess. 23 (1987).

[29]   "If a licensee's determination is *reasonable* and arrived at in good faith the...[FCC] will not disturb it." Fairness Report, 48 F.C.C. 2d 1, 13 (1974).

presented a controversial issue, the FCC would refrain from indicating whether it considered the issue in question to be controversial. Instead, the FCC would limit itself to a determination of whether it was reasonable for the licensee to conclude that the relevant issue was not controversial.

Through the Fairness Doctrine, the FCC attempted to promote viewpoint diversity over the airwaves in a way that would not undermine the delicate balance necessary for broadcasters properly to carry out their dual functions as public trustees and as journalists. The obligations imposed by the Fairness Doctrine were designed to secure broadcaster's compliance with their duties as public trustees, while the FCC's largely indirect and relatively remote methods of oversight were crafted to minimize interference with broadcaster's performance of their journalistic functions. Without significantly relying on granting the public direct access to the media,[30] the Fairness Doctrine devised means for broadcasters to provide a greater diversity of viewpoints for the benefit of their audience. Moreover, to the extent that issues relating to minorities have tended to be controversial in the United States, the Fairness Doctrine could be plausibly viewed as enhancing the opportunities for the airing of minority viewpoints. Indeed, issues such a racial discrimination, racial integration and affirmative action involving preferential treatment of racial minorities have been hotly controverted issues in the United States. And, though conceivable, it seems unlikely that a broadcaster could fulfill its duty to present contrasting views on such issues without any recourse to minority viewpoints. For example, it is hard to imagine that in a community divided by allegations of police brutality against certain minorities, a broadcaster would devote programming to the subject of police brutality without presenting any minority viewpoint on the issues relating to the controversy.

For all its prophylactic features, however, the Fairness Doctrine proved highly problematic, as its implementation required much more government involvement regarding the merit of particular issues than had been originally expected. On the surface, the determination of whether it would be reasonable to maintain that a particular issue is non controversial may seem fairly simple and unproblematic. To use the FCC's own hypothetical example, suppose a controversial proposed law is before the Congress and a licensee has allowed its advocates to

---

[30]   The Fairness Doctrine permits the broadcaster to select spokespersons for contrasting view and does not provide for a right of access save in cases involving personal attack. See 47 C.F.R. §§ 73, 123, 300, 598, 679 (1975).

broadcast their views while denying access to any of its opponents. Under these circumstances, the FCC would have no trouble deciding that the broadcast licensee had been unreasonable, without considering the merits of the proposed law.[31] Nevertheless, upon further reflection, this example is misleading to the extent that it refers to a situation in which the controversial nature of the subject under consideration is self-evident. In contrast, in many cases the very determination of whether a subject is controversial is itself a controversial matter. Indeed, there are cases in which the context of a statement makes it unclear whether it addresses a controversial issue, and others where the ultimate determination as to whether a particular subject should be deemed controversial depends, to an important extent, on the political, ideological, cultural and emotional biases of those who are ultimately responsible for the decision.

An example of a situation where the context left it unclear whether a particular statement addressed a controversial issue is provided by the fairness complaint relating to cigarette advertising on television.[32] The broadcast licensee claimed that the advertisement did not raise a controversial issue as it merely asserted that cigarette smoking is pleasurable. Based on that interpretation, the licensee's determination that the advertisement does not raise a controversial issue seems reasonable. If, however, one interprets the advertisement as implicitly asserting that cigarette smoking is desirable as well as pleasurable, then it would be unreasonable to claim that the advertisement does not address a controversial issue.

Even more disturbing are those cases in which the determination of whether an issue should be deemed controversial depends, in the last analysis, on the political biases of the decision-maker. For example, at the height of the Vietnam war, when Americans were deeply divided over the use of the armed forces in an unpopular undeclared war, an anti-war activist group filed a fairness complaint against certain radio and television stations which had broadcast armed forces recruitment messages as a public service.[33] According to the complaints, the recruitment messages raised

---

[31]   13 F.C.C. at 1256.

[32]   *WCBS-TV* 8 F.C.C. 2d 381, stay and reconsideration denied, 9 F.C.C. 921 (1967), *aff'd sub. nom. Banzhaff* v. *FCC*, 405 F.2d 1082 (1968). *cert. denied*, 396 U.S. 842 (1969). Subsequently, the United States Congress banned cigarette advertisement from radio and television. See Public Health Cigarette Smoking Act of 1969, § 6, 15 U.S.C. § 1335 (1970).

[33]   *San Francisco Women For Peace*, 24 F.C.C. 2d 156 (1970).

a controversial issue since many people did not believe that it was beneficial for the individual or for society to join the armed forces, and since it was impossible to divorce the recruitment advertisements from the war in Vietnam where most recruits were likely to be sent.[34] The licensees, on the other hand, denied that the military recruitment ads raised a controversial issue, and a majority on the FCC concluded that the licensees had not been unreasonable. Moreover, in reaching this conclusion, the FCC majority reasoned that the military recruitment ads were much like similar recruitment ads for policemen, firemen and others, and noted that the government's power to raise an army had not been questioned. Rather, the complaint objected to the use made of the armed forces, an issue not raised by the broadcast of the recruitment messages, according to the FCC majority.[35] In the estimation of the dissenting FCC Commissioner, however, the recruitment messages could no more be separated from the Vietnam war than could the cigarette advertisements from the health hazards associated with smoking.[36]

In view of the political atmosphere prevailing in the United States in the late 1960's and early 1970's, it seems fair to assume that the answer to the question of whether military recruitment messages could be divorced from the Vietnam war would, to a large extent, depend on the political views of the person to whom the question is addressed. To one who supported the war, or was indifferent to it, or was even mildly against it, it would most likely be reasonable to separate military recruitment from pursuit of the Vietnam war. To one vehemently opposed to the war, on the other hand, it would virtually certainly seem unreasonable to consider military recruitment as if it occurred in a void, when the main motivation for such recruitment, and the principal upshot of it, was undoubtedly the pursuit of military operations in Vietnam.

In as much as Fairness Doctrine determinations hinge on political biases, and as FCC Commissioners, who are Presidential appointees, can be expected to represent mainstream political views, the Fairness Doctrine looms as an inadequate vehicle for the proliferation of viewpoint diversity. As an illustration, consider the following hypothetical example relating to minority views. Because of their disparate

---

[34]   Id.

[35]   Id. at 157-158.

[36]   Id. at 161 (Johnson, Commissioner, dissenting).

experiences, blacks and whites in the United States are likely to have different perceptions of the system of criminal justice. While both blacks and whites agree that justice is not served in all cases, whites are likely to view the system of justice as basically fair, with a few aberrant cases. Blacks, on the other hand, would tend to view the system of justice as inherently racially biased, and hence, as loaded against them. Given these circumstances, the portrayal of the United States criminal justice system on television as being basically fair, would most probably not be viewed by the vast majority of whites as raising any controversial issue. Consistent with this, broadcasters would be prompted to assert that the issue is non-controversial, and government regulators, who are by and large white, would be predisposed to deem the broadcasters' assertions as being reasonable. And, the upshot of all this would be, in all likelihood, a failure to provide greater access to the media to minority viewpoints.

In the last analysis, the Fairness Doctrine may foster greater diversity of viewpoints in connection with controversies among mainstream groups, or between mainstream and more marginal groups, so long as those in the mainstream acknowledge that the subject over which there exists disagreement is controversial. But where mainstream beliefs are so entrenched that those who share them do not perceive that their political, ideological or cultural positions are open to controversy, the Fairness Doctrine as actually implemented by the FCC seems largely inefficient. Accordingly, although the Fairness Doctrine conforms to the mixed substantive and procedural model of regulation, which seems particularly well suited to broadcasting, it ultimately needs to be supplemented or replaced. Moreover, going beyond the Fairness Doctrine is all the more urgent in a stage three society where, as already pointed out, the greatest threat to freedom of expression is the listening public's lack of exposure to dissonant, marginalized and unpopular viewpoints. With this in mind, let us now turn to an examination of affirmative action as an alternative (or a supplement) to the Fairness Doctrine, for purposes of increasing the dissemination of minority viewpoints in the media.

V. Promoting Minority Viewpoint Access Through Affirmative Action in the Allocation of Broadcast Licenses

V.1. The FCC's minority preference policies

Nearly a decade before it abrogated the Fairness Doctrine,[37] the FCC concluded that minority viewpoints were inadequately represented over the airwaves, and undertook to change this state of affairs through the implementation of preferential treatment in favor of minorities.[38] Stressing that "[a]dequate representation of minority viewpoints in programming serves not only the needs and interests of the minority community but also enriches and educates the non-minority audience,"[39] the FCC adopted its "enhancement for minority ownership" policy.[40] This policy comes into play when the FCC conducts a comparative hearing to select one among several qualified applicants who compete for a single license to use a particular broadcast frequency. Pursuant to the "enhancement for minority ownership" policy, the FCC is supposed to count minority ownership and participation in management as a "plus" factor in its determination, on the basis of a comparative hearing, of which one among the competing applicants should be awarded the coveted broadcast license.[41] Thus, all other factors being equal, an applicant who is under minority ownership or management should be awarded the broadcast license consistent with the "enhancement for minority ownership" policy. Moreover, FCC practice has included awards of licenses to minority owned applicants even where competing

---

[37]   See supra note 19.

[38]   See FCC Statement of Policy on Minority Ownership of Broadcasting Facilities, 68 F.C.C. 2d 979 (1978).

[39]   Id. at 980.

[40]   Id. at 982. The FCC also adopted other affirmative action policies which will not be discussed here.

[41]   Id. Moreover, besides minority ownership and participation in management, the FCC considers six other factors at a comparative hearing for the award of a new license: "diversification of control of mass media communications, full time participation in station operation by owners (commonly referred to as the 'integration' of ownership and management), proposed program service, past broadcast record, efficient use of the frequency, and the character of the applicants." *Metro Broadcasting, Inc.* v. *FCC*, 110 S. Ct. 2997, 3004 (1990).

applicants should have clearly been awarded the contested license based on a fair consideration of all the other relevant factors.[42] The "enhancement for minority ownership" policy together with the six other factors considered in comparative hearings relating to broadcast license applications conform to the mixed procedural and substantive model of regulation. Indeed, all seven factors weighed by the FCC constrain the competition for broadcast licenses, without directly impinging on broadcast operations. Thus, whereas minority ownership is accorded significant weight in the competition for licenses, the FCC imposes no direct obligations on broadcasters to air minority viewpoints. Because granting a broadcast license to a minority owned applicant does not guarantee an increased airing of minority viewpoints, the "enhancement for minority ownership" policy is clearly a less efficient (as well as less direct) means towards the intended governmental objective than would be the imposition of a flat duty on broadcasters to air minority viewpoints. The latter alternative is foreclosed, however, because it would smack too much of state control over the flow of ideas.

Recourse to preferential treatment is prompted by concern for free speech and for the journalistic integrity of broadcasters, but it raises important concerns of its own. Chief among these, are concerns about efficiency, equality and liberty. These concerns, moreover, were vigorously debated in the context of the litigation that led the United States Supreme Court in a closely divided 5-4 decision to uphold the constitutionality of the FCC "enhancement for minority ownership" policy in the 1990 case of *Metro Broadcasting, Inc.* v. *FCC.*[43]

V.2. Minority preferences and efficiency

Focusing first on efficiency, granted that awarding broadcast outlets to minority owned applicants is less efficient than requiring the broadcast of minority viewpoints or awarding such outlets to applicants committed to present minority viewpoints regardless of the racial or ethnic make-up of the ownership, there is still a serious debate as to whether one can establish any reliable correlation between minority

---

[42]   See *Metro Broadcasting*, 110 S. Ct. at 3005-06 (stating that license to operate a new television awarded to Rainbow which was ninety percent Hispanic-owned in spite of competitor Metro's local residence and civic participation advantage).

[43]   Id. at 2997.

ownership and the presentation of minority viewpoints. A bare majority on the United States Supreme Court concluded in *Metro-Broadcasting* that a sufficient nexus between minority ownership and the presentation of minority viewpoints could be established,[44] but the dissenting justices rejected that conclusion, emphasizing that it was based on racial stereotyping and on an underestimation of the role of market forces in shaping program content decisions.[45] More specifically, those who believe that no sufficient nexus exists between minority ownership and minority viewpoints are prone to argue that any assumption that all members of a racial or ethnic group share the same perspective is stereotypical and demanding as it negates the individuality, autonomy, and ability of individual members of the group in question to think for themselves. Furthermore, to the extent that program content decisions are driven by market forces, the racial or ethnic origin of the decisionmaker would appear to play an insignificant role in the determination of what is to be broadcasted. American broadcasters are engaged in a competitive business where profitability hinges on success in the sale of airtime to advertisers, which, in turn, depends principally on the size of the broadcast audience. Accordingly, competition would appear to constrain broadcasters' programming choices in terms of what is likely to appeal to the largest possible segment of the broadcast audience. Under these circumstances, even if a minority owned broadcaster were inclined to propagate minority viewpoints, presumably such broadcaster's economic interests would strongly militate against a course of action which would forgo maximizing the size of the broadcast audience.

Proponents of the view that a sufficient nexus exists between minority ownership and viewpoints, on the other hand, can plausibly defend their position without having to fall prey to racial or ethnic stereotyping and without ignoring the important role of market factors. Leaving aside any mechanistic one-to-one correlation between the ethnic origin of a person and the views which he or she holds, one may often detect minority views in the sense of being held by a large proportion of a given minority while being held but by a small number of persons belonging to other groups. For example, in the context of a trial for an interracial crime in the United States, it would not be surprising if a large majority of African-Americans were to believe that the system of justice was racially biased, while a

---

[44]   Id. at 3017.

[45]   Id. at 3040.

similarly large proportion of whites were to believe just as firmly that there was no such bias. Moreover, even where no homogeneity of views may be detected among the members of a minority group, they may well generally converge towards the same perspective. The existence of a distinct perspective - which may be embraced with varying degrees of intensity by individual members of the minority group - is likely to be attributable to common cultural, religious, national or historical experiences that differentiate the affected minority from other groups in society.

While it seems undeniable that group experience plays a significant role in molding an individual member's perspective - such as the experience of slavery which has left a palpable imprint on the perspective of African-Americans - it should not be forgotten that individuals typically belong to more than one group, so that even if views and perspectives were strictly correlated to group affiliation, there would still be many overlaps. For example, while American blacks and whites belong to two different groups for purposes of the history and politics of race relations, they might well form part of the same group - both in terms of a convergence of views and of perspectives - in relation to an economic policy of a foreign country which had a serious adverse impact on the United States economy. In the last analysis, ignoring the complex and dynamic nexus between views and group affiliation seems as objectionable as crudely postulating a one-to-one correlation between them. Assuming that a person harbors a particular view *because* he or she is black or white, Jewish or Hispanic degrades by disregarding the equal worth and dignity of that person. But insisting on disregarding an individual's group affiliation can equally degrade - for the same reason - to the extent that such an individual relies on the well of common group experiences to formulate views and to forge a distinct identity.

Turning to the role of market forces in the determination of broadcast program content, proponents of the sufficient nexus thesis can invoke two distinct and mutually consistent propositions: First, market forces are sufficiently complex, dynamic and flexible to accommodate a series of variables, including increases in the expression of minority views; and, second, as the FCC has asserted, broadcast content "is not purely market driven".[46]

The market forces that play a significant role in the context of broadcasting are hardly simple, mechanistic or objective (in the sense of being inexorably imposed from the outside on broadcasters). Indeed, programming demand is not

---

[46]   Id. at 3012.

likely to be completely impervious to the forces of production.[47] Rather, as the broadcasting audience's wants are to a large extent uncertain and ill-defined, broadcasters seem bound to have a significant hand in shaping programming demand. Moreover, from the standpoint of programming, American broadcasting involves not one but several markets. For example, the market for national network television programming is likely to be quite different from that for local radio programming. Whereas network television may depend for success on finding the largest possible common denominator for a national audience, a radio station that is local in scope and that operates in a crowded field may only remain viable by appealing to a large proportion of a discrete, targeted group whose current programming needs are inadequately served. Consistent with these observations, while the FCC's minority ownership policies have led to increased minority oriented programming both in radio and on television, such policies have thus far had a greater impact on radio programming than on television programming.[48]

Broadcast content seems not exclusively shaped by market forces, on the other hand, in that it involves the expression of ideas, and that trading in ideas is not the equivalent of dealing in many other commodities. A business may be indifferent to selling textiles instead of metals, so long as both would equally maximize profits. The same, however, is much less likely to be true of the broadcasting of ideas. For example, in the face of a strong demand for the broadcast of anti-Semitic views, it would be highly unlikely that Jewish broadcasters would rush to meet that demand to maximize profits. It seems fair to surmise that most broadcasters in a similar situation would rather forgo profits than propagate views which they personally find threatening or abhorrent. In any event, broadcast programming options consistent with market constraints are generally sufficiently diverse to allow a broadcaster to allocate a certain portion of airtime to the presentation of personally held views without significantly affecting the profitability of his or her station.

The preceding observations support the conclusion that a sufficient nexus between minority ownership and increasing the presentation of minority viewpoints can be established in order to justify the FCC's "enhancement for minority ownership" policy from the standpoint of efficiency. Even the most ardent

---

[47]   Cf. John Kenneth Galbraith, *The Affluent Society*, 127 (1976) (consumer wants are to a large extent created by producers).

[48]   See *Minority Role in Broadcasting Yields Far Bigger Effect on Radio Than TV*, New York Times, Aug. 1, 1990, at B6, col. 4.

proponents of this policy could not seriously contend that it does more than significantly boost the odds for increased presentations of minority viewpoints over the airwaves. But, given that more direct means which would undoubtedly be more efficient, such as imposing an obligation on broadcasters to air minority viewpoints, are foreclosed for reasons spelled out above, the "enhancement for minority ownership" policy might well be the most efficient means to promote viewpoint diversity consistent with the constraints that surround broadcast regulation. Nevertheless, endorsement of this policy could not be justified unless one could adequately deal with the concerns it raises in relation to liberty and equality.

V.3.   Minority preferences, liberty and equality

The concerns raised by the FCC's minority preference policies in relation to constitutional liberty and equality are closely intertwined. This follows from the fact that the principal conceptions of political liberty depend to an important extent on the stand they adopt towards equality. Indeed, from the broader perspective of the philosophical debate about the relationship between liberty and equality, two principal positions have emerged. According to some, liberty and equality are essentially antagonistic, so that increases in equality can only be obtained at the cost of decreases in liberty.[49] According to others, however, liberty and equality are not antagonistic, but complementary, and there can be no genuine liberty where inequality prevails.[50] Now the FCC's minority preference policies can be attacked both from the standpoint of liberty and from that of equality. For example, proponents of negative liberty who view equality as antagonistic to liberty would undoubtedly tend to view the FCC's minority preference policies as interfering with the functioning of a genuinely free marketplace of ideas. Similarly, for those who conceive of equality as predominantly justified in terms of equal treatment rather

---

[49]   See, e.g. David Hume, *An Enquiry Concerning the Principles of Morals, in Hume's Enquiries 194* (3rd ed. 1975); Friedrich A. Hayek, *The Constitution of Liberty*, 87 (1960).

[50]   For a systematic defense of this position see Richard Norman, *Does Equality Destroy Liberty in Contemporary Political Philosophy* (Keith Graham ed. 1982); see also John Rawls, *A Theory of Justice*, 225 (1971) ("The liberties protected by the principle of [political] participation lose much of their value whenever those who have greater private means are permitted to use their advantages to control the course of public debate.")

than equal result or fair equality of opportunity, the very creation of a preference based on race or ethnic origin would undoubtedly be illegitimate.[51]

A proper assessment of attacks on the FCC's minority preference policies from the standpoint of liberty or equality lies beyond the scope of the present undertaking. Accordingly, I shall focus on the more manageable task of attempting a justification of the preferential policies in question in terms of one particular conception of the relationship between liberty and equality as it relates to broadcasting in its role as a forum of public debate on important issues. This conception endorses the proposition that liberty and equality are, for all relevant purposes here, intertwined in such a way that there cannot be any genuine liberty in the absence of equality. Remembering that the most important liberty involved is that of the broadcast audience to make choices based on access to all the relevant information and ideas; and that the electronic marketplace of ideas cannot accommodate - at least in so far as it is to serve as a viable forum for public debate - all those who wish to express their views or all available viewpoints; it seems imperative that there be some equality of access to the airwaves. Indeed, if only the views of the most powerful, or of the majority, were to find their way to the electronic marketplace, the broadcast audience would lack some of the tools necessary to the full enjoyment of their liberty of political participation.[52] And this is especially true in a stage three society where liberty is particularly threatened by conformism and close mindedness.

Even conceding that the broadcast audience's liberty of political participation cannot be reduced to a mere negative liberty, and that it depends on the institution of some kind of equality in the electronic marketplace of ideas, there remain several questions concerning liberty and equality which must be addressed before settling on the legitimacy of the FCC's minority preference policies. In a nutshell, these questions are: Whose liberty? Which liberty? And, which equalities?

From the standpoint of free speech rights, other liberties besides the collective liberty of the broadcast audience are implicated in the context of regulation

---

[51] For an extended discussion of these issues in the context of preferential treatment policies, see Michel Rosenfeld, Affirmative Action and Justice: A Philosophical and Constitutional Inquiry (1991); for same in connection with the FCC minority preference policies see Michel Rosenfeld, *Metro Broadcasting v. FCC: Affirmative Action at the Crossroads of Constitutional Liberty and Equality*, 38 UCLA L. Rev. 583 (1991).

[52] See note 50 supra.

of access to the media. These liberties include the liberty of the broadcaster as a journalist, the liberty of all those who wish to broadcast their views but do not have a right to access to the media, and the individual (negative) liberty of members of the broadcast audience against being subjected, through government action, to views which they would prefer to avoid. Moreover, from the standpoint of constitutional equality, minority preferences must withstand challenges from those who would have succeeded in obtaining a license to broadcast but for the operation of such preferences. Also, to the extent that an adequate electronic marketplace of ideas depend on some form of equality among viewpoints, the latter equality should be susceptible of reconciliation with equality among persons. Finally, since under the relevant conception pursued here, liberty is equated with equal liberty, access to the media for some, but not all, viewpoints and for some, but not all, willing spokepersons should be rejected unless it can be reconciled with a plausible road map towards equal liberty.

V.3.a. Free speech as equal liberty

While there is hardly a consensus on this issue, several American constitutional scholars regard equality as playing a central role in shaping free speech rights,[53] thus lending support to a conception of free speech as implying equal liberty as well as equal respect and equal dignity. Consistent with this conception, free speech should guarantee to every person an equal right to self-expression[54] and equal access to the information necessary for an autonomous human being to make responsible decisions concerning his or her personal, social and political destiny.[55]

---

[53] See, e.g., Bollinger, supra note 2, at 45; David Richards, *Toleration and the Constitution*, 217-18 (1986); Lawrence Tribe, *Constitutional Choices*, 192-98 (1985); Kenneth Karst, *Equality as a Central Principle in the First Amendment*, 43 U. Chicago L. Rev. 20, 21 (1975).

[54] See, e.g., Karst, supra note 53, at 26 (equal liberty of expression is essential to sense of self-respect, as means of "staking a claim to equal citizenship").

[55] See, e.g., Rawls, supra note 50, at 225 ("All citizens should have the means to be informed about political issues" and "should be in a position to assess how proposals affect their well-being and which politics advance their conception of the public good").

Under the conception of free speech as equal liberty, ideally, everyone would have the same opportunity for self-expression and for exposure to all the information which might be relevant to shaping one's personal and political destiny. Moreover, while it is obvious that broadcasting is a limited medium that could not satisfy the entire demand for self-expression and for disseminating information, this is not troubling in and of itself, to the extent that there are several other means of communication, and that not all kinds of intended messages are well suited for the broadcast medium.[56] But even if these facts are properly taken into account, there would still remain more persons who wish to express themselves in the broadcast medium than available airtime, and more relevant viewpoints seeking to compete in the electronic marketplace of ideas than opportunities for such viewpoints to receive sufficient exposure to vie for the viewing and listening public's attention. Because of this, satisfaction of the equal liberty requirement associated with freedom of speech depends on implementation of a course of action compatible with the preservation of equal respect and equal dignity where it is not possible to fulfill all presumably equally legitimate claims.

There are at least two normatively justifiable ways of upholding equal respect and dignity in the face of scarcity of some good that ideally ought to be allocated equally to all. One of these involves recourse to the principle of equality of opportunity;[57] the other relies on a ranking of claims by their relative order of importance, with all claims in the most important category having to be satisfied before satisfying any of the claims in the next category.[58] Also, both of these can play a useful role in the endeavor to achieve equal liberty in broadcasting. Indeed, to the extent that not all viewpoints can be equally accommodated over the airways, equal liberty can nevertheless be upheld through the promotion of equality of opportunity among viewpoints. Furthermore, to the extent that broadcasting gives rise to a clash between the self-expression claims of broadcasters, those of would be

---

[56] For example, communicating one's affection to a loved one may be of utmost importance in terms of a person's need for self-expression, but few would claim that broadcasting would be a desirable medium for such communication.

[57] For an extended discussion of the relation between equality of opportunity and equality of result, see Rosenfeld, *Affirmative Action*, supra note 51, at 22-29 (1991).

[58] For an extended discussion of the egalitarian claim that everyone's most important needs must be satisfied before any need that does not rank as high is satisfied, see Thomas Nagel, *Mortal Questions*, 111-18 (1979).

broadcasters who enjoy no access rights, and the claims of the broadcast audience to receiving relevant information through the broadcast media, this clash seems susceptible to resolution through implementation of an order of priority. Specifically, in accordance with this order of priority, the claims to information of the broadcast audience rank higher than the self-expression of broadcasters and non-broadcasters alike. In justification of this order of priority, moreover, one can advance the following argument: whereas overall claims to self-expression and those to information are of equal rank, in the context of the broadcast media rights to information should rank higher than rights to self-expression. This is because whereas broadcasting plays a particularly important role in the dissemination of information crucial to the public debate that circumscribes democratic self-government, it is often not the best - and almost never the only - medium for self-expression. Accordingly, in broadcasting the collective free speech interest information should prevail over the individual free speech interest in self-expression.[59]

V.3.b. Equality of opportunity among viewpoints and the priority of collective speech interests

Endorsing equality of opportunity among viewpoints and according priority to collective rights to information over individual rights to self-expression, however, does not automatically lead to the conclusion that the FCC's minority preference policies are consistent with the principle of equal liberty. First, it is not obvious that such minority preferences are consistent with equality of opportunity among viewpoints. And second, upon closer examination, the line between the collective interest in information and the individual interest in self-expression is not as sharp as might be initially thought.

Focusing on the second of these concerns to begin with, there are various reasons why information interests cannot be neatly separated from self-expression interests. First, the proposition that the former are collective in nature while the latter are individual does not consistently hold up. Indeed, the collective interest in

---

[59] This last conclusion seems especially justified in a stage three society where self-expression rights are presumably fairly safe while exposure to a wide range of diverse viewpoints remains a paramount concern.

the broadest possible exposure to diverse viewpoints can easily clash with individual interests in not being exposed to certain viewpoints. Thus, it is quite likely that a significant portion of the broadcasting audience would actually prefer not to be confronted by a large number of views that it regards as personally, morally or politically disturbing, threatening or repugnant. Moreover, the greater the audience that wishes to avoid certain views, the more likely it seems that a purely market driven broadcasting industry would fail to air such views. On the other hand, self-expression emerges upon reflection as being as much a collective interest as an individual one. For example, self-expression becomes a collective concern when the members of an identifiable national, ethnic, cultural, or political group widely share certain beliefs or views that they wish to express to obtain the attention, sympathy, respect, or collaboration of the larger community.[60] Under such circumstances, what is paramount for the individual members of the group is not that each person be given an individual right of self-expression, but that representatives of the group who can adequately express the commonly held belief be heard. To the extent that one seeks self-expression to communicate one's feelings, beliefs, and aspirations to others, transmission of a commonly shared message to the intended audience by an acknowledged spokesperson should usually prove an acceptable alternative to individual access to an overly crowded forum. In short, not only is there an overlap between individual and collective interests in viewpoint dissemination, but in some cases - such as when an individual achieves vicarious self-expression through a spokesperson - individual and collective interest coincide, while in others - such as where a large portion of the audience wishes to avoid exposure to viewpoints that are relevant from the standpoint of democratic self-government - these interests collide.

Another reason why it is difficult to disentangle self-expression interests from interests in information has to do with the broadcaster's dual role as journalist and as a public trustee. Viewed in her capacity as a trustee, the broadcaster's duty to meet the audience's need for information clearly remains paramount even if it can only be fulfilled at the cost of thwarting her own self-expression needs. From the standpoint of the broadcaster's role as a journalist, however, her ability to satisfy her audience's need for information depends to a large extent on the preservation of her

---

[60] See, e.g., *Report of the National Advisory Committee on Civil Disorders*, 210 (1968) which stressed that the existing media "have not communicated to whites a feeling for the difficulties and frustrations of being a Negro in the United States".

uninhibited right to self-expression. Indeed, a broadcaster who fears government interference with her ability to express her own views is less likely to labor vigorously to inform the public about the workings of their government. Accordingly, protection of a broadcaster's right to uninhibited self-expression is necessary, not primarily for its own sake, but rather as the best possible guarantee that the broadcaster will endeavor to meet the audience's collective interest in information and criticism relating to its government.

The preceding analysis does not invalidate the basic proposition that in broadcasting collective free speech interests ought to be given priority over their individual free speech counterparts. Based on that analysis, however, it becomes necessary to broaden the notion of collective interests and to understand the limitations inherent in certain forms of government regulation, albeit that such regulation is genuinely intended to promote an agreed upon objective. Keeping in mind that equal liberty is supposed to foster equal respect and democratic self-government, the collective interests which ought to be accorded priority in broadcasting are both the dissemination of a wide array of diverse views and the propagation of vicarious self-expression. These two collective interests are, moreover, closely related as viewpoints primed for vicarious self-expression are also highly likely to be important from the standpoint of the collective free speech interests of the broadcast audience. For example, vicarious self-expression through the broadcast media of a widely held minority view to the effect that the majority is insensitive to minority concerns would provide the broadcast audience with highly relevant information which ought to be taken into account in the decisionmaking process associated with democratic self-government. On the other hand, regarding limitations on the exercise of governmental regulatory powers, it seems obvious that protection of broadcasters in their capacity as journalists precludes direct government intervention to promote underrepresented viewpoints over the airwaves, and renders problematic even some indirect regulatory devices such as the Fairness Doctrine.

Keeping in mind the dual nature of the collective interests to be persued by broadcasting and the above mentioned constraints on certain kinds of governmental regulation, it is now necessary to take a closer look at whether the FCC's minority preference policies are well suited to promote equality of opportunity among viewpoints consistent with adherence to the equal liberty principle. To begin with, the notion of equality of opportunity among viewpoints requires some elaboration since it is not self-explanatory. Moreover, even the more familiar concept of equality of opportunity among persons is a complex one that admits of several different meanings.[61] For present purposes, however, suffice it to note that equality of opportunity among persons usually requires that some factors that would influence the result of a competition among such persons be neutralized so that the outcome of the competition become the function of other factors. For example, if existing laws favor certain would-be competitors over others giving the former a great advantage in the pursuit of a coveted scarce good, instituting equality of opportunity may require amending such laws to remove law as a factor, so that the competition could be decided on the basis of other factors, such as intelligence, hard work, etc.

A distinction is often drawn between "formal" and "fair" equality of opportunity (among persons). Formal equality of opportunity has been defined as follows: "X and Y have equal opportunity in regard to A so long as neither faces a legal or quasi-legal barrier to achieving A the other does not face."[62] Fair equality of opportunity, on the other hand, requires that "those with similar abilities and skills should have similar life chances... irrespective of the income class into which they are born".[63] In other words, formal equality of opportunity is achieved when legal and quasi-legal factors are neutralized, whereas fair equality of opportunity is realized when differences among competitors owing to social and economic advantages as opposed to natural capacities are neutralized.

To the extent that equality of opportunity involves neutralizing certain factors in order to accentuate others in relation to competition for a scarce good, it focuses on the means or instruments available to those who compete for the good in question. There is also another kind of equality of opportunity which has to do with a competitor's probability of success rather than with the means at his or her disposal. For example, in the context of a fairly conducted lottery for a coveted prize, it can be said that each lottery participant enjoys equality of opportunity in the sense of having the same probability of winning the prize as every other participant.[64]

---

[61]   For an extended discussion of the concept of equality of opportunity, see Rosenfeld, *Affirmative Action*, supra note 51, at 22-29; Rosenfeld, *Substantive Equality*, supra note 8, at 1687.

[62]   Robert Fullinwider, *The Reverse Discrimination Controversy*, 101 (1980).

[63]   Rawls, supra note 55, at 73.

[64]   See Douglas Rae, et al. *Equalities*, 65-66 (1981) (distinguishing "means-regarding" equality of opportunity from "prospect-regarding" equality of opportunity).

Turning now specifically to the concept of equal opportunity among viewpoints, it is true that, in some sense, every person has a distinct viewpoint. Accordingly, it is conceivable to collapse equality of opportunity among viewpoints into equality of opportunity among persons. In the sense relevant here in terms of the collective interests to be served by broadcasting, however, viewpoints should be generally conceived as essentially collective in nature. This follows from the fact that these viewpoints seem bound to represent, at least in part, the cultural social, ethnic, religious and/or political position of a particular group in society.[65] One important consequence of the fact that one cannot count on a one to one correlation between viewpoints and persons is that equality of opportunity among viewpoints cannot be produced through a lottery. A lottery would provide a particularly desirable procedural regulatory device in as much as it could be implemented without risk of governmental biases permeating the selection process. Because of the lack of correspondence between viewpoints and persons, however, a lottery among persons would not produce equality of opportunity among viewpoints. On the other hand, conducting a lottery among viewpoints would require a criterion to determine what constitutes a distinct viewpoint as opposed to mere utterance of a view that may be shared by a large number of speakers. But since no such criterion could be purely objective, government biases would inevitably play a role in decisions concerning what ought to count as a distinct viewpoint.

Given that there appears to be no possibility of instituting any completely neutral regulatory scheme leading to genuine equality of opportunity among viewpoints in the context of broadcasting, the focus should turn to minimizing governmental bias instead of attempting to eliminate it. Moreover, to the extent that it is impractical to give every viewpoint vying for expression in the broadcast media an equal probability of success, attention should be given to the removal of certain barriers to access to the media. Formal barriers are presumably not an issue in the United States, as any one is, in theory at least, free to enter the market competition among would-be broadcasters. Formal equality of opportunity among viewpoints, however, is inadequate at least in so far as it has failed to yield sufficient exposure

---

[65]   This is not to preclude that a particular viewpoint relevant to the collective interests associated with broadcasting might be held only by a single individual, such as a prominent author or artist. It is rather to emphasize that at least some relevant viewpoints which should be disseminated to the broadcast audience are bound to be widely held among the members of a certain group, such as a political organization or an ethnic or racial group.

in broadcasting for minority viewpoints to satisfy the collective free speech interests associated with the equal liberty principle.

Just as fair equality of opportunity for persons requires neutralizing advantages stemming from social class differences to foster competition on the basis of natural abilities, fair equality of opportunity among viewpoints would seem to call for neutralization of all factors which prevent or inhibit competition among ideas on the basis of their intrinsic qualities. Thus, fair equality of opportunity among viewpoints should yield a scheme of dissemination for ideas which would produce a competition yielding winners and losers on the basis of the persuasiveness of arguments advanced in support of specific ideas rather than, say, on the basis of the financial ability of an idea's proponent to widely distribute it for broadcasting to the exclusion of other ideas presumably equally deserving of consideration.

Whereas fair equality of opportunity among ideas may be desirable in theory, it raises a series of vexing problems in practice. A major such problem stems from the difficulty inherent in any cogent attempt to separate intrinsic from extrinsic qualities when it comes to ideas and viewpoints. Suppose, for example, that Neo-Nazi views do not find their way on television because none of the powerful business corporations ultimately responsible for television programming decisions are willing to provide access for such views. Now, it may well be that this result is due not to the corruption of ideas by money, but rather to a sound judgement that given the lack of intrinsic worth of Neo-Nazi ideology, it ought not take the place on the crowded television spectrum of other ideas and viewpoints which are patently more worthy of serious consideration. On the other hand, suppose that no access to television is provided for the view that justice requires extensive redistributions of corporate wealth. In this latter case, it seems quite likely that the economic interests of broadcasters rather than the intrinsic merits of the proposed view could be held ultimately accountable for the exclusion.

Another problem in relation to the collective interests associated with equal liberty stems from the fact that whereas all views on a single subject stand *prima facie* on an equal footing (i.e. before they are subjected to the public deliberative process which is supposed to assess them in terms of their intrinsic qualities), not all subjects are of equal importance. For example, subjects like health care, economic policy and military affairs clearly seem more important from the standpoint of democratic self-government than the use of magic healing potions, proclaimed useless by all serious scientists, as a cure for all of society's physical and spiritual ills. Consistent with this, fair equality of opportunity among viewpoints

80

should result in accommodating a wide array of views on the most important subjects confronting society before making the airwaves available to views on subjects of lesser importance. Two troubling difficulties arise, however, in connection with any attempt to establish a hierarchy among subjects of public debate: First, there are not incontestable criteria for setting such a hierarchy, with the consequence that any government intervention in the process of setting the requisite hierarchy poses a grave risk of government manipulation of the flow of ideas that reaches the electronic marketplace. Second, even if the requisite hierarchy could be established without controversy, there could still be vigorous disagreement over which subject is addressed by a particular utterance. Returning to the view about magic healing potions, is the subject addressed magic - in which case it could be properly cast as of relative minor importance to a contemporary industrial democracy - or is it health or religion, both subjects of major importance in terms of the collective interests associated with equal liberty.

Even if one remains mindful of these difficulties, which cannot be addressed at greater length here, the FCC's minority preference policies can nevertheless be defended as justified under the principle of fair equality of opportunity among viewpoints. Given the dramatic underrepresentation of minority viewpoints in American broadcasting, there is little question that minority viewpoints on all subjects, including the most important ones, have not been granted comparable opportunities for access on the electronic media as have non-minority viewpoints. Moreover, the paucity of minority views over the airwaves is detrimental both to the vicarious self-expression needs of the minority audience and to the information needs of the broadcast audience as a whole. Also, this frustration of self-expression needs is compounded by the distorted view of minorities that the holders of certain non-minority viewpoints (who have achieved wide exposure for their views in broadcasting) have projected through insensitive stereotyping of certain minorities.[66] Indeed, negative stereotyping seems a worse affront to equal respect than a mere failure to afford sufficient opportunities for self-expression. In addition, the combination of negative stereotypes and gross underrepresentation of minority viewpoints skews the information presented to the broadcast audience as a whole in a way that fosters and perpetuates prejudices against minorities.

Affording a fair opportunity for self-expression to those who have been portrayed as inferiors should rank as a priority for anyone who interprets freedom

---

[66]   See *Metro Broadcasting, Inc. v. FCC*, 110 S. Ct. 2997, 3021 (1990).

of speech as entailing equal liberty.[67] From the standpoint of increasing viewpoint diversity, the highest priority in broadcasting should be accorded to the voices of those who have not only been largely left out, but also widely typecast in ways that belie their entitlement to equal respect. This highest priority seems fully justified, even though it accords precedence to minority viewpoints over other viewpoints on the same subjects or on other subjects of equal importance.

A significant reason for wishing to communicate one's viewpoint to others is frequently the hope of persuading one's audience to embrace it, or at least to take it seriously. By affording an equal opportunity for the presentation of diverse viewpoints, a public forum may provide to each of its speakers an equal opportunity to convert listeners to the speakers' viewpoint. If a viewpoint is excluded from a public forum, its proponents lose the opportunity to persuade members of that audience. But if, in addition to being excluded, a viewpoint or its proponents are relentlessly attacked or demeaned, then it is likely that hostility against this viewpoint will grow to such a degree that merely lifting a ban against it would not put it on par with a viewpoint introduced to the forum for the first time. Thus, the formerly excluded and demeaned viewpoint will most likely enjoy a lesser opportunity of being persuasive (for reasons other than its intrinsic worth) than a viewpoint that was similarly excluded but not demeaned, or a viewpoint competing for attention for the first time. Because of this added handicap, giving the excluded and demeaned viewpoint priority enhances its opportunity of finding converts without depriving other viewpoints of an equal opportunity to do the same.

So long as minority viewpoints remain severely underrepresented in broadcasting, the FCC's minority preference policies appear to be consistent with the promotion of fair equality of opportunity among viewpoints. An important issue remains, however, namely whether fair equality of opportunity among viewpoints can be satisfied notwithstanding denial of access to the viewpoint which would have found its way over the airwaves but for application of the FCC's "enhancement for minority ownership" policy. To the extent that the viewpoint displaced by the FCC's minority preference policy is already represented in broadcasting, the denial of access seems unproblematic. Moreover, even if the viewpoint in question would have been presented for the first time over the airwaves, its exclusion in favor of a minority viewpoint would still be justifiable in terms of fair equality of opportunity

---

[67]   Cf. Karst, supra note 53, at 26.(self-assertion is a way for the disadvantaged to stake a claim to equal citizenship).

among viewpoints, provided that neither the excluded viewpoint nor its proponents have been vilified and demeaned like the minorities accorded preferential treatment.

V.3.c. *Equality among persons*

Having indicated how the FCC's minority preference policies can be consistent with freedom of speech inasmuch as it requires equality among viewpoints, there remains to be determined whether these policies can be reconciled with equality among persons. To begin with, whereas equality among persons is distinct from equality among viewpoints, the two are nonetheless to a significant extent related. Thus, for instance, viewpoint equality, as it concerns vicarious self-expression, is ultimately predicated on equality among persons, in as much as such collective self-expression is a means to assert the claims to equal respect and dignity of every person who vicariously partakes in the respresentative's utterances. Furthermore, to the extent that no person enjoys a right to access to the media for purposes of individual self-expression, neither the overall scheme of broadcast regulation in the United States, nor the exception created by the FCC's minority preference policies, appear violative of equality among persons. That leaves the equality rights of those who compete for a broadcast license, and in particular of those who would have obtained such license but for the FCC's "enhancement for minority ownership" policy. Two principal arguments may be advanced on behalf of the latter: First, minority preferences impose a stigma on those who are excluded on account of the preference; and, second such preferences deprive the non-preferred competitors of equal opportunity rights. The first argument tracks a well known argument against non-minority preferences, frequently invoked in the United States in the context of racial segregation and of laws and policies designed to disadvantage African-Americans. The original argument emphasizes that racially conscious policies that disadvantage minorities are based on an (at least implicit) assumption that such minorities are inferior and undeserving, and thus impose a stigma through negative stereotyping. The parallel argument, on the other hand, stresses that, because minority preference policies distinguish on the basis of race or ethnic origin, the non-minorities whom they disadvantage are just as stigmatized as the minorities disadvantaged by racist laws.

This latter argument is hardly persuasive, however, because whereas both racist laws and minority preference policies treat persons differently in relation to their race, the two situations are by no means equivalent. Thus, for example, an African-American denied employment because of racism is likely to be stigmatized in as much as there is a widespread racist belief that African-Americans are not as capable and as industrious as whites. On the other hand, a white job applicant denied employment on account of a preferential treatment policy does not risk being perceived as lacking in capability or industriousness *because* of his race. Similarly, as the majority opinion in *Metro Broadcasting* indicated, the non-minority would-be broadcaster who would have obtained a license but for the FCC's minority preference policies cannot be seriously considered to have suffered any stigma.[68]

The second argument relating to equality among persons is that the FCC's minority preference policies deprive non-minorities of an equal opportunity to obtain a broadcast license, and hence violate such non-minorities' right to equal respect. Even if one were to concede that preferential treatment in the competition for employment is violative equality of opportunity among persons,[69] the FCC's minority preference policies could still be defended as being consistent with equality among persons. Indeed, although equal opportunity among persons ranks as important, it is not an ultimate moral value in the way that equal respect is. Accordingly, equal opportunity rights may be limited so long as the limitation does not contravene anyone's right to equal respect. Consistent with this, in job allocation where the primary objective is to maximize economic efficiency, denying any applicant an equal opportunity to compete for a job is likely to be both counterproductive and violative of equal respect. In broadcasting, however, one of the key objectives is to increase viewpoint diversity in accordance with the dictates of the equal respect principle, and the rights of broadcasters (and would-be broadcasters) are clearly subordinate to those of the audience. Therefore, requiring certain parties competing for a broadcast license to absorb some decreases in their chances of success arguably does not appear to deny equal respect to anyone.[70]

---

[68]   *Metro Broadcasting, Inc. v. F.C.C.*, 110 S. Ct. 2997, 3025 n.49 (1990).

[69]   For an extended argument to the effect that preferential treatment in the allocation of scarce jobs is not necessarily violative of equal opportunity rights, see Rosenfeld, *Affirmative Action*, supra note 51, at 284-96.

[70]   According to the Supreme Court's majority in *Metro Broadcasting* the decreases in opportunity for non-minorities as consequence of FCC's minority preference policies upheld in that case were virtually imperceptible. See 110 S. Ct. at 2997, 3026-27 (1990).

Another defense of the FCC's minority preference policies as consistent with equality among persons centers on the proposition that equality of opportunity cannot be extended to all coexisting spheres of interaction, since pursuit of equality of opportunity in one sphere is likely to conflict with its realization in another. Consistent with this approach, broadcasting is partly a competitive business operating in the economic marketplace, and partly a public forum devoted to maximizing viewpoint diversity. To the extent that it is a competitive business, broadcasting should abide by equality of opportunity among persons; to the extent that it is responsible for viewpoint diversity, broadcasting should abide by equality of opportunity among viewpoints. When these two forms of equality of opportunity clash, however, arguably equality among viewpoints should be given priority over equality among persons. This is because, from the standpoint of equal respect, (vicarious) self-expression and exposure to viewpoint diversity are more important than achieving any particular success in the economic marketplace.[71] Accordingly, the FCC's minority preference policies are compatible with the realization of equality among persons.

So long as liberty and equality are regarded as complementary and jointly embodied in the principle of equal liberty, the FCC's minority preference policies seem fully consistent with freedom of speech and constitutional equality. Moreover, although equality of opportunity among viewpoints is bound to clash on occasion with equality of opportunity among persons, it is possible to resolve such clashes in a way that respects both equality among viewpoints and equality among persons.

VI.   Conclusion

The justification of preferential treatment in the competition for broadcast licenses, as a means to enhance minority viewpoint access to the airwaves consistent with plausible criteria of liberty, equality and efficiency, underscores the virtues of the mixed substantive and procedural model governmental regulation. The problem of access for minority viewpoints to the American broadcasting media illustrates the difficulties raised when neither a purely procedural, nor a substantive model, of state

---

[71]   This assumes that the losers in the competition for a broadcast license, due to a reduction in their probability of success attributable to the pursuit of viewpoint diversity, can find suitable business alternatives capable of satisfying their material needs.

regulation are adequate to bring about a desired objective. In the context of American broadcasting, as the subject of minority access plainly indicates, a purely procedural market-type regulation is inadequate both in terms of efficiency and in terms of the free speech requirements of a stage three society. On the other hand, regulation based on the substantive model, whereby the state would command broadcasting certain views in order to enlarge the spectrum of views available to the broadcast audience, would have to be rejected as incompatible with adequate protection of free speech rights. Furthermore, even if the state were not tempted to suppress views it considered highly inimical to, or threatening against, its vital interests, state selection of viewpoints for broadcasting could be inefficient to the extent that the projection of state biases into the process of choosing among competing views would lead to a less diverse array of viewpoints than would market competition or some other means of selection. Finally, given the complex interplay of interests and values relating to the achievement of viewpoint diversity in broadcasting, the mixed substantive and procedural model of regulation seems most likely to combine a sufficient degree of efficiency with adequate safeguards for both freedom of speech and equality rights. Also, in as much as the FCC's minority preference policies seem better poised to succeed in spreading minority viewpoints over the airwaves than would reliance on the Fairness Doctrine, it appears that more indirect forms of mixed substantive and procedural governmental regulation are more desirable than their more direct counterparts. In sum, the vindication of the FCC's minority preference policies indicates that, at least in certain cases, the use of market regulatory mechanisms partially constrained by principles that embody well defined substantive values is bound to be both more legitimate and more efficient than reliance on either the market or a set of substantive directives standing alone. The lesson to be drawn from this is that, for a complex contemporary society, solutions may increasingly lie neither with the market nor away from the market, but with the proper circumscribing of market forces in accordance with cogent and well defined norms derived from widely recognized substantive values.

BUILDING A FREE PRESS

by Owen M. Fiss

The year 1989 marked a new beginning. The Berlin Wall fell and with it the Soviet empire. East Germany was soon absorbed by the Federal Republic of Germany, but other nations in Central and Eastern Europe long held in captivity by the Soviet Union proclaimed their independence. In 1991, history took still another turn. The Soviet Union itself disintegrated, and from its ruins a large number of new nations emerged in Central Asia and Eastern Europe.

All the nations that once constituted the Soviet Union and its empire are now engaged in a reconstructive process of considerable scope and intensity. One dimension of this reconstructive process is economic: The great socialist experiment, in which all the means of production were owned by the state, has been declared a failure. The production of goods and services under socialism did not keep up with that of capitalist societies, and in the name of economic efficiency reformers are now transferring the ownership of state enterprises to private hands. Another facet of the reconstructive process is political. Many, but not all, of the countries from the Soviet bloc have denounced their totalitarian past and have, in one way or another, often through the adoption of a constitution, committed themselves to democratic principles: to making a government responsive to the desires and wishes of the citizens, not the other way around.

In many respects, the two facets of the reconstructive process are consistent with one another. Indeed, the economic reforms may facilitate the establishment of democracy and are often justified in those terms. Removing the power over economic decisions - say jobs and income - from the hands of government officials not only improves efficiency but also deprives these officials of a powerful instrument of control over the public. Citizens will feel freer to criticize and disagree. Of course, state officials can still retaliate against citizen-critics by launching criminal prosecutions, but such sanctions are more visible and thus perhaps harder to deploy than deciding not to hire or promote someone. In any event, criminal sanctions were available even under a socialist economy.

From this perspective, the task of building a free press in one of the new democracies is rather straightforward: Transfer ownership of all the state-owned media - both the newspapers and the electronic media - to private interests. Sell assets like printing presses or broadcast facilities or, simply give them away. Allow

87

A. Sajó (ed.), Rights of Access to the Media, 87-108.

free entry of new enterprises. In some domains, licenses, for example, may be necessary to avoid interferences on broadcasting frequencies due to spectrum scarcity, but such licenses can be awarded to the highest bidders or through a lottery. Aside from the economic gains, such a program of rapid privatization would enhance the independence of the print and electronic media from government officials, and thus create a structure that would permit the media to provide the citizens with information and opinions that are fiercely critical of state officials. For the first time citizens would be in a position to choose their representatives in an informed manner and to make state officials responsive to their desires.

One hitch may arise from the fact that the reporters and journalists working for the newly privatized media are likely to be the same ones who worked for the state-owned media in the past. Changes in ownership do not immediately produce a change of staff. Account must, therefore, be taken of the numbering consequences of life in a totalitarian society - the critical faculties of the journalists who served the dictatorship are likely to have been dulled or destroyed.[1] Every effort must, therefore, be made to encourage reporters and journalists to use the privileges of freedom purchased for them by private capital. This may require the self-organization of journalists and the elevation of journalism into an honorable profession, one that sees itself as independent of the state and devoted to making government policies responsive to the citizen's desires.

In time, state officials might retaliate or sanction the outspoken critics of the newly privatized press. Such actions might take various forms, some criminal, others civil. State officials might charge particular journalists or broadcasters with lessening the esteem of the state (seditious libel), destroying the reputations of individual public officials (defamation), disclosing state secrets (subversion), or even fomenting unrest (inciting a breach of the peace).[2] Such state actions should not be assumed to be mean-spirited or simply vindictive; they often are intended to protect legitimate state interests, for example, maintaining public order or insuring the smooth functioning of government. Nevertheless, in order to permit the press to freely criticize government - to provide what we in the United States call "breathing

---

[1]   See Jiri Pebe et al., *The Media in Eastern Europe*, Radio Free Europe/Radio Liberty Res. Rep., May 1993, at 22, 22-23, 26, 28, 29, 31 and 32.

[2]   For a discussion of the various ways in which the state may interfere with the free functioning of the press, see Harry Kalven, Jr., *A Worthy Tradition*, 3-73 (1988).

space"[3] - these retaliatory actions by the state against the newly privatized media should be strictly confined or bounded.

Imposing these limits on state power may require the development of a strong and independent judiciary - an institution that can stand above the fray of partisan politics and interpret and enforce principles of freedom that are not easily amended or changed.[4] The United States Constitution guarantees freedom of the press and has been read by the Supreme Court to give the press - almost entirely privately owned - a measure of autonomy from state regulation. In looking to this experience, however, 89'ers should bear in mind that though the autonomy guaranteed to the press in the United States is indeed admirable, it is not absolute. It varies from context to context and depends on the weight and significance of the countervailing state interest involved. The Supreme Court has been generous in its protection of the press when nothing more than the reputation of such officials was at stake,[5] but of an entirely different mind when the press was about to disclose a state secret regarding, for instance, the construction of nuclear weapons or a troop movement.[6]

---

[3] *New York Times Co. v. Sullivan*, 376 U.S. 254, 272 (1964).

[4] Although the democracies emerging in the former Soviet Empire continue to struggle in carving out an independent role for their judiciaries, on specific occasions the Russian and Hungarian Constitutional Courts have lent a measure of protection to the press and have kept hostile government officials at bay. See Frances H. Foster, *Izvestiia as a Mirror of Russian Legal Reform*, 27 Vand. J. Transnat'l L. 675 (1993); Andrew Arato, The Hungarian Constitutional Court in the Media War (paper presented at Central European University conference "The Development of Rights of Access to the Media", June 21, 1993.

[5] See *New York Times*, 376 U.S. at 279-83 (barring a "public official" from recovering damages for defamatory falsehood absent a showing of actual malice); *Curtis Publishing Co. v. Butts*, 388 U.S. 130 (1967) (a majority of the Court agreeing to extend the New York Times test to apply to "public figures" as well as "public officials").

[6] See, e.g., *Near v. Minnesota*, 283 U.S. 697, 716 (1931) (prior restraint of speech might be justified to prevent publication of sailing dates of transport ships or the location of troops in time of war); *New York Times v. United States*, 403 U.S. 713, 725-27 (1971) (Brennan, J., concurring) (prior restraint could be justified in peacetime to suppress "information that would set in motion a nuclear holocaust"). See also *United States v. Progressive*, 467 F. Supp. 990 (W.D. Wis. 1979) (enjoining a magazine from printing the instructions for building a hydrogen bomb), appeal dismissed, 610 F.2d 819 (7th Cir. 1979) (publication elsewhere of similar material made issue moot). See generally Fiss, *Free Speech and the Prior Restraint Doctrine: The Pentagon Papers Case*, in *The Supreme Court and Human Rights* 49 (Burke Marshall ed. 1982).

Underlying the general strategy I have been outlining - of privatizing the press, encouraging journalists to see themselves as members of a profession, and creating for the press a constitutionally protected zone of autonomy from state regulation - is an assumption that the state is the natural enemy of democracy. Indeed, aside from the purely economic considerations, privatization recommends itself so strongly as a strategy for building a free press simply because it takes control of the press away from the state. Such an assumption about the unfriendly posture of the state is most understandable in a transitional democracy, where people have lived under a state dictatorship for many years and are now trying to escape from that horror. However, the transition will not last forever and in any event should not obscure the full dimensions of the reconstructive process. For more than two hundred years we in the United States have had a continuous democracy, and in this setting we have learned that the state can have two faces - sometimes it acts as an enemy of democracy, but sometimes as its friend. Initially, this may seem paradoxical, a replay of the double-talk that characterized the socialist dictatorships of the not-too-distant past, but not once we acknowledge that the market is itself a structure of constraint and that the state might be needed to counteract those constraints placed on the press by the market. The newly constituted press might be called "free" because the papers or radio or television stations are not owned or controlled by the state, but they do not operate in a social vacuum. The owners seek to maximize their profit by maximizing revenue and minimizing costs, and their capacity to maximize revenue is curbed by competitive pressure. These are the iron laws of capitalist economics, which hold true for the newly privatized media as much as they do for any other business.

No social actor is completely autonomous. Everyone is embedded in a social structure and is restrained by it. A question must therefore be raised whether the constraints imposed by the market on the media are of any special source of concern from a purely political perspective. It may safely be conceded that the market constrains the media, but some would argue that this constraint is not inconsistent with democratic goals and indeed might actually further such goals. The desire to maximize revenue will drive publishers and broadcasters to increase the attractiveness of their product to the public, and thus make the coverage and method of presentation responsive to consumer desires. The public gets what it wants. There is much force to this vew, as aconomic theory and the American experience teaches, but I do not believe it conveys the whole story.

First, the capacity of the newly privatized media to respond to consumer desires will be limited by costs. The businessman seeks to maximize profits. That requires minimizing costs as well as maximizing revenues, and thus the media may well offer the public considerably less than it wants. Overwhelmed by the costs of newsgathering or producing high quality documentaries, the temptation has been great in the television industry, for example, to rely on the reruns of "sit-coms" or "soap operas".

Second, reliance on advertising as the method of generating revenue - as typically is the case where the press is privatized - will introduce a number of distortions. One stems from the obvious fact that regardless of how desired a program or series of articles might be by the public, these programs or articles will not be underwritten by advertisers unless they are likely to enhance the sales of the would-be advertisers' products. It was reported, for example, that coverage of the Gulf War in the United States was slighted by the commercial television networks because advertisers did not want their products associated with scenes of death and destruction. Similarly, a prominent feminist magazine ("Ms") found it difficult to find advertisers, especially those selling beauty products for women, because the articles did not reinforce the image of women presented in the advertisements or otherwise induce women to buy the advertised products.

The dependence on advertising also leads publishers and broadcasters to discriminate among potential views and readers in determining what they present and how it will be presented. Particular "target audiences," not the public in general, will be of concern to the privately owned press, and these audiences are defined in terms of purchasing power and susceptibility to advertising. Far from the democratic norm of one person, one vote, those with large disposable income will see their own tastes reflected in the media.

Third, while a certain segment of the public may govern the content of broadcasts and newspapers through ordinary market processes, these individuals do not deliberate collectively. The radio or television program that individuals choose in the privacy of their home, after dinner and a day's work, might well be different than programs they might choose after fully discussing and debating all the options. The same is true regarding the daily purchase of a newspaper. Admittedly, democratic theory does not require all social decisions to be a product of collective deliberation, but the normative force of any claim made in the name of "the public" - here it would be about the coverage of the press - often presupposes such deliberation.

92

Thus, there is good reason to doubt that the newly privatized media will give the public all that it wishes, or that the coverage or broadcasts determined by the market - what I will call "market-determined speech" - can be viewed as the rough approximation of "democratically-determined speech" - the broadcasts and coverage that would be chosen by a people after full deliberation, unconstrained by costs, and with full respect to the principle of one person, one vote.[7] There may, however, be a deeper source of concern: Should the ideal or standard by which one judges the output of the market be what I have called democratically-determined speech? Democracy involves a choice by a people, but perhaps that choice does not extend to the views that they hear or the positions that they must confront. Perhaps the aspirations should be even higher.

Democracy is a system of government that assigns the ultimate responsibility to the public to decide how it wishes to live, but presupposes that the public is fully informed when it makes that judgment. Democracy requires that the public have all the relevant information and is aware of the contending or conflicting points of view on any issue. A free press is to make this supposition a reality. One way of expressing this is to say that in a democratic system the mission of the press is to produce on matters of public importance a debate that is "uninhibited, robust, and wide-open".[8] Suppose the people decide, however, that they are sick and tired of "robust public debate," but are only interested in mind-dulling entertainment or with newspapers or television programs that give expression to their sexual fantasies. Would a democracy be required us to respect that choice? I think not, no more than a commitment to contractual freedom requires one to respect a contract in which someone sells himself or herself into slavery.

A distinction should thus be drawn between "democratically-determined speech" and what I have called "robust public debate", and the latter should be seen as the standard against which we should measure the output of the market. Such a view may seem alien to the system of liberties we have enjoyed in the United States

---

[7] Writing on the Polish experience, Karel Jakubowicz makes a similar distinction between what he terms "free communication" and "democratic communication," arguing that in the emerging democracies of Central and Eastern Europe, greater emphasis has been placed on the libertarian, market-oriented concept of "free communication" than on communication which is representative of the community at large. See Karol Jakubowicz, *Freedom vs. Equality*, E. Eur. Const. Rev., Summer 1993, at 42.

[8] *New York Times Co. v. Sullivan*, 376 U.S. at 270.

and that has been used as a model for many in Eastern and Central Europe and Central Asia, but this is not so. The United States Bill of Rights, including the protection afforded to the press in the First Amendment, is often spoken of as a protection of "minority rights" or "individual rights"- or as a bulwark against "tyranny of the majority".[9] In protecting the press against state interferences, the Supreme Court never assumed that in trying to muzzle the press the state was acting autonomously from, or in disregard of, popular desire or majority will. On the contrary, the Court knew all too well that more often than not state officials, whether legislative or executive, were acting as instruments of popular will, yet took upon themselves a responsibility to preserve the robustness of public debate - in a word, to protect democracy from itself.

In a similar vein, then, nation builders should be concerned with constraints imposed by the market, not simply because market-determined speech will be a poor approximation of democratically-determined speech, but rather because it may well depart significantly from the more abstract, largely idealized standard - robust public debate. Once the media are privatized, programming and coverage will be largely determined by the confluence of numbers of factors - marginal cost and marginal revenue - that have no discernible relationship to needs of a democratic polity. As businessmen, the owners of the media will have their minds on profits, not on the task of supplying the public with the information and various opinions it needs in order to exercise its sovereign prerogative.

Even on this view, some may treat state constraints on public debate as a wholly different plane than those emanating from the market. To some extent, this view stems from precise wording of the United States Constitution ("Congress shall make no law abridging the freedom of speech, or of the press"). The First Amendment freedom of the press consists of a prohibition on one branch of the state (Congress). But such a detail about the American experience should not restrain those who are now actively engaged in the process of building new democratic societies, drafting new constitutions, or interpreting constitutional provisions that may be worded in other more affirmative terms. For example, the new Hungarian constitution, following the European tradition, provides: "The Republic of Hungary

---

[9]   In *The Bill of Rights as a Constitution*, 100 Yale L.J. 1131, 1147-52 (1991), Professor Akhil R. Amar challenges the conventional wisdom that the First Amendment freedoms of speech and press are essentially aimed at protecting minorities, and argues that the "structural core" of the First Amendment seeks to protect popular majorities from hostile Congressional action.

shall recognize and protect freedom of the press." In any event, my own impression is that the distinction often drawn in American circles between market constraints and state constraints rest on grounds that are more philosophic than textual, though in the end, they too are less than fully persuasive.

One such ground for drawing a distinction between the two types of constrains stems from a narrow conception of the domain of public debate, confining it to speech that pertains to the election for public office or the work of government.[10] The democratic mission of the press, so the argument runs, is to assist the public in choosing government officials and evaluating their work; the principal danger to be concerned with is that government officials will use the power at their disposal to retaliate against those who dare to criticize them. In my view, however, there is no reason to construe the democratic mission of the press so narrowly: yes, the press would "check" governmental officials, to borrow Professor Blasi's term,[11] but it also has a responsibility to address large questions of economic and social structure, such as the distribution of wealth and the role of workers in the management of their firms. All such subjects are within the jurisdiction of the demos.

Moreover, even if the domain of public debate be conceived narrowly, thereby limiting it to criticism of government officials and their policies, there may be reason to be wary of market constraints, because they have the effect of favoring certain governmental policies and the officials who implement them. Imagine the position a newly privatized press will take on a candidate for government urging a radical redistribution of wealth or the institution of worker control.[12] Not every government policy is market-sensitive in this way, but many are and thus there is reason to be concerned with the impact of market constraints on public debate even if that exception be narrowly and artificially confined to reach only speech that considers governmental affairs.

---

[10] See, e.g., Robert H. Bork, *Neutral Principles and Some First Amendment Problems*, 47 Ind. L.J. 1 (1971).

[11] See Vincent Blasi, *The Checking Value in First Amendment Theory*, 1977 Am. B. Found. Res. J. 521.

[12] For a discussion of the ways in which the Western press has failed to cover the "grand issues", including social structure and distribution of wealth, see Charles E. Lindblom, *Politics and Markets*, 204-207 (1977).

State constraints and market constraints have also been sharply differentiated because of the difference in the method by which the two are enforced. The state has a monopoly over the legitimate use of force and can throw those who violate its edicts in jail.[13] A press mogul enforces his demands by excluding an article, shaping a show in a certain way, or firing a reporter who turns in copy that does not sell papers. In actual practice, this distinction between the methods of enforcement may be less clear-cut. The state can enforce its constraints through civil remedies (e.g., damage awards or denial of licenses), and if the United States is any guide, such remedies may well turn out to be commonplace. A question can also be raised about the presumed difference in the harshness of the sanctions. How much worse is it to throw someone in jail than to be fired or to have a business fail? Even granting these distinctions, however, the difference in the method by which the state and market enforce their edicts is of no special moment from democracy's perspective. What is crucial is not the moral quality of the means used to enforce a constraint nor the hardship suffered by the individual who bears the brunt of the sanction, but rather the effect of the constraint on public discourse.

To be sensitive to the constraints placed on public debate by the market in this way is not to urge that the media in the democracies emerging from the shambles of the Soviet Union and its empires should be owned by the state. Privatization does seem an overall sensible strategy. It has already been pursued with the newspapers and I would extend that strategy to television and radio. They too should be sold to private interests. Such a strategy may be justified in terms of the immediate past history of these new nations, where the press was used by the Soviet dictatorship and its puppet governments as an instrument of control. Rapid privatization is needed to destroy the habits of subservience that the dictatorial practices of the past may have instilled, or at least to convince the citizenry that things have changed and that the press can be believed. A general policy in favor of privatization may also be premised on a more calculating judgment-market constraints should be taken seriously, but they are more diffuse and thus less threatening than those emanating from the state. Such a view seems supported by the American experience, which has its pluses and minuses, but, after all, has produced the most stable if not the most vibrant democracy the world has ever known. For

---

[13] See Charles Fried, *The New First Amendment Jurisprudence: A Threat to Liberty*, 59 U. Chi. L. Rev. 225, 235-37 (1992).

more than two hundred years the newspapers in the United States have been privately owned and we have had private ownership of radio and television ever since those technologies became available.

A decision as to the basic structure of ownership does not, however, preclude a series of supplemental or interstitial state interventions founded on the idea that the market is a structure of constraint and that left to itself may well limit or skew public debate. Once again, the United States experience is instructive. We have the most thoroughgoing system of private ownership of the media in the world, yet over the years we have adopted a wide number of interstitial strategies to counteract the constraining effect of the market. Doubts can be raised, and have been raised, as to whether these measures have been fully effective. Some have urged that they be strengthened, yet few - aside from the most orthodox, who see the nose of the camel everywhere - would contend that these forms of state intervention are inconsistent or incompatible with a decision to privatize the basic structure.

One category of supplemental state interventions might be called "program regulation." Within this category I would include the Federal Communications Commission (FCC) regulation - referred to as the fairness doctrine - that required broadcasters to cover issues of public importance and to do so fairly.[14] Laws allowing persons who are subject to a personal attack or political editorializing to respond and a requirement that the networks give adequate coverage to presidential elections might also be considered to be program regulations.[15] At one time an effort was made by public interest groups to have the FCC require networks to air "editorial advertisements."[16] This too might be considered a program regulation.

A second category of state intervention is more structural. The aim is to alter the content of newspapers and broadcasts by altering the structure of ownership, once again, not to reverse the overall judgment in favor of private ownership, but rather to intervene interstitially within the capitalist structure to

---

[14] For a discussion of the background and content of the fairness doctrine, see *Red Lion Broadcasting v. F.C.C.*, 395 U.S. 367, 369-71 (1969). See also Randall Rainey, *The Public's Interest in Public Affairs Discourse, Democratic Governance, and Fairness in Broadcasting*, 82 Geo. L.J. (1993).

[15] See *Miami Herald Publishing Co. v. Tornillo*, 418 U.S. 241 (1974); *CBS v. F.C.C.*, 453 U.S. 367 (1981).

[16] See *CBS v. Democratic Nat'l Comm.*, 412 U.S. 94 (1973).

enlarge the domain of public discourse. Antitrust might be considered an example of such a structural regulation, but it is only a limited one, since it seeks to perfect the market rather than to counteract or supplement it.[17] Another variant can be found in the "cross ownership" rules of the FCC, which prohibit the owner of a newspaper from acquiring a television or radio station in the same market.[18] The assumption is that such acquisitions could not be barred on purely economic grounds.

An even more robust form of structural regulation could be found in the decision of Congress in the 1960's to establish and fund a public broadcasting network to supplement rather than supplant the commercial networks. A public broadcasting system could cover issues likely to be slighted by the commercial networks but which are nevertheless vital to democratic self-government.[19] Mention should also be made of the policy of the FCC to give preference to racial minorities in the award of licenses.[20] To some extent that policy could be understood as a way of improving the social status of minorities, but it also has a speech dimension and could be considered a form of structural regulation. The assumption is that race is a proxy for viewpoint and that these new owners would exercise discretion allowed

---

[17]   Despite antitrust laws and enforcement in the United States, 98 percent of all American cities with a daily newspaper had only one as of 1986. See Robbie Steel, *Joint Operating Agreements in the Newspaper Industry: A Threat to First Amendment Freedoms*, 138 U. Pa. L. Rev. 275, 277 (1989). See generally William E. Lee, *Antitrust Enforcement, Freedom of the Press, and the "Open Market": The Supreme Court on the Structure and Content of Mass Media*, 32 Vand. L. Rev. 1249 (1979).

[18]   See Second Report and Order, Rules Relating to Multiple Ownership of Standard, FM, and Television Stations, 50 F.C.C.2d 1046 (1975). The FCC's "cross ownership" rules were at issue in the recent case *News America Publishing v. F.C.C.*, 844 F.2d 300 (D.C. Cir. 1988).

[19]   See Public Broadcasting Act of 1967, 47 U.S.C. §§ 390-399; Carnegie Commission on Educational Television, Public Television: A Program for Action (1967).

[20]   The United States Supreme Court upheld the constitutionality of this policy in *Metro Broadcasting v. F.C.C.*, 497 U.S. 547 (1990). Two years later, however, the United States Circuit Court of Appeals for the District of Columbia Circuit invalidated a similar FCC policy giving preference to women in the licensing process. *Lamprecht v. F.C.C.*, 958 F.2d 382 (D.C. Cir 1992). The author of *Lamprecht*, Clarence Thomas, is now a justice of the Supreme Court. Two of the five justices on the majority in *Metro Broadcasting*, Justices Brennan and Marshall, have since retired.

to them by the market in favor of diversifying programming and thus enriching public debate.

Many of the regulatory measures that I have described are aimed at television and radio, as opposed to newspapers, but now and then the state has tried to regulate newspapers. In some instances the United States Supreme Court has looked upon such regulation with great disfavor and has built into the law a distinction between electronic and print media. Most notably, it invalidated a Florida right-to-reply statute in a context in which it was assumed that such a regulation would be constitutional if applied to television or radio.[21] However, as recognized by most constitutional law scholars, there is no basis for the distinction in the Constitution and scarcely should be emulated.

In the United States television and radio stations are licensed by the state, to avoid interferences on the broadcast frequency, but they are as much part of the press as newspapers. They too shape public discourse and inform people of the world that lies beyond their immediate experience. The place of television and radio as part of the working press has been recognized in other areas of the law, such as libel, where broadcasters are endowed with the very same privileges and responsibilities that belong to newspapers. Admittedly, the obscenity standard has been adjusted to permit greater state control of the electronic media,[22] but that is premised on the fact that it is harder to shield unwitting or especially vulnerable audiences (e.g., children) from radio or television broadcasts, not on the idea that television or radio are not part of the press. Admittedly, the property rights of a television or radio station have their origins in a deliberate, allocative decision of government, specifically an award of a license. The property rights of newspapers have a more diffuse origin; they come from the common law and state policies that apply to all businesses. But the special constitutional status of the press derives from the function of that institution in society, to inform the public, and should not be

---

[21]   *Miami Herald Publishing Co. v. Tornillo*, 418 U.S. 241 (1974).

[22]   See *F.C.C. v. Pacifica Foundation*, 438 U.S. 726 (1978) (holding that the FCC
         may constitutionally sanction radio and television stations for the broadcast of
         "indecent" or "offensive" material even if that material would not be considered
         "obscene" under standards established for printed material).

made to turn on the source of its property rights or the particular dynamics that gave rise to them.[23]

The supplemental state interventions I have described and that seek to enrich public debate are generally referred to under the category of the "right to access." This term was introduced by an influential article in the late 1960's by Professor Jerome Barron.[24] The expression seeks to capitalize on the mystique that surrounds "rights-talk" in the United States, but for that very reason is misleading. Most of the rights that figure in contemporary constitutional debates, for instance the right to procreative freedom, further some individualistic value, but this is not true of Barron's "right to access." That right does not seek to protect the self-expressive interests of an individual citizen seeking access, but rather is intended to further a collective goal: the production of robust public debate. A more apt expression - and the one I will use to refer to the entire panoply of program and structural regulation intended to enrich public debate - is "access regulations."

Even with this emendation an ambiguity persists. People speak of access, but do not specify access to what. Since in my view the purpose of access regulations is to enrich public discourse, rather than to give vent to some self-expressive interest of an individual, what must be guaranteed is access to the public, not to a media. Access to a radio or television station or newspaper is provided only as a way of affording access to the public, and any access regulation should be judged accordingly. That explains why the so-called public access channels on cable T.V. - allowing the citizen to appear on camera at 3:00 A.M. - are inadequate. Such appearances play no more role in public deliberations than having a book deep in the stacks of a university library. Of course, the determined citizen can seek out the viewpoint, but one must be realistic about the public's inquisitiveness. On the other hand, as long as the viewpoint or information is in general circulation and thus fully available to the public, no further demand for access remains. The predicate for regulation dissolves, or to put it differently, to insist upon access in these circumstances would be unnecessary, perhaps even vindictive. To use a metaphor

---

[23]   Access regulation of yet another form of media, cable television, is currently at issue in a case pending before the United States Supreme Court, see *Turner Broadcasting System v. F.C.C.*, No. 93-44.

[24]   Jerome A. Barron, *Access to the Press - a New First Amendment Right*, 80 Harv. L. Rev. 1641 (1967). Professor Barron further developed the issue of the "right to access" in his book, *Freedom of the Press for Whom? The Right of Access to Mass Media*, (1973).

of Charles Fried, it would be "a way of showing off power by hoisting flags on other people's flagpoles".[25]

Subject to these limitations, the access regulations or the package of program and structural interventions I have sketched - and there are many variants[26] - should be seen as having an important role to play in any scheme trying to establish a free press. Access regulations are not inconsistent with the decision to privatize the media, but rather can serve as a supplement intended to lessen some of the constraints of the market for the purpose of enriching public debate. Of course, such forms of state regulation need to be reinforced by the development of a professional ethos by journalists that emphasizes the democratic rather than the economic goals of the enterprise they work for. Far from dampening the evolution of such an ethos, or being redundant, access regulations might actually facilitate the evolution of that ethos and give it some vitality. They confer the state's imprimatur on what the journalists are trying to achieve for themselves. Similarly, recognition of a measure of autonomy for the press from state interference is not inconsistent with such supplemental regulations. Both editorial autonomy and access regulations have the same purpose - allowing the press to fulfil its democratic mission. The line between state interferences that will be disallowed (e.g., prosecutions for seditious libel) and those allowed (e.g., the fairness doctrine) is defined in terms of the same metric: robust public debate. The disallowed constrict public debate; the allowed enhance it.

During the 1960's and 1970's, these distinctions were readily understood. While the domain of editorial autonomy was broadened and the press became increasingly professionalized, access regulations flourished. But during the late 1970's and 1980's - as America became more and more obsessed with the wonders of the market and the activist state fell into disfavor - the law took a somewhat different course. Access regulations became suspect. Aside from the decision invalidating the Florida right-to-reply statute, the Supreme Court refused to require networks to accept editorial advertisements and made it clear that the fairness

---

[25] Fried, supra note 10, at 253. Fried applied this metaphor to all program regulation, what he refers to as "forced programming," on the questionable hypothesis that the public will always tune out.

[26] See Ilana Dayan-Orbach, *Beyond the Marketplace of Ideas: Corporate Reorganization of the Media*, 278-346 (1993) (unpublished manuscript, on file with the author, setting forth proposals to reorganize the boards of directors of press corporations to strengthen their democratic mission).

doctrine was a matter of administrative discretion.[27] In 1987 the FCC renounced the fairness doctrine,[28] and a Congressional effort to restore it was vetoed by President Reagan.[29]

To be sure, not all access regulations were invalidated during this period. Regulations requiring the networks to cover presidential elections were allowed to stand.[30] Also, in the late 1980's the Supreme Court upheld - in a close vote - the policy of the FCC that gave preference to minorities in the award of broadcast licenses.[31] Still, as a general matter, it is fair to report that during the 1970's and 1980's the right of access and the entire idea of regulating the press in the name of democracy came under increasing attack. As a consequence a strong doubt now exists in the minds of many as to whether access regulations are consistent with our commitment to a free press. The timing of this turn of events is, at least to my mind, particularly unfortunate, for it coincided with the collapse of the Soviet empire and the beginning of the reconstructive enterprise that is the subject of this essay. The risk is great that, like all politicians, 89'ers will have a short time horizon and confuse the Reagan years for the whole of American experience.

During the 1970's and 1980's many objections were raised to access regulations. One expressed the doubt whether such regulations actually enriched public debate. The argument was made that the fairness doctrine made the networks more careful of what they broadcasted, for fear that if they carried a show on some controversial issue they would need to allow time for a response. The effect of regulation was, so some claimed, a form of self-censorship - grey speech. On the other side, it was argued that certain features of the regulatory program - for example, the affirmative requirement to cover issues of public importance - might guard against the risk of grey speech. It was also pointed out that the judgment about

---

[27]   See *CBS. v. Democratic Nat'l Comm.*, 412 U.S. 94 (1973).

[28]   See *Syracuse Peace Council*, 2 F.C.C.R. 5043 (1987) (concluding that "the fairness doctrine, on its face, violates the First Amendment and contravenes the public interest"), *aff'd on narrower grounds*, 867 F.2d 654 (D.C. Cir. 1989), *cert. denied*, 493 U.S. 1019 (1990).

[29]   23 Weekly Comp. Pres. Doc. 715 (June 19, 1987) (President Reagan vetoing the Fairness in Broadcasting Act of 1987).

[30]   *CBS v. F.C.C.*, 453 U.S. 367 (1981).

[31]   *Metro Broadcasting v. F.C.C.*, 497 U.S. 547 (1990). See supra note 17.

the efficacy of the fairness doctrine or other access regulations must be made on a comparative basis: Even assuming some self-censorship due to regulation, broadcasting might be more varied and more keyed to public issues than if the regulation did not exist at all. To fully assess the impact of access regulations, one must not simply look to the incidents of self-censorship, but should consider the whole program of access regulations and imagine how it would be if these regulations did not exist. Only then would we know whether they enriched or impoverished public debate.

This objection to access regulations turned on empirical judgments about the likely consequences of access regulation, but others were more principled. One such objection involved the principle against content regulation and argued that access regulations, by their very nature, were not content neutral. This principle is founded on the idea that the choice over public issues should be left in the hands of the public and that it is wrong for state officials to decide what ideas are good or bad or even to favor one side over another in a public debate. State officials must be neutral on these issues and let the people decide. Such a requirement of state neutrality seems attractive, firmly rooted in democratic theory and the entire First Amendment tradition,[32] but I do not see it as barring access regulations.

Admittedly, content judgments are indeed made when the state regulates in the name of democracy. With program regulation, content judgments are made directly; with structural regulation, indirectly. Given the scarcity of resources and the multiplicity of viewpoints, state officials must make judgments as to what views or positions are to be favored, either when it awards a subsidy, grants a preference to some group in the licensing process, or determines that a broadcaster must cover an issue of public importance. However, these content judgments and the others made in fashioning or enforcing access regulation are not to determine outcome, but only to protect the integrity of the deliberative process. In all these cases the state is acting like a parliamentarian, trying to make certain that the public is fully informed, and makes content judgments in order to properly discharge that function. It is as though the state were saying, "Let's hear from the other side", or "We have heard that point several times now". In making these calls the state qua parliamentarian is obviously looking to the content of what is said, but should not

---

[32]   See T.M. Scanlon, Jr., *Content Regulation Reconsidered, in Democracy and the Mass Media*, 331 (Judith Lichtenberg ed., 1990); Geoffrey R. Stone, *Content-Neutral Restrictions*, 54 U. Chi. L. Rev. 46 (1987). See generally Kalven, supra note 1.

be barred from doing so by the rule requiring content neutrality, for properly understood, that rule bars only those content judgments that have no other justification than to determine or shape outcome. Of course, any regulation of process will necessarily have an impact or effect upon outcome, but the choice that democratic theory seeks to insulate from state influence or control is one preceded by full debate, not one that is uninformed or ill-considered. A fully informed citizen is likely to make a different decision than an uninformed one, but the state's role in educating the citizen and thus producing a different outcome is not to be condemned from the perspective of democracy.

Sly politicians can always say they are not regulating process when in fact they have no other purpose or justification than the manipulation of outcome. The danger of such manipulation should call for institutional arrangements that take program or structural regulation out of the hands of those most intensely interested in political outcomes and place it in the hands of agencies that are relatively removed from politics. We in the United States had some experience with independent administrative agencies in the early part of the 20th century and wisely placed the administration of the fairness doctrine and control over the licensing process in the hands of such an agency (the FCC), rather than the President or Congress. Similarly, an independent public corporation - the Corporation for Public Broadcasting - was established to administer the Congressionally funded radio and television networks. That corporation is still dependent on annual appropriations, but otherwise is insulated from direct control by Congress or the President.[33] The emerging democracies of the East obviously have no such tradition to fall back on, so that it would be necessary to create analogous institutions afresh. The difficulties inherent in such a task, especially given a recent past of totalitarianism, which politicized all institutions, are indeed formidable, but the creation of the institutions of advanced capitalism - a banking system or a securities market - out of shambles of state socialism was no less daunting.

---

[33] By statute, the Corporation for Public Broadcasting is largely independent of control by Congress or the executive; 47 U.S.C. § 398(a) prohibits "any department, agency, officer, or employee of the United States [from exercising] any direction, supervision, or control over public telecommunications, or over the Corporation or any of its contractors, or over the charter or bylaws of the Corporation. . . ." Measures have also been taken to remove the Corporation from the influence of partisan politics. The members of the Corporation's board are appointed by the President and confirmed by the Senate, but 47 U.S.C. § 396(c)(1) provides that no more than six of the ten members may be from the same political party.

Even with such independent agencies or institutions, the risk still persists - as it does in the United States - that the power to make content judgments will not be used to preserve the integrity of public debate, but to skew the debate in favor of one outcome. That risk can be minimized, but can never be eliminated altogether. On the other hand, it should be realized that by adopting a strong prophylactic rule - one denying state officials any power whatsoever to make judgments based on content - would simply allow the debate to be wholly shaped by the market, which, of course, is not neutral as to content. The biases of the market are not the product of deliberate decisions of government officials, but rather derive from businessmen competing with one another. Nevertheless, from democracy's perspective, the concern should be no less. Democracy requires full and open debate in all issues of public importance and is threatened by any interference or constraint on that debate, regardless of the identity of the interfering agency or the precise nature of the dynamic that brings it into being.

Access regulations not only require government to make content judgments, but also sometimes - as in the case of program regulation - require some newspaper or television or radio station to carry a message or article that the owners of the enterprise find odious. The purpose of such a requirement is not to punish the newspaper or station for having engaged in some scandalous reporting, or even to humble it, but rather to broaden the public's understanding. Still, a question has been raised as to whether such compulsion is consistent with a principle - rooted in the 1943 decision of the Supreme Court in *West Virginia Board of Education v. Barnette*[34] that guarantees to the individual freedom not to support or affirm an idea that he or she finds offensive.

In its original context the *Barnette* decision seems to constitute a powerful affirmation of freedom of conscience or religious liberty. The Supreme Court refused to capitulate to patriotic fervor then sweeping the country and protected young school children from being compelled to salute the American flag. These children were Jehovah's Witnesses and found the pledge of allegiance inconsistent with their faith. The Court's decision did not seem to have any bearing on the various regulations of the type I am recommending, and in fact access regulations were never challenged on that ground during the period they were first developed. However, in the late 1980's the Supreme Court ripped the right not to speak from its original context and used it to invalidate an access regulation developed by

---

[34]   319 U.S. 624 (1943).

California. In the case in question, *Pacific Gas & Electric*,[35] the challenged regulation required a power company to allow a public interest organization to use the so-called extra space in a billing envelope to reach the public. The extra space consisted of the space in a billing envelope that could be used to place an insert without increasing the minimum postage charge. That space had been used in the past by the power company for distributing its own newsletter and was now being allocated by the utility commission to the public interest group to use four times a year. However, the Supreme Court invoked *Barnette* and concluded that the utility commission had violated the free speech guarantee of the First Amendment.

The significance of *Pacific Gas & Electric* for program regulation of the press was immediately recognized. The author of the plurality opinion, Justice Powell, made reference to the earlier decision of the Court invalidating the Florida right-to-reply statute to support his decision, and in 1987 in *Pacific Gas & Electric* was used by the FCC as one of the grounds for invalidating the fairness doctrine.[36] If it violates the First Amendment to require a utility company to carry in its billing envelope a message that it finds offensive, it should be equally violative of the First Amendment, so the FCC reasoned, to require a network to broadcast a show that it finds objectionable. In my view, both the Supreme Court's decision in *Pacific Gas & Electric* and the FCC's extension of it to the press seem questionable.

In a society in which the press is privately owned, it must be immediately acknowledged that program regulation or state-mandated access entails a compromise of property rights and a loss of the economic values associated with those rights. The mandated message or program will displace the article or program a station or publisher deemed more profitable. The displaced message can only be carried if extra pages are added or the broadcast day somehow extended. The economic loss may be small or of limited significance, but its reality cannot and should not be denied. A little loss is still a loss.

Some may see this economic loss as giving rise to a duty of compensation by the state, under the theory that property is being taken for a public use. The United States Constitution provides that no property shall be taken for public use without compensation. However, a claim of compensation founded on this provision

---

[35] *Pacific Gas & Electric Co. v. Public Utilities Comm'n of California*, 475 U.S. 1 (1986).

[36] *Syracuse Peace Council*, 2 F.C.C.R. 5043, 5057, 5070 n.227, 5071 nn.241-46.

106

was rejected by the Supreme Court in a case involving still another type of access regulation - California required shopping center owners to allow political activists to enter upon their property for purposes of reaching the public.[37] The Supreme Court ruled that the economic loss caused by this act of the state (protest activities may induce shoppers to stay away) was not a taking, but only a regulation, of property. In reaching this conclusion, great stress was placed on the generality of the regulation.

Wisely, this ruling was left unquestioned in the *Pacific Gas & Electric* case. No member of the Court thought the regulation by the utility commission was a taking of the property of the power company, and presumably the result would be the same in a press case or some business without a government conferred monopoly. If the economic loss occasioned by a grant of access to a shopping center or a billing envelope is not a taking, neither is the economic loss suffered by the press when access is granted to it. There is an economic loss, but that is true of most government regulation of business and none of the special conditions that transform regulations into takings are present.

The free speech claim does not arise from the economic loss simpliciter, but rather from the fact that the owners of the power company or the newspaper or radio or television station are being compelled to support financially views or ideas that they do not subscribe to and may actually detest. It is hard, however, to turn this objection into a viable principle of constitutional law without dismantling the modern democratic state. The entire taxation system of the modern state is predicated on the idea that money taken from citizens may be used to support activities they detest, such as war, parades, particular lectures at state universities, or many of the books in public libraries. Such compelled financial support is seen as an obligation of citizenship, necessary to serve community purposes, which in the case of access regulations consists of the preservation of the democratic process itself. Having one's property or wealth used to support activities a citizen detests is but a price of democracy.

This idea was faintly acknowledged in *Pacific Gas & Electric*. Justice Powell readily admitted that the power company could be taxed or assessed for purposes of supporting the public interest group.[38] But if that is so, it is hard to

---

[37]   *Prune Yard Shopping Center v. Robbins*, 447 U.S. 74 (1980).

[38]   *Pacific Gas & Electric*, 475 U.S. at 19.

understand what the objection could be to directly giving this public interest group access to the billing envelope. There is no functional difference between, on the one hand, giving the public interest group the space ordinarily used by the power company and then requiring the company to spend the extra money (the extra postage) to get its message out and, on the other hand, taxing or assessing the power company and then giving the money collected to the public interest group to disseminate its ideas. For constitutional purposes, there is no difference between property and its economic value, or to put the point more generally, between program and structural regulation.

Of course, when access is given to some specific items of property - a shopping center, mailing envelope, newspaper, radio station or television channel - there is a risk of false attribution not present with taxation. Some readers or viewers might think the message conveyed is that of the publisher or station rather than the person or organization given access. That is why the right claimed in *Pacific Gas & Electric* is variously described not as a right not to speak (as in the original *West Virginia Board of Education v. Barnette* case), but as a right against forced association. But as is evident from the shopping center cases, it is doubtful that anyone would falsely attribute the ideas presented as belonging to the utility company or the publisher or the television station. In any event, the danger of false attribution should require a disclaimer - not a denial of access altogether. Forcing someone or some organization to issue a disclaimer - for example, "the ideas presented are not those of the station" - forces someone to speak, but not in the way that the child in *West Virginia Board of Education v. Barnette* was forced to speak. This speech does not perpetuate an orthodoxy, but rather makes its opposite possible.

Like the rule against content regulation, the rule protecting the right not to speak should be read as a bar to access regulations. Both rules have an important role to play in democratic societies, whether of a transitional or continuous variety, but the proper domain of these rules has to be carefully delineated. They should not be read by the reformers as precluding a system of state regulation intended to broaden public debate and thus to complete the democratic mission of the press. A question can always be raised as to whether those regulations are working as intended, or even whether they are being used as a pretext to silence critics of the state. But that question can only be answered in a context-specific manner, based on the facts and the experience lived under the regulation, and even then, the failures and abuses of a system of access regulations must be compared with the condition of public discourse that might arise if the press is left totally and completely to the vicissitudes of the market. Privatization of the most rigid and unrelenting variety, denying any role for access regulation whatsoever, may be a step beyond the dictatorships of the past, but still a far, far way from the dreams of 1989.

ACCESS TO THE MEDIA IN WESTERN EUROPE

by Eric Barendt

I.   Introduction

In this paper I propose to discuss the ways in which the law in some Western European countries attempt to protect pluralism of voices in the media. The paper is confined to the laws in the United Kingdom, France, Germany and Italy, though I will make one or two comparisons with important principles and leading court decisions in the United States.[1] I will for the most part confine my account to an exposition of the most important rules in these countries, without attempting an expert critique of their relative effectiveness in achieving their goals, explicit or implicit.

Some important points should be made at the outset. First, the press and broadcasting media have entirely different legal histories and structures. This is true of every country, even the United States of America where broadcasting is now very lightly regulated. The press is unlicensed and is generally not subject to controls over its contents, save for those imposed by the general laws of defamation, privacy, obscene publications, public order and so on. On the other hand, most continental countries, but not Britain, do have special press laws, some provisions of which will be discussed later in this paper.

In contrast, a licence must be obtained before broadcasting is allowed, and there are a number of controls over the contents of broadcasting which go beyond those imposed by the general criminal and civil law. For example, in most European countries (the Netherlands being a notable exception) broadcasting companies are not allowed to editorialize and are required to be impartial between political parties and groups in their selection of programmes and in the views expressed in those programmes. Moreover, there are positive obligations to show programmes of quality and merit, to broadcast news and current affairs programmes, original drama and films, and now under the Broadcasting Directive and Council of Europe Transfrontier Television Convention to devote a majority of transmission time to

---

[1]   This limit is not imposed because the law in these countries is necessarily the best developed or most interesting, but owing to my ignorance of the position in other countries.

A. Sajó (ed.), Rights of Access to the Media, 109-120.
© *1996 Kluwer Law International. Printed in the Netherlands.*

"European works".[2] In contrast, there are few special controls now on the contents of radio and television programmes in the United States.

A second point is that the requirement of plurality of voices, or, as it is sometimes termed, the plurality of the sources of information, is still a developing notion in the legal systems of Western Europe. It has been recognized as an attribute of freedom of expression in the broadcasting (and press) decisions of the French Conseil Constitutionnel,[3] and as an aspect of broadcasting freedom by the German Constitutional Court[4] and the Italian Constitutional Court.[5] Their general argument is that legislation must ensure that the media are open to a variety of views and must not be dominated by private media monopolies or oligopolies. In its 1988 decision, for example, the Italian Constitutional Court repeated a requirement in its earlier rulings[6] that Parliament enact strong anti-trust rules before private broadcasting is permitted at the national level. The Conseil Constitutionnel required the competition rules in the French 1986 broadcasting bill to be made stricter in several respects before the measure could be judged constitutionally valid, while the German Constitutional Court in its *Fourth Television* ruling insisted that state licensing authorities consider whether an application for a broadcasting licence was likely to exercise a dominant role in the market before awarding permits.

A constitutional requirement of plurality of opinion, regarded as a necessary attribute of freedom of expression, could logically be applied to the press. The Conseil Constitutionnel in two decisions has taken this step (see 3 below). But this is exceptional. Generally legal systems are hesitant to take positive steps to protect press pluralism, largely because the press has a different history and traditionally is not subject to special contents regulation. If the requirement of plurality were

---

[2]   Directive of 3 Oct. 1989, 89/552/EEC, O.J. EUR. COMM. L. No. 298/23, art.4; Council of Europe Convention on Transfrontier Television, art.10.

[3]   In particular, see Decision 86-217 of 18 Sept. 1986, Debbasch, *Les Grand Arrêts du Droit de l'Audiovisuel*, 245 (Paris 1991).

[4]   See the *First Television* case,, 12 BVerfGE 205 (1961) and the *Fourth Television* case, 73 BVerfGE 118 (1986).

[5]   Decision 225/74 [1974] *Giur. cost.* 1775 and Decision 826/88 [1988] *Giur. cost.* 3893.

[6]   In addition to the ruling in 1974, supra note 5, see Decision 148/81 [1981] *Giur. cost.* 1379.

applied, the door might be opened to arguments that there should be enforceable rights of access to the newspaper columns and perhaps even restrictions on the freedom of newspaper owners and editors to adopt their own line on political questions, at least where the exercise of that freedom leads to an overall imbalance in the range of opinions presented to the public. But the goal of plurality of views is sometimes stated in legislative provisions; for example, the United Kingdom Fair Trading Act 1973 requires the Monopolies and Mergers Commission to report on whether a newspaper merger is contrary to public interest, "taking into account all matters which appear in the circumstances to be relevant and, in particular, the need for accurate presentation of news and free expression of opinion".[7]

A third introductory point is that the goal of pluralism in the media can be pursued in a number of ways. One method is the imposition of content controls, for example, precluding the use by the owner of a broadcasting station to project his own political opinions, requiring impartiality and fairness, and conferring rights of access for political parties, social groups and individuals. This method has been adopted in the case of public broadcasting channels, and to a lesser extent their private competitors, but not newspapers and other printed media. Secondly, private access to the broadcasting media is now allowed through the abolition by legislation, sometimes under pressure from constitutional court rulings, of the traditional public broadcasting monopoly. It is, of course, questionable how far the grant of licences to a handful of commercial operators really increases the range of opinions disseminated on the broadcasting media. But the Italian experience shows that the development may be valuable. Before the late 1970's RAI, the public broadcasting monopoly, was controlled by the Christian Democrats. The decision of the Constitutional Court in 1976 held the monopoly at the local, though not national, level contrary to freedom of expression, and subsequently a variety of local stations and then de facto networks sprung up. Although for years there was chaos on the airwaves, at least the RAI Christian Democrat monopoly was at an end.

Another development is the requirement now found in many broadcasting laws that a certain proportion of transmission time be allocated to independent producers. In Britain this step has been taken for the last few years, largely it should be said for economic reasons. The Thatcher government considered the "comfortable duopoly" of the BBC and the ITV regional channels inefficient as both sectors were overmanned. Requirements on both BBC and the commercial sector to allocate 25%

---

[7]   S.59(3).

of transmission time to the apparently more efficient independent producers have been imposed by the Broadcasting Act 1990. Article 5 of the 1989 Broadcasting Directive now requires all EC states to reserve at least 10% of their transmission time (excluding that devoted to news, sports and game shows) for "European works created by producers who are independent of broadcasters". A further very general requirement is that an "adequate proportion" (of what?) should be reserved for "recent" works, that is, those transmitted within 5 years of production. The objective of these provisions is to stimulate new sources of television production, especially in medium and small-size enterprises, and to provide outlets for creative artistic talent.

Finally, there is the use of anti-trust and cartel rules and merger control laws to prevent the accumulation of broadcasting licences and to limit the growing phenomenon of cross-media ownership. There are considerable doubts about the effectiveness of these rules on their own in securing a real plurality of opinion. Anti-trust rules may prevent one company owning, say, more than three national licences for national television or radio services, but diversity of ownership does not guarantee a diversity of programmes. For instance, there have been quite strict anti-trust rules in the USA for a long time, but programs there are still very homogenous. At most it can be said that the application of anti-trust rules law is a necessary, but not sufficient condition for program diversity, and even that can be questioned.

In the main part of this paper, I want to concentrate on two types of plurality rule: first, access rules, and secondly, anti-trust and merger control rules. The former are really only relevant to the broadcasting media, though associated rights of reply may be claimed against the print media and (I think) in Germany against the cinema. On the other hand, competition and merger rules generally apply to the press, and many countries now have distinctive cross-media ownership rules to limit interests of the press in broadcasting and vice versa.

II.   Rights of Access

A right of access may loosely be defined as a right of an individual or organization to use a particular medium - a newspaper, radio or television channel - to put over an opinion in the form of an article, a broadcast for a few minutes or even to make a programme. It can be stated with some confidence that no right of access exists in the case of the press. It is viewed everywhere as incompatible with the traditional liberal "freedom of the press", frequently protected in constitutions, such as the First Amendment or Article 5 of the German *Grundgesetz*. Some powerful arguments have been made for a different approach, which would regard the press as a "public forum", required like, say, parks and open spaces, to be available for the use of free speech.[8] But this is very much a minority view. It should be added that the German Press Council has recommended in non-binding guidance to editors that they should provide information from a wide variety of sources, whether they share the viewpoint of the newspaper itself or not. The principle should be given particular weight during election periods. There is no equivalent principle, however, in the United Kingdom Press Complaints Commission Code, though there is one requiring editors to provide a fair opportunity for reply to factual inaccuracies.

On the other hand, some rights of access to broadcasting media have been granted by legislation. It has even been argued that there may be a *constitutional* access right to use radio/television under a free speech clause: the argument is usually that since these media are constitutionally regulated to serve the interests of viewers and listeners, as well as professional broadcasters, it is reasonable to ensure that minority views enjoy access opportunities. But the argument has been rejected by a majority of the Supreme Court in the USA[9], to some extent on the ground that the broadcasting media are entitled to exercise the same "editorial freedom" to draw up their program schedule as are press editors. The 1974 decision of the Italian Constitutional Court required Parliament to make provision for access opportunities for political, religious and social groups representative of important strands of opinion, but in contrast to *the right of reply* also required by the ruling, it is doubtful whether the Court had in mind a constitutional right enforceable by individuals.[10]

On the other hand, legislation in a number of countries provides statutory access rights for the benefit of defined groups. For example, in Germany *Laender* (state) legislation typically gives the Churches and Jewish communities rights to have

---

[8]   See Jerome Barron, *Access to the Press - a New First Amendment Right*, (1967) 80 Harv. L. Rev. 1641.

[9]   *CBS v. Democratic Nat'l. Comm.* 412 US 94 (1973).

[10]   Decision 225/74 [1974] *Giur. cost.* 1775. In two later cases the Court has refused to hear references raising the question whether there is an individual right of access: Decision 139/77 [1977] *Giur. cost.* 1822 and Decision 194/87 [1987] *Giur. cost.* 1437.

religious services and other religious programs transmitted; sometimes the obligation binds private, as well as public, broadcasting corporations. In France too, Churches enjoy a right to have religious services transmitted, though this is binding only on France 2, the major public channel. A small amount of time is also reserved on the public channels for broadcasts by professional groups and trade unions: the time is quite limited (only 6 hours a year, for broadcasts of not more than 10 minutes). In all these cases the transmission costs are paid for the broadcasting organizations.

Much the most comprehensive provision is in Italy, where the law of 1975 conferred a right of access to political parties represented in Parliament, trade unions and other political associations, cultural, ethnic, religious and linguistic organizations, and all other socially relevant groups which request access. It should be noted that only groups, not individuals, enjoy access opportunities, and that the determination of access claims is to be resolved, not by the courts as one might expect, but by the Parliamentary Commission, which is in effect the supreme regulatory authority for RAI. The Constitutional Court has refused to decide the question whether this jurisdiction is compatible with the terms of its ruling in 1974, which had led to the access provision, while the Corte di Cassazione in 1983 rejected the view that that ruling contemplated the institution of a right enforceable by the ordinary courts.[11]

In contrast to the relative rarity of general access provisions, it is normal for political parties to enjoy access rights, particularly during election periods, to use the broadcasting media. This is even now the case in Britain[12], where otherwise there are no access rights at all. There are such rules in France, Italy and the German states. These party political and election broadcasts are provided free, and are controlled by the parties themselves, though the broadcasting authority may retain some legal control to ensure that the broadcast does not offend legal rules, e.g., that it is not libellous nor does it incite racial hatred.

These party political broadcasts must be distinguished from political advertising, which is forbidden in some countries (such as Britain and France) and for which the parties themselves pay. The claim that there is a right under Article 10 of the European Convention to make political broadcasts has been rejected by the

---

[11]   Decision 1072/84 [1984] *Giur. cost.* 175.

[12]   Broadcasting Act of 1990, s. 36.

Commission, though it did indicate that it might take a different view if, say, a claim by a major party for fair access during election campaigns was turned down.[13]

Also in contrast to the absence of general access rules (apart from Italy) is the usual provision of right of reply laws. These vary considerably from one country to another, and they also vary from one medium to another. For example, in France there is a very wide right of reply to the press.[14] It may be claimed by anyone referred to in an article, whether or not it is alleged to contain a mistake of fact or not or whether it asserts a matter of fact or opinion. In contrast in Germany the right of *Gegendarstellung* under state press and broadcasting laws may only be claimed when it alleged that *false factual* statements have been made, and two broadcasting laws (Sudwestfunk state treaty and Hesse law) provide such a right only when it is proved that a false statement was made. The European Community Broadcasting Directive (Article 23) requires member states to provide a right of reply to assertions of incorrect facts, a formulation which appears to take a narrow view of the right. Recently the EP has called for the right to be extended to radio broadcasts and to the press.

Rights of reply laws are not true access rules, since they only arise when the right is triggered by a previous program or article, and generally they are confined to the correction of false statements of fact. They are as much, probably more, concerned, with the protection of the individual's right to protect his reputation and dignity as they are with providing the public with a complete and balanced picture of a controversial story.

It is worth asking why access rights, so frequently claimed by left-wing and minority groups, have rarely been granted. One answer is that it is difficult to enforce them without complicated administrative regulation and oversight, and without interference with the broadcasters' entitlement to draw up their own program schedule. They are, moreover, not necessarily the most effective means for securing a wide range of balanced programs. It is in comparison relatively easy to formulate and apply rules for the access of political parties and for rights of reply. One exception to this negative impression of the access argument is in the context of cable. With the large number of cable channels available, some of them unused or nut fully used by the operator, access requirements are quite common. They are

---

[13]   4515/70, *X and Assoc. of Z. v. UK.*, 38 Coll. Dec. 86.

[14]   Law of the Press 1881, art. 13.

standard in the United States and in Germany, but have not been imposed in the United Kingdom.

Access programs, whether made as of right or under concession from the broadcasting company, have rarely proved popular. That may be because they are made without professional skills, or because they are scheduled by the broadcasting body at off-peak times when few people are likely to hear or watch them. In any event they are not now, for better or worse, an important topic of media discussion in European countries.

III.   Competition and Mergers Law

There is in contrast increasing interest in the part these rules may play in preventing the emergence of monopolies and oligopolies which threaten pluralism in the press, broadcasting and in other media. The French Conseil Constitutionnel in two rulings has held that pluralism of sources of information in the press is a principle of constitutional status, a necessary corollary of the freedom of expression guaranteed by Article 11 of the 1789 Declaration of the Rights of Man.[15] It is clear that the law must protect pluralism; it is not just an option. On the other hand, the means by which this is done is a matter of legislative discretion, and there is no necessity for rules on transparency and financial accountability - though these rules do exist in the French legislation. The earlier decision of 1984 invalidated large parts of a relatively tough anti-concentration law. The Conseil made it clear that the rule limiting the market share of national daily papers to 15% of the market could not apply retrospectively. Divestiture orders, it seems, would be regarded (for reasons not clearly explained in the decision) as contrary to press freedom and freedom of enterprise. Moreover, the law should be construed only to cover attainment of that share through mergers and acquisitions, not through increased circulation.

Doubts about their constitutionality with respect to the press freedom protected by Article 5 of the Basic Law have prevented the formulation by the states in Germany of strict merger control rules and other laws designed to promote pluralism, e.g., rules limiting the market-share of certain publishers, circulation limits on acquisitions, etc. On the other hand, the Bundeskartellamt has intervened on some occasions to prevent press mergers. But still the Springer group enjoys

---

[15]   Decision 84-181 of 11 Oct. 1984; Decision 86-210 of 29 July 1986, Rec. 110.

about 30% of the daily newspaper market, as does Hersant in France, and News International in the UK. As already mentioned, the UK Fair Trading Act requires the Monopolies and Mergers Commission (MMC) to take into account the impact of a press merger on freedom of expression. The effectiveness of the legislative provisions is considerably weakened, however, by the discretion enjoyed by the Secretary of State not to refer a proposed merger to the MMC where he is satisfied that the newspaper concerned in the transfer is not economic as a going concern, and that if it is to continue as a separate newspaper the case is one of urgency.[16] The discretion not to refer has been frequently exercised, most notably when Rupert Murdoch's News International took over *The Times* and *The Sunday Times*.

In general press merger laws and other controls designed to prevent domination of the media by a handful of press barons have proved relatively ineffective. Even the 1984 Press Law in France, to some extent diluted in 1986 (for example the acquisition ceiling was raised to 30% of the market), was unable to stop the remorseless expansion of the Hersant Empire. One reason is that the laws themselves tend to be too weak; another is that they are ineffectively implemented by politicians and monopolies commissions. An underlying explanation is the strong commitment to a traditional view of press freedom. That view considers all regulation of the ownership and control of newspapers contrary to the freedom; government in other words has no business trying to promote press freedom. That view is, however, not upheld now by the Conseil Constitutionnel in France. Perhaps a more important reason is that politicians and governments are terrified of the press, more so than they are of the broadcasting media. Newspapers are free to express their political bias at elections, and no government wishes to antagonise what is ex-hypothesi a powerful newspaper group by toughening up anti-concentration laws. The alliance, for example, between the Conservative government in Britain and the Murdoch papers is one reason for the former's continued electoral success.

In complete contrast, anti-concentration measures in the broadcasting media are now standard. They are designed, inter alia, to limit shareholdings in broadcasting enterprises, to prevent the accumulation of licences in both one sector of the broadcasting media and between the sectors of radio, television and cable, and to control the rising phenomenon of cross-media ownership. For example, the

---

[16]   Fair Trading Act 1973, s.58(3).

United Kingdom Broadcasting Act 1990, supplemented by regulations,[17] has detailed rules which prevent the accumulation of more than two regional television licences, a certain number of local radio licences, or, say, a licence for regional television and more than a 20% interest in national radio. There are also cross-media ownership rules, introduced for the first time in this legislation. They provide, for example, that the proprietor of a national or local newspaper may not hold more than a 20% interest in a body holding a licence for a national or regional television service or a national radio service. The same rule applies in the converse situation, where a broadcasting licensee holds an interest in the press. There are similar rules for local cable and radio services and local papers. One controversial omission from the legislation is that there is no control over the cross-ownership of what are termed non-domestic satellite services, in effect Rupert Murdoch's BSkyB, and national papers. There is little doubt that this was deliberately designed to help a prominent supporter of the government.

There are similar French and Italian rules in their broadcasting legislation. Interestingly, the provisions in the legislation in both countries were introduced, and in the case of France made stricter, after rulings of the constitutional tribunals had indicated that this was necessary in order to safeguard pluralism of information. The Italian rules are particularly bizarre, in that they were clearly intended to satisfy the Constitutional Court's demands and at the same time to enable Berlusconi to keep his national networks, provided he surrendered his newspaper interest. On the other hand, the rule forbidding anyone holding even one national television licence, if he publishes a daily paper, the circulation of which exceeds 16% of the daily circulation of papers in Italy in effect excludes the entry of Fiat into the broadcasting market - Fiat controls *La Stampa* and *Corriere della Sera*. Some, but by no means all, of the German state broadcasting laws, contain cross-media ownership restrictions, while typically they contain provisions restricting the accumulation of licences and imposing limits on the amount of capital which an individual may control in a private broadcasting licensee.

These media specific rules may be supplemented by the country's general competition and mergers law. Sometimes this could rise to confusion. There may be jurisdictional conflict between the powers of a monopolies commission and those of the regulatory broadcasting body. This is evidenced in Italy and Germany, particularly the latter where there may be conflicts between the jurisdiction of the

---

[17]   SI 1991/1176.

federal cartel authority and the *state* broadcasting authorities. Another difficulty now is whether there is scope for EC action in this area. The Community Merger Regulation of 1989 does not contain any rules specific to the media, but enables national authorities to apply their own measures to protect certain interests, including "plurality of the media", even where there is a Community dimension.[18]

A recent Commission Green Paper has reviewed whether there is a need for Community action.[19] It does not see the need for it to preserve pluralism as such, because it considers, perhaps too optimistically, that national governments are able (and willing) to do that, where appropriate. But it does think that the disparity of the cross-media ownership and other competition rules may inhibit the effective working of the internal market. Disparate laws might inhibit a company which on economic grounds would prefer to enter a particular national market from doing so. For example, from 1994 any EC company is free to take over a company which holds a Channel 3 television licence in the United Kingdom. But in Portugal the rule is that the sole object of a television licensee must be television activity. So an Italian or German consortium which has general industrial as well as media interests may be induced to enter the British rather than the Portugese market, when it might be more efficient for it to have chosen the latter. On that ground the EC Commission rather hesitantly concluded that there is a powerful case for Community legislation.

Interestingly the Green Paper appreciates the limits of competition and mergers law in guaranteeing pluralism. This is particularly evident in the context of cross-media ownership, where it can be argued that newspapers and broadcasting constitute entirely different markets, so there is no place for competition rules. Yet undeniably the control of substantial interests in both these sectors, or in one of them and videos or films, significantly reduces the variety of information and ideas available to the public. In support of the Green Paper the European Parliament has expressed a strong desire for EC action to harmonize national provisions and to guarantee "diversity of opinion and pluralism where the proposed concentration is on a European scale."[20]

---

[18] Reg. 4064/89, art. 21,3. O.J. EUR. COMM. L. No. 395/1.

[19] *Pluralism and Media Concentration in the Internal Market*, 480 final (1992).

[20] Resolution of 16 Sept. 1992 on Media Concentration, art. 27, O.J. COMM. L. No. 284/44.

IV.   Conclusion

Neither access entitlement nor competition law seems by itself an adequate tool by which to secure the goal of plurality of information and ideas. In the broadcasting context (though not that of the press) as much, perhaps more, is achieved by the traditional contents controls of impartiality, fairness and the requirement to show a wide range of programs. These latter are still imposed rigorously on public broadcasting, but have been weakened in most countries for the private sector. There can be little doubt that the goal of plurality of information is only very imperfectly achieved: the principal reason for that is surely that we do not try hard enough to achieve it. And that perhaps is because there is a more than lingering doubt about the entitlement of government and the law to bring this about, when the attempt may infringe the classic liberal theory of media freedom.

THE CONSTITUTIONAL CONCEPT OF THE PUBLIC SPHERE ACCORDING TO GERMAN BASIC LAW WITH SPECIAL CONSIDERATION OF THE BOUNDARIES OF FREE SPEECH

by Ulrich K. Preuss

I.   Introduction

Among the constitutional rights of Germany's Basic Law the individual rights to communication laid down in Article 5 are of utmost importance. Following a general understanding of basic rights according to which they are not so much to be understood as means of the individual to separate himself or herself from society but rather have been created in order to serve the citizen's participation in the differentiated web of social life, the Court attributes a prominent role to the rights to communication.

Thus, the German Constitutional Court, since its very origination has been emphasizing that the right to freely express one's opinion is "absolutely constitutive of the free democratic order" and therefore restrictions upon this right are subject to severe requirements of justification. Before I elaborate on this issue in more detail, it seems appropriate to give a rather sketchy overview of the Basic Law's conceptual framework, of what in Germany has widely become to be called "communicative freedoms". Therefore, the second part of this paper will deal mainly with the questions of licensing, regulation, and public interest standards for the access to electronic media and their underlying theoretical assumptions. The third part will treat the problem of the limitations to which the communicative freedoms are subject according to the Basic Law and its interpretation through the Federal Constitutional Court. Finally, in the fourth part, I shall briefly turn to the German constitution's stand on the issues of hate speech and "lustration".[1]

---

[1]   There is, of course, an abundance of jurisprudential and constitutional legal literature to all three subjects in German language. Rather than trying to give an exhaustive account of the manyfold differentiations and subtleties in these fields, in this article, I have restricted myself to giving the English-speaking reader a rough overview over the main ideas of the German constitutional protection of mass and individual communication.

121

A. Sajó (ed.), *Rights of Access to the Media*, 121-138.
© 1996 *Kluwer Law International. Printed in the Netherlands.*

II.   Access to Electronic Media

II.1.   The institutional dimension of the freedom of communication

To begin with, it should be mentioned that Article 5 of the Basic Law contains the constitutional guarantees of different communication rights. Similar to the First Amendment of the American Constitution which comprises the freedoms of speech and of the press, the German Basic Law includes freedom rights both to individual and to mass communication. The former category includes the rights to freely express and disseminate one's opinion in speech, writing, and picture and to inform oneself from generally accessible sources. The latter class encompasses the freedoms of the press, of broadcast, and of films.

Like so many stipulations of the Basic Law this seemingly detailed enumeration of communicative freedoms must be understood as a reaction to the Germans experience not only with Goebbels' "Ministry of Propaganda", but with the entire elimination of plurality in all mass media by the Nazi government. This experience may explain why both in the adjudication of the Constitutional Court and in the professional constitutional debates, an "institutional understanding" of the freedoms of communication has been prevalent.

An "institutional understanding" of the freedoms of communication refers to the importance of these basic rights not only for the individuals' interest in participating in the public sphere, but for the flourishing of civil society as well. In other words, the democratic society itself is essentially interested in the existence and smooth operation of a democratic public sphere, (i.e., of a sphere in which all relevant opinions, values, interests, perspectives can be and in fact will be expressed). The constitutional rights, and particularly the rights to freedom of communication, do not exist exclusively for the sake of the individuals, but for the well-being of society itself.

In view of our experience that such an ideal pluralist public sphere is not likely to emerge spontaneously, the constitutional guarantee of the right to communication has not only the limited meaning of obligating the state to forswear any kind of interference with the individuals' freedom. Rather, it involves the constitutional responsibility of the state - primarily of the legislature, but of the executive and the judicial branches as well - to promote the development and sustainability of a pluralist public sphere. This includes the duty to create the basic conditions which enable the individuals to make use of their communicative freedoms.

Thus, it is widely recognized in Germany that the legislature has the obligation based on Article 5 of the constitution to prohibit an excessive economic concentration in the press business because it is prone to restrict unduly the pluralist character of the public sphere. However, this does not mean that the basic communicative freedoms of the constitution give the state the constitutional authority to abolish market structure in the press business altogether (as some authors claimed several years ago). Rather, the "institutional" or "objective" concept of basic rights that is continually developed by the Constitutional Court implies the understanding (which, to be sure, is not shared by all constitutional authors in Germany) that in modern complex societies *freedom has to be organized*. This concept also includes the notion that it is the state which has to promote the realization of individual freedoms by creating the appropriate institutional schemes. To give another example, this institutional approach lead the Constitutional Court to recognize rather far-reaching rights of the press, such as a constitutional defense for the acts of acquisition of information (including the protection of the anonymity of informers) or the protection of the physical distribution of newspapers.

It should be emphasized, however, that this constitutional doctrine has had rather little influence on the real conditions of the press market. Although German antitrust law contains a handful of regulations with special regard to the press, this market does not display any particularities which could be interpreted as the result of the constitutional call for communicative pluralism. Hence, despite rather demanding constitutional precepts, access to the press is open according to criteria not considerably different from the requirements for access to the market at large.

II.2. The concept of "organized freedom" in the area of electronic mass media

The opposite is true with regard to the electronic mass media, (i.e., to radio and television). In order to understand the constitutional particularities of the electronic mass media it should be noted that in Germany the electronic media, in contrast to the printed media, were state-owned and governmentcontrolled at their origination during the 1920's. The original electronic media were utilized recklessly and skillfully by the Nazis as instruments of ideological domination and seduction.

As stated above, this nightmarish experience was the main reason why the drafters of the Basic Law and the founders of the Federal Republic after World War II created and constitutionally guaranteed a state-independent radio system. However, the constitutional freedom of broadcast could not simply imitate the traditional freedom of the press. This is because two main conditions of broadcasting were entirely different from those of printed newspapers. First, the scarcity of air waves did not allow the right to broadcast to be treated as a freedom accessible to everybody but rather as a scarce good which had to be rationed. Second, the amount of capital necessary for the performance and emission of radio and television programs was so huge that this served as an unsurmountable barrier against an ordinary citizen's access to this medium. Although it was conceivable that a financially powerful business company would be able to raise the funds necessary for establishing a private broadcast network, this was largely regarded as undesirable. Such private networks were considered undesirable because this created the danger that the public sphere would be controlled by economic forces that did not represent the full range of the pluralist public sphere.

Torn between the equally undesirable alternatives of a state-controlled or a capital-dependent broadcast system, the founders of the Federal Republic of Germany, strongly supported by the American, British and French occupying powers, established a broadcast system that circumvented both variants. It was public, but also independent from state control. Until the end of 1983, broadcast in Germany was exclusively performed by public broadcasting corporations having legal capacity and being organized according to the principle of what is normally called "internal pluralism".

The principle of internal pluralism requires that the plurality of the opinions, values, interests and perspectives existent in society has to be represented in the different committees and in particular in the governing boards of public broadcasting corporations. These internal-pluralist committees devise the guidelines according to which journalists perform their editorial tasks. This institutional device has caused much dissatisfaction because it has lead to a kind of a proportional representation of the three leading political parties and caused a "balanced journalism" which in the view of many people leaves the impression that indeed this system is state-run.

This is certainly an overstatement, but it is undeniable that the idea to mirror, as it were, society's pluralism in the organic structure of the public broadcasting corporation has largely been interpreted by the political parties as an invitation to behave as the main representatives of civil society. In particular, political parties have been rather successful in wielding an almost dominant influence on the assignment of the top positions to their respective real or alleged supporters.

However, financing of public broadcasting corporations might be an even more important factor. The system was rather simple: whoever possesses a radio or a television set is legally presumed to make use of it (i.e., to receive radio or television emissions). For this "use", the individual is taxed, the tax being determined by state law. In the meantime, the tax contributions of the recipients are supplemented by a considerable amount of revenues from advertising, so that it is justifiable to speak of a mixed public-private system of financing.

As I already stated, this purely public system ceased to exist at the end of 1983, when the first private broadcasting corporations were admitted.

Today an individual living in Germany and making use of cable and satellite radio and television could probably receive up to thirty programs, at least half of them being transmitted by private suppliers. This has given rise to the question of whether it is still justified to presume that the owner of a radio or television set receives the programs of the German public broadcasting corporations and hence has to pay a monthly tax. Until now the issue is only being discussed in small circles, but it can easily be anticipated that in the course of ever more fierce competition between the public and the private suppliers of radio and television programs for the resources of the advertising industry this discussion will soon come up in political debates.

This question leads back to the German particularities of the constitutional guarantees of the freedom of broadcast.[2] As long as the public broadcasting corporations had both the factual and the legal monopoly on transmitting programs the constitutional objective to protect the plurality of the public sphere was more or less perfectly achieved by the "internal-pluralist" structure of the public broadcasting corporations. As a consequence, "freedom of broadcasting" consisted mainly of the rights of the public broadcasting corporations to be protected against government interference with their editorial work.

---

[2] The opinions of the German Constitutional Court regarding the freedom of broadcast are the following ones, the first dating back to 1961, the last having been issued as late as 1991 (the first number refers to the volume, the second to the first page of the official publications of the opinions of the Court): 12/205; 31/314; 57/295; 73/118; 74/297; 83/238.

Freedom of broadcasting did not include the individual right of a media *entrepreneur* to receive a broadcasting license, much less the negative right not to be curbed by the state in establishing a broadcasting business and transmitting programs. In other words, what is and has been an essential element of the freedom of the press, namely the freedom to print and to disseminate a paper without any kind of prior consent, authorization, or license of the state, did not apply to the freedom of broadcast. When the technical situation which, in addition to the large capital requirement (for establishing broadcasting systems), that prompted this institutional concept, gradually changed at the beginning of the 80's, with the development of broadcast satellites, cable television, and of new frequencies, the Constitutional Court had to modify its concept of freedom of broadcast.

Some authors drew the conclusion that in this new technical situation, which was paralleled by the Europeanization and even internationalization of the media market, the freedom of broadcasting involved everybody's right to broadcast radio and television programs. Others reject this suggestion with the argument that the freedom of broadcasting requires first of all the guarantee of a free communicative process in which the plurality of existent opinions has to be represented.

This principle does not exclude the admission of private radio and television program suppliers, but it requires that the legislature determine the institutional framework within which the transmission of broadcast programs, public and private, can happen. Also, private broadcasting needs legislative regulation to ensure that the private suppliers of programs have to satisfy some minimum requirements of providing balanced, impartial and fair programming. In other words, they are not only subject to the imperatives of the market but have to meet the standards of a democratic public in a mass society as well. Again, here we are faced with the idea of "organized freedom" as a concept of individual liberty in the age of highly interdependent social relations.

However, the Constitutional Court acknowledged that the lawgivers may set lower standards of program quality for the private suppliers because they have to collect their funds through advertising. This requires a more or less permanent mass audience which cannot watch programs which are primarily devoted to serious information and to cultural entertainment. At present, we speak of a "dual broadcast system" in Germany, consisting of a public column and a private column. The public system is assigned the task of the so-called basic supply of information, instruction, and entertainment.

This does not mean that public broadcasting corporations are becoming an extinct species. To the contrary, the Court has specified that they have the constitutional right to exist and to develop and that the state has to provide the necessary institutional and financial means. In particular the legislature has to secure the predominance of their public funding through taxes (which is at the same time a protection of the private suppliers against an excessive competition of the public corporations on the tight advertisement market).

The private broadcasting corporations have to apply for a license which is normally granted for ten years with the option of prolongation. The media laws (which fall into the jurisdiction of the *Laender*) stipulate that private broadcasting involves the execution of a public task which has to be performed according to special principles which apply to the program. Besides the principles of fairness and impartiality already mentioned, the private broadcasting corporations have to fulfill additional requirements which aim to provide a minimum level of program quality, such as the prohibitions against allotting more than 20% of the daily transmission time to advertising, or to interrupt a single program of no more than 60 minutes for advertising. Other legal restrictions pertain to the protection of minorities and of the youth. Such restrictions also forbid the incitement of racial hatred, the transmission of cruel and inhumane violence in a manner that expresses its acclamation, the glorification of war, and the showing of pornography.

Finally, there is still the governmental plurality directive that governs the whole mass communication system of Germany and therefore, applies also to private broadcasting corporations. According to the legal standards that the *Laender* have set in an inter-state treaty, concluded in 1991, the pluralist character of the privately broadcast programs can be obtained either by an external- or an internal-pluralist scheme.

The existence of external pluralism is presumed if each of three programs produced in Germany by three different private broadcasting corporations and broadcast nation-wide (at a given time) can be received by more than half the population in Germany. In this case, special state broadcasting agencies which supervise the private license holders have to work toward the realization of the goal that the entirety of the three programs is pluralistic. In other words, the entire programming must articulate a plurality of opinions and voice the views of the relevant political, ideological and social forces and groups of civil society. If this condition does not apply, (i.e., if less than three different private programs are broadcast at a given time), the plurality directive has to be fulfilled by the internal-pluralist rule.

In this second case, (which presently does not apply) every single private program has to meet the plurality requirements. As I stated already, the *Laender* has established special broadcast agencies which oversee the private broadcasting corporations' compliance with these legal precepts. Obviously it is no easy task to check whether a program is pluralistic or whether it is biased or unfair. When can one make the unequivocal statement that a movie is pornographic or glorifies inhuman violence?

Nevertheless, the State broadcast agencies have to cope with this dilemma and particularly with the difficult task to be the guardian of communicative plurality in the sphere of the electronic mass media. Not the least problem is the fact that the sanctions which the agencies can enforce are either too weak or too strong to be efficient. They can express admonitions if they believe that the private broadcasting corporation has violated the law, and request forbearance. If this proves unavailing, they can suspend the license. Ultimately, they can, and under certain circumstances they must, revoke the license.

In view of the huge investments which are at stake, and taking into consideration the potential effects of a revocation of the license on the regional and state labor market, an agency is not likely to utilize this ultimate instrument of legal supervision. The private broadcasting corporations are of course fully aware of this dilemma of the state. Therefore, it is not surprising that, although there is now widespread dissatisfaction with the performance of the private broadcasting corporations, the German public has more or less surrendered to its self-incapacitation.

III. Constitutional Limitations of Communicative Freedoms

III.1. The conceptual principle of "legal proviso"

Despite this critical assessment of the Constitutional Court's success in its attempt to limit the effects of the market on the performance of the electronic mass media, it cannot be denied that the idea of the constitutive significance of the right to free and public communication is well established in German constitutional discourse. This premise has had a considerable impact on the determination of the limitations to which these freedoms are subject. A few remarks about the general structure of the basic rights doctrine may be appropriate beforehand.

The concept of basic rights is based on the assumption that an individual's freedom is only limited by the like rights of all other individuals and by the requirements of prevailing public interests. This then raises the question of who is authorized to define these limitations. Obviously, this depends on the perception of who is likely to jeopardize the individuals'. freedom. In the continental European tradition with its powerful tradition of state absolutism, (i.e., the single antagonist of freedom was the executive branch of the state), the state was synonymous with the monarchical executive (police, army, bureaucracy).

This anti-executive tradition has survived the monarchy and has remained powerful even after the collapse of the monarchy and the establishment of the democratic republic. But there has not only been an anti-executive, but also a pro-legislature tradition. If the executive was the "natural" enemy of freedom, the people, or, for that matter, the representative of the people, the freely elected parliament has been regarded as the "natural" defender of freedom. It has been assumed that the people itself, at least its representatives cannot be interested in curtailing their own freedom or the freedom of their constituency respectively, and hence parliament became the natural, as it were, protector of the constitutional freedoms of the individuals.

It need not be elaborated here that obviously the Anglo-American constitutional tradition is quite different and far less optimistic about the people's capacity to preserve its own freedom than the Continental-European. In this tradition, the smooth operation of institutional devices which, like an "invisible hand", produce beneficial effects is given priority over the integrity and enlightenment of the people. As a result, the main guardian of individual rights are the courts, whereas the legislature is part of the problem, not the solution. Thus, the First Amendment puts constraints on the United States Congress, because Congress is regarded as a potential threat to individual freedom.

Under German constitutional law, which is mainly influenced by the continental European tradition the authority to impose limitations to the basic constitutional freedoms is reserved to the legislature. The technical term in German is "*Gesetzesvorbehalt*", which means "legal reservation" or "legal proviso". This term circumscribes the requirement of a specific enactment if constitutional rights shall be restrained.

130

The requirements are defined in the respective constitutional rights themselves. In some cases the legislature has a rather broad discretion in restraining a right for the pursuit of public interests (as is the case with regard to the freedom of assembly). In other instances, as with regard to the freedom of conscience and of religion, or the freedoms of art and science, any restraint imposed by the legislature is prohibited altogether. These freedoms which are exempt from the legal reservation may only be limited by similar constitutional rights of other individuals or by public interests that possess constitutional significance themselves, such as the security of the state, the rule of law or the social state principle.

III.2. The limitation through the provision of "general statutes"

Having depicted the constitutional framework for limitations of basic freedoms in a rather sketchy manner, I want to give a brief account of the particular constitutional device of the freedoms of expression and communication. According to the legal reservation (or legal proviso) of Article 5 paragraph 2 of the German Constitution, "[t]hese rights find their limits in the provisions of general statutes, in statutory provisions for the protection of youth, and in the right to respect for personal honor".

In other words, the legislature is entitled to restrain the freedom of expression and communication through statutes under three alternative conditions. Under the first condition, freedom of communication may be restrained in order to protect a person's honor and reputation against defamation, for instance by civil and criminal laws on action for libel. In the second instance, restraints may be used in order to protect youth against the harmful effects of the publishing and dissemination of representations and illustrations of violence, pornography, crime, racial hatred or the glorification of war. Under the third condition, restraints may be imposed in order to pursue any other public interest if, and only if the law is neutral vis-à-vis information and ideas. Thus, with the third condition, a law is considered neutral if it neither restricts ideas nor restricts or discourages the expressions of ideas by the implementation of the law.[3]

This is essentially the meaning of the constitutional wording of "general statutes". A statute is "general" (as opposed to being "special") if it pursues public

---

[3]   In the United States we refer to this as a "content-neutral" statute.

interests and has effects other than the suppression or restriction of the intellectual content of ideas and information. Thus, a law that aims at the prevention of certain ideas (or of ideas at large) or at restraining the reception of such ideas or information would be an unconstitutional "special" law.

One should note that the requirement of generality only applies to laws which pursue legitimate goals other than the protection of reputation and of youth. In other words, special laws that aim at the protection of youth and reputation are permitted, whereas, according to the wording of the constitutional right to expression and communication, special laws for the protection of, say, the security of the state, the safety and respect of minorities, or religious or political peace are constitutionally prohibited.

This jurisprudential approach to the problem of limitations on the freedom of expression has a striking similarity with the distinction between the "absolutist" and the "balancing" approach discussed in American debates about the meaning of the First Amendment. Put into this framework, the constitutional provisos for the protection of reputation and of youth would fall into the category of a balancing approach, while the legal reservation of "general statutes", (i.e., the strict prohibition of any legal stipulation aiming at the intellectual content of ideas or information) would amount to an absolutist approach. I leave it open whether this analogy will bear closer examination, because the German Constitutional Court has developed a line of reasoning which interprets the meaning of "general statutes" in terms of a balancing approach.[4]

Theoretically, the German Legislature is not impeded by the Constitution in protecting any public good against potential impairment through ideas and information, because, unlike the implication of the absolutist approach, there is no domain of communicative freedom that is *a priori* exempt from balancing. On the other hand, the Court has established standards of balancing which give the communicative freedoms rather strong weight in any balancing test.

First of all, before passing laws which restrict the communicative freedoms for the sake of public interests the legislature must scrutinize: (i) whether the restriction serves a legitimate, constitutionally acknowledged public goal, (ii) whether the restriction is an appropriate means for the protection of this public goal,

---

[4]   The leading opinion, the so-called *Lueth* case, is published in 7/198, 205 of the official publications of the opinions of the Court. *Lueth* has been followed by many other similar decisions. See, e.g., 66/116, 150; 71/206, 214.

(iii) whether, it is a necessary means for the specific end,[5] and (iv) whether the restriction of communicative freedom stands in reasonable proportion to the relevance of the stated public goal. This is essentially the content of the principle of proportionality which applies to all enactments which restrain basic constitutional rights.

But this principle is of particular importance for communicative rights, because the Court emphasizes the absolute significance of this category of individual rights for the public sphere. Thus, a law which prohibits the distribution of leaflets on public streets in order to avoid the additional costs for the street-cleaning would neglect the weight of public debate and reasoning for a democratic society and would fail the balancing test.

A second proviso says that the laws which restrict the communicative freedoms in order to protect public interests have to be interpreted by the courts and the executive and administrative branches in a restrictive manner such as to save as much of the substance of the communicative freedoms as possible. According to the wording of the Court, the restraining laws have to be interpreted "in the light of the paramount significance of the communicative freedoms". Third, the Court also invokes the principle of "benevolent interpretation" of freedom of communication. Whenever a public act of communication is ambiguous and can be interpreted in different ways, the courts and state agencies are obliged to base their legal judgement on that understanding which does not collide with another protected interest.

IV.   The Cases of Hate Speech and Lustration

Having outlined a sketchy framework of the jurisprudential understanding of the boundaries of Free Speech Rights, let me turn to two special cases which are of major political importance, namely the instances of hate speech and of so-called lustration.

---

[5]   With regard to this criterion, the Legislature must consider whether its goal (in passing the law) can be reached by alternative means which constrain the communicative freedoms less.

IV.1. Hate speech

The Federal Criminal Code of Germany contains several punishable acts which pertain to what in the American context is frequently called "hate speech" or "fighting words". The criminal offense of "incitement of the people" (for national, racial, or religious reasons) includes communicative acts through which hatred against parts of the population is stirred up or through which they are defamed and disparaged.[6] The distribution of writings which incite racial hatred and that depict cruel and inhumane acts of violence against humans in a manner that either glorifies or plays down the inhumane character of these acts is also a criminal offense.[7] Section 86 of the Criminal Code penalizes the production, distribution and use of means of propaganda and of symbols of Nazi organizations.

Obviously, in all three cases the law prohibits the public expression of particular ideas and information. According to the wording of Article 5 of the Constitution, mentioned above, interference with the intellectual content of communication through special laws is only permissible for the protection of personal reputation and of youth. The criminal offenses I have enumerated clearly transcend these limitations. However, the constitutionality of these criminal provisions is beyond any reasonable doubt. It is certainly indicative of this contention that the constitutionality of the aforementioned sections have not yet been challenged before the Constitutional Court.

The Constitutional Court has frequently held that criminal laws that aim at the protection of the constitutional and legal order are general laws and hence constitutional, even if this implies the prohibition of the expression of ideas. One could possibly reason that the prohibition of the incitement to racial, national etc. hatred does not refer to the intellectual *content*, but to the *mode* of expressing one's opinion. But this distinction will not always grasp the problem, because frequently it is not the form, in which an idea is presented, but its very substance that is entirely abhorrent and unbearable in a democratic society. A suggestion to deprive certain parts of the populations of their rights as citizens or even to kill them, even if this suggestion is presented in a "civilized" manner is an example of such an abhorrent idea. This is why the Federal Constitutional Court balances the value of

---

[6]   Section 130 of the Criminal Code.

[7]   Section 131 of the Criminal Code.

134

the freedom of expression against the merit of the protected interest. The test that a law must pass is the following one: Does the punishable act intentionally aim at the expression of a particular opinion, or does it seek to protect a public interest, irrespective of a particular opinion and its content? Although this test is not always fully satisfactory, it is appropriate in most cases.

To use the example of the punishable act of incitement of the people against certain parts of the population:[8] the right of the entire population to enjoy a peaceful life is a public interest which has to be protected against all kinds of potential impairment. There is no reason to hold that this protection should be less effective if the threat is carried through the means of public expression. In this instance, the law is not intended to suppress particular opinions in favor of other opinions, but rather to protect a public interest against any kind of assault, be it physical, be it intellectual. This is what then is called the "generality" of the law. The law is not created specifically to suppress speech but rather to protect the public.

This argument is not fully immune to critical objections. One may ask whether the essence of the constitutional protection of free speech is to give the expression of ideas and information priority over all other kinds of human behavior. Furthermore, would this not require us to make a clear distinction between acts and opinions, so that physical assaults on parts of the population would be punishable, whereas intellectual attacks would enjoy the constitutional protection of intellectual freedom?

Although this criticism certainly bears some truth, it is equally apparent that in some cases intellectual attacks can have effects very similar to physical assaults - in fact, frequently they precede and instigate physical attacks. Thus, a theoretical approach which delivers a clear-cut criterion for the distinction of deeds and opinions is required. But even if this can be found, one needs to focus on "dangerous opinions", and the corroborating effects that mass media may have on such opinions. It is obvious that under the conditions of modern mass society the optimistic judgements of the eighteenth and nineteenth centuries about the thoroughly beneficial effects of the public expression of opinions, notwithstanding their content, needs critical scrutiny.

---

[8]   Section 130 of the Criminal Code.

IV.2.   "Lustration"

It has become a commonplace assumption that the press, or, for that matter, the mass media at large, has become the fourth branch of government in societies that allow an independent public sphere. As current events in democratic countries of Europe show, the publication of indecent behavior or other immoral acts of politicians in the mass media very often is the first step toward their resignation. In recent times, the mass media has frequently operated as a method of political purge. If this method is utilized in a systematic manner, we may speak of a strategy of "lustration". This term refers to the public exposure of persons who have been compromised by their close relation with the old regime and who now, after the transformation, seek the protection of anonymity.

In Germany the strategy of lustration is of lesser significance, because the unification treaty includes legal instruments to exclude former collaborators of the regime, particularly those who have worked for the former state security agency (the "Stasi") and who have violated human rights, from employment in the public service. Similar rules apply for the admission to the bar, and they have even had some influence on the right of private employers to dismiss former proponents of the old communist regime. Moreover, urged by civic groups of the former opposition, the German *Bundestag* has enacted a law which regulates the rather unobstructed access of individuals who had been victims of the regime's oppressive measures and of the media to the large files of the state security agency of the GDR (the *"Stasi-Akten"*).

Although the mass media have already "lustrated" some prominent figures of the former GDR (with limited consequences for their present political or economic standing), the main effect of the law on the access to the files of the Stasi is its bureaucratic function. Whenever a former citizen of the GDR is considered for employment in the public service, a routine request is made with the so-called *"Gauck-Behörde"* (Gauck is the head of the agency which is in charge of the files of the Stasi; he was one of the leading actors in the opposition of the GDR). Thus, in Germany up to now lustration has not become and is not likely to become a systematic strategy of sanctioning and punishing the exponents of the old regime.

However, there is one particular case of lustration which took place before the enactment of the law on the files of the "Stasi" and which is now pending before the Federal Constitutional Court. A newspaper that had been founded by some prominent members of the opposition of the GDR soon after the collapse of the old regime published some two thousand names of individuals under the headline: "The Full-Timers. The Top Two Thousand on the Payroll of the Stasi". This list was a correct and authentic list of all individuals who received their salary from the Stasi. But not all individuals included in this list were formally employed with the Stasi, (i.e., not all had formal labor contracts with the Stasi). Some of them, among them the plaintiffs of this case who were medical doctors, had contracts with the famous and notorious sports club "Dynamo". Dynamo was well renowned as the Stasi-sports club. The head of the Stasi, Mielke, has been president of this club for more than thirty years. There is abundant evidence for the conclusion that this club is nothing but a special branch of the Stasi.

Despite this evidence, the civil courts, in two instances, granted the plaintiffs an injunction to cease the publication of their names under the aforementioned headlines. While the renunciation of naming the respective individuals was the immediate effect of the Courts' decisions, the indirect effect was worse. The costs of the proceedings, including the fees of the plaintiffs' attorneys, by far exceeded the financial means of the paper, which in the meantime had become bankrupt. This, too, was a small victory for the old communist elites over the opposition which pushed them out of power. This time they did not utilize the means of communist dictatorship, but the opportunities of the *"Rechtsstaat"*.

The legal question at stake is the following. As I already mentioned, the constitution allows the stipulation of boundaries of free speech through special laws if they further the protection of reputation. But here, too, the special law must not underrate the significance of free speech and indiscriminately give the individual's right to reputation preference over the right to free speech (which includes the right to critical assessments of a person's behavior, character, performance etc.).

Thus, the necessity of balancing between two competing protected interests arises. Whereas the Court excludes invectives from the constitutional protection of Article 5, its balancing of free speech against personal reputation is rather generous in favor of the former. This is particularly so if the person who feels unduly attacked by the press or by any other kind of public speech is himself or herself a public figure and has given sufficient cause for debating his or her actions, behavior, or character. Some critics even contend that in Germany the protection of reputation against public attacks has been abolished altogether. This is of course an overstatement, but it shows that indeed the right to free speech is not overly restrained by the right to reputation.

However, this holds true only for the expression of opinion and for the critical assessment of a person's behavior or character. This generosity does not apply to false factual statements. Hence the well-known difficulty of differentiating between facts and evaluations is of major importance. To a certain degree, it is part of the democratic game that individuals have to endure "false" critiques, (i.e., evaluations that they deem extremely unjustified but that simply reflect the subjective view of their fellow-man).

It is far less plausible to accept that one's reputation is exposed to wrong factual contentions and that everybody has to bear this as a necessary burden of a democratic society. Evidently, a person's reputation is more vulnerable to the public expression of negative facts than to negative evaluations - the former pretend to be objective, the latter are purely subjective. This is, of course, not the case with facts: contradictory facts cannot be equally true. Consequently, the distinction between facts and opinions plays an important role in the judicature of the Federal Constitutional Court.

According to this jurisprudence, the constitutional guarantee of free speech applies only to evaluating statements, not to the communication of pure facts (like statistics). It should be mentioned that this line of constitutional reasoning is disputed among constitutional scholars. However, until now the Court has stuck to its opinion. The underlying idea of this judgment is that Article 5 of the Basic Law protects the integrity of the intellectual dispute or the exchange of ideas. Hence, only evaluating reasoning, not factual statements contribute to the kind of public sphere that the constitution presupposes and intends to promote. The communication of facts is only covered by this constitutional guarantee if they relate to the formation of opinions (i.e., if they are evaluating and assessing statements). False and misleading facts can never be regarded as a valuable contribution to the formation of public opinion. This is why they do not enjoy the protection of Article 5.

In order to enjoy the constitutional guarantee of Article 5 a defendent must contend that his or her public speech, which is subject to the request for an injunction, has not been a factual, but an evaluative statement. The petitioner, in contrast, who feels that his or her reputation was unduly attacked will try to establish that the statement consisted entirely of factual elements which he or she can prove to be untrue. Given the experience that it is frequently difficult or even impossible to draw a clear and objective line between the factual and the evaluative elements of a statement, the Court has specified its in judicature that it determines that the drawing of this distinction is itself subject to constitutional scrutiny. Roughly

138

speaking, this means that in all cases of doubt the courts have to judge the case on the basis of an evaluative rather than a factual statement.

In the pending case of the publication of the pay-roll of the Stasi, the key question had been whether the head line "The Full-Timers. The Top Two Thousand on the Payroll of the Stasi" was a factual statement, and if so, whether it was a false factual statement. This had been the contention of the claimants, whether it was a predominantly evaluative and critical assessment of the role of certain categories of persons.

Whichever way the case is finally decided, it demonstrates that the institutional devices of the *Rechtsstaat* equally protect the just and the unjust - both the former opposition against the communist regime that ultimately overthrew it and the proponents of this very regime themselves. The *Rechtsstaat* makes no political distinctions whatsoever, and therefore, a politics of lustration is either restrained by the normal operation of the Constitution, or it is a particular kind of revolutionary justice which is acknowledged as such. What is damaging both for the revolution and for the newly acquired *Rechtsstaat* is the use of lustration as a means of revolutionary justice, but disguised as a normal method of public debate in a democratic society. The exposure of individuals to public contempt without giving them all guarantees of the due process of law is only justifiable in the short period of and after the revolution. Within the framework of normal politics of a *Rechtsstaat*, it is not tolerable.

ACCESS TO THE MEDIA AND DEMOCRATIC COMMUNICATION: THEORY AND PRACTICE IN CENTRAL AND EASTERN EUROPEAN BROADCASTING

by Karol Jakubowicz

"Free communication" and "democratic communication" are - perhaps paradoxically - two different concepts, arising out of two different social philosophies of communication and what Denis McQuail[1] calls "basic communication values": freedom in the first case and equality in the second. The interesting thing about Central and Eastern European countries is that in passing from the opposition to the government their political elites of today practically abandoned their old goal of promoting "democratic communication" in favor of espousing, without really saying so, the ideal of "free communication", with its quite different notion of "access" to communication on a society-wide scale.[2]

I.   Different Types of Communicative Democracy

The concepts of "free communication", "freedom of the press", "free speech" are essentially expressions of the libertarian theory of the press in which access to communication is free in the sense that there are no legal and administrative barriers to becoming a receiver of messages and, theoretically, to becoming a sender of them. This, then, is negative freedom, simply that of expressing oneself without prior restraint, but with no assurance of the ability to exercise this freedom in social discourse. It is founded upon the free market economic system and entails economic freedom for media to operate in their public role and in their private business

---

[1]   D. McQuail, *Media Performance: Mass Communication and the Public Interest*, London (1992).

[2]   B.R. Webster, *Technology and Access to Communications Media*, Reports and Papers on Mass Communication, No.75. Paris, UNESCO (1975). Webster classifies types of access to communication and the media from several points of view: in numerical terms (individuals, small groups, communities, masses); in functional terms (learning, social, official, political); and those of the communication mode (passive, feedback, interactive, participatory).

139

A. Sajó (ed.), *Rights of Access to the Media*, 139-163.
© 1996 Kluwer Law International. Printed in the Netherlands.

capacity. It is accordingly based on what Denis McQuail[3] calls the market model, based in part on the assumption that diversity of media content reflecting social diversity would be ensured by the law of supply and demand. In other words, that media would reflect the demands of would-be receivers, whether these are expressed directly in the audience market or indirectly through the advertising market. However, as John Keane argues extensively, the market model by no means ensures diversity or indeed freedom of communicator entry into social discourse:

> "[C]ommunication markets restrict freedom of communication by generating barriers to entry, monopoly and restrictions upon choice ... there is a structural contradiction between freedom of communication and unlimited freedom of the market ... the market liberal ideology of freedom of individual choice in the marketplace of opinions is in fact a justification of the privileging of corporate speech and of giving more choice to investors than to citizens. It is an apology for the power of king-sized business to organize and determine and therefore to *censor* individuals' choices concerning what they listen to or read and watch."[4]

In this situation, non-corporate speech has a chance to be heard mainly from alternative media which occupy a relatively marginal position.[5] This is confirmed by the West German situation, where "the counter-elites ... and the alternative public ... [aiming] at changing political and social structures especially through more and new forms of political participation"[6] have at their disposal only the alternative press, "a marginal, yet politically relevant part of the media system" which seeks to use multiplier and spill over effects to bring "counter-issues" ignored by the establishment media to general notice.

Awareness of the shortcomings of the media systems based on the principle of negative freedom of speech, offering no realistic prospect of playing an active role in social, particularly mass communication, led early on to calls for some

---

[3]   McQuail, *Media Performance*, supra note 1.

[4]   J. Keane, *The Media and Democracy*, Cambridge, Blackwell, 89, (1991).

[5]   See, e.g., J. Downing, *Radical Media: The Political Experience of Alternative Communication*, Boston, South End Press (1984); J. Downing, *The Alternative Public Realm: The Organization of the 1980's Anti-Nuclear Press in West Germany and Britain*, Media Cult. & Soc. 2, 163, (1988).

[6]   D. Mathes & B. Pfetsch, *The Role of the Alternative Press in the Agenda-Building Process: Spill-over Effects and Media Opinion Leadership*, 1(6) Eur. J. Comm., 33-62 (1991).

guarantees of a positive freedom to communicate and to putting major stress on equality as a main value of public communication. Equality is understood here as both equal access to media channels for everyone, and equal or fair reflection in media content of society in all its diversity of interests, lifestyles, beliefs and ideologies.[7]

As far as equal access to media channels and opportunities to communicate is concerned, Brecht argued in his *Theory of Radio* already in 1932 that the medium must be changed from a means of distribution to one of communication, "allowing the listener not only to hear, but to speak". In later formulations, this found an echo in "the right to receive" and "the right to transmit" as "the basis of any democratic culture",[8] in "each receiver a potential transmitter",[9] and in "the right to communicate is ... a fundamental human right",[10] later supplemented by the view that "a right to communicate includes a right to *telecommunicate*.[11] This positive freedom to communicate is seen by its supporters to involve a fundamental entitlement, a right to communicate whose recognition involves an obligation on the part of society to guarantee its exercise.[12] From Willliams to Keane,[13] this has been interpreted to mean an obligation on the part of society to promote equality of access by developing structures, financed out of public funds, to enable all (even minority) social groups to express their views and join social discourse.

The difference between negative and positive freedom to communicate may be extended into the concepts of *formal* and *full communicative* democracy. For the

---

[7]   McQuail, *Media Performance*, supra note 1.

[8]   R. Williams, *Communications*, Hamondsworth, Penguin Books, 120 (1968).

[9]   H.M. Enzensberger, *Constitutents of a Theory of Mass Media, in* Sociology of Mass Communications, 99-116. (D. McQuail ed.), Harmondsworth, Penguin Books (1972).

[10]   D. Fischer & L.S. Harms, eds., *The Right to Communicate: A New Human Right*, 19. Dublin (1983).

[11]   L.S. Harms. *The Right to Communicate: What a Small World*, The Third Channel 2, 158-172 (1985).

[12]   Fischer & Harms, supra note 10.

[13]   Williams, supra note 8; Keane, supra note 4.

latter concept to be put into practice, communicative democracy would have to be seen as an integral element of political democracy and as an essential part of the process of democratic governance. In other words, equality in communication would have to become a goal of public policy, resulting in the creation of some publicly-funded mechanism ensuring exercise of the right to communicate in practice.

As the idea of the right to transmit (or communicate) gained acceptance, and as new research showed communication to be a process of exchange rather than an act of one-way transmission of content,[14] the nature of social communication was redefined in a way consistent with the spirit of interactive, participatory communication.[15]

The original four theories of the press did not include one of democratic communication. It was only later, on the crest of 60's dissent to established social and also communication structures, that they came to be supplemented with such a theory, first developed by Raymond Williams,[16] and then elaborated upon by Denis McQuail who proposed the democratic-participant media theory as a new normative press theory.

McQuail also mentions the category of Western models a distinctive "social democratic" version of press theory which provides legitimation for public intervention into the communication processes, including even collective ownership of the media, so as to achieve socially desirable ends, such as true independence from vested interests, access and diversity of opinions. Proposals by Williams and Keane, mentioned above, clearly fit into this category.

Theoretical work was coupled with a practical interest in devising ways reforming existing media institutions, especially broadcasting systems.[17] Jouet's

---

[14] O.A. Wiio, *Open and Closed Mass Media System and Problems of International Communications Policy*, Studies of Broadcasting 13, 67-90 (1981); E.M. Rogers, *Future Directions in Mass Communciation Research: Towards Network Analysis and Convergence Models*, 122-136 *in* New Structures of International Communication? The Role of Research, Leicester, IAMCR (1982).

[15] L.R. Beltran, *L'adieu a Aristotle: la communication horizontale*, Paris, UNESCO (n.d.).

[16] Williams, supra note 8; D. McQuail, *Mass Communication Theory: An Introduction*, London (1987).

[17] A.W. Branscomb & M. Savage, *The Broadcast Reform Movement at the Crossroads*, 4 J. of Comm., 24-34 (1978).

early typology of the three levels and degrees of media democratization (access, participation, social management of the media) is characteristic of the work of many authors,[18] seeking to propose the kind of communication policy and media structures needed to ensure feedback,[19] access[20] or "participatory programming".[21] Important work has been done on criteria for judging pluralism and diversity in mass communication,[22] with Jacklin,[23] and McQuail and van Cuilenburg[24] perhaps coming closest to defining them.

Another area of debate has dealt with the general social context. Especially representatives of critical theory have studied macro structural determinants affecting the operation of broadcasting because they saw democratization of communication (as forming) part of a broader process of distribution of social power and influence in society" allowing "all sectors of the population to contribute to the pool of information that provides the basis for local or national *decision-making* and the basis for the allocation of resources in society.

---

[18] J. Jouet, *Community Media and Development: Problems of Adaptation*, Working paper of the UNESCO Meeting on Self-Management, Access and Participation in Communication, Belgrade (1977), *reviewed in* N.W. Jankowski, *Community Television in Amsterdam*, Amsterdam, University of Amsterdam (1988).

[19] *Broadcasters and their Audiences*, Vol.1. Torino, ERI (1974).

[20] F.J. Berrigan, ed., *Access: Some Western Models of a Community Media*, Paris, UNESCO (1977).

[21] B. Groombridge, *Television and the People: A Programme for Democratic Participation*, Harmondsworth, Penguin Books (1972).

[22] J.G. Blumler, *The Social Character of Media Gratifications*, 41-60 in Media Gratifications Research Current Perspectives, K.N. Rosengran, et. al., eds., Beverly Hills, London, New Delhi, Sage Publications (1985); W. Hoffman-Riem, *National Identity and Cultural Values: Broadcasting Safeguards*, in Journal of Broadcasting and Electronic Media 3, 57-72 (1987).

[23] P. Jacklin, *Representative Diversity*, 2 J. of Comm., 85-88 (1978).

[24] D. McQuail & J.J.van Cuilenburg, *Diversity as a Policy Goal: A Strategy for Evaluative Research and a Netherlands Case Study*, Gazette 3, 145-162 (1983).

144

Efforts to define democratic communication[25] have led to a broad agreement that it should remove the distinction, built into many communication patterns, between the sender and the receiver. Elimination of the difference between the sender and the receiver, allowing everyone to be a sender at will, would amount to putting into practice the ideal type of communicative democracy which might be called *direct communicative democracy* where everyone would be a "sendceiver" engaged in participatory horizontal communication, incorporating immediate response and feedback.

Direct communicative democracy is, however, an all but impossible dream as far as mass communication is concerned: "in large-scale societies *representative* mechanisms in the field of communications cannot be bypassed... some will necessarily communicate on behalf of others, if only for a time."[26]

If so, then we need to distinguish another ideal type - that of *representative communicative democracy*. It would prevail in a situation in which all segments of society could own or control their own media or have adequate access to them for the purposes of communicating to their own members and to society at large. Few of their members would need be active mass communicators in their own right. Still, the group's views, ideas, culture and world outlook would enter social circulation at a level appropriate to the group's size and scale of operation (i.e. through the intermediary of national or regional, local or community media), would be known to the community at large and could potentially influence its views, policies or outlook.

In this context, let us note Scannell's concept of "communicative entitlements" as part of the traditional Western system of mass communication. These presuppose "communicative rights" (the right to speak freely, for example). However, usually it is the role of the mass communicators, acting "on behalf" of the public, to "entitle" it to speak and serve as gate-keepers in the process. It is thus a system in which, as Scannell puts it, "power accrues to the representatives, not to

---

[25] Various definitions or attempts to formulate them are reviewed in A. Screberny-Mohammadi, n.d., *Community and Democracy Directions in Research*, Leicester, IAMCR (n.d.).

[26] J. Keane, supra note 4.

those whom they represent".[27] The question therefore becomes, as Keane[28] has pointed out, precisely "how to render 'media representatives' accountable to the reading and listening publics" and how to make media content representative of what the public thinks and how it feels.

To some extent, an answer is provided in the ideal type of *representative participatory communicative democracy*. This refers to a situation when groups or movements which control particular media are structured and organized in a truly democratic way; then all or most of their members are able to influence the operation of their media and participate in the determination of their goals, even if only a few of them are communicators *per se*. However, the structures and mechanisms of representative participatory communicative democracy have so far been found mostly in groups, communities and organizations. It is uncertain whether they can be replicated at the societal level.

II.   The "Solidarity" Ideal of Democratic Communication

To gain some insight into the thinking of Central and Eastern European dissident movements of the 1980's on the issue of social communication, let us look at some of the concepts developed by Solidarity in Poland.

The key concept in 1980-1981, when Solidarity first formulated its views on the subject[29] was *socialization*, meaning direct social control over the media operating in the interest of society. A second major concept was *access* to the media, understood broadly enough to be almost equivalent to "the right to communicate". "Social access to the media" was a widely used phrase, meaning that the media should be at the disposal of society for the purpose of free, equal and pluralistic communication. Hence a determination to abolish all monopolies in this sphere and

---

[27]   P. Scannell, *Public Service Broadcasting and Modern Public Life*, 11(2) Media Cult. & Soc., 136-166 (1989).

[28]   J. Keane, supra note 4, at 44.

[29]   Cf. K. Jakubowicz, *Between Communism, and Post-Communism: How Many Varieties of Glasnost? in* Democratization and the Media: An East-West Dialogue, (Splichal, Hochheimer, Jakubowicz, eds.), Ljubljana, University of Ljubljana (1990).

introduce a system of horizontal, participatory communication ("society talking to itself").

The ideologues of the new information order in Poland saw communication as *empowerment*, as the exercise of a right, and satisfaction of the need, to communicate by "speaking with ones' own voice", without the need for spokesmen and intermediaries. It was seen as a precondition of *subjectivity*, i.e. dignity and master of one's own fate. In general social terms, this approach springs from what might be called a *substantive* understanding of democratic communication as an element of "communicative democracy", i.e. as a way of satisfying a fundamental human and *social* need, and as a prerequisite of democracy and self-government.

This view that communications and information are central to the exercise of full and effective citizenship adds - as Murdock and Golding point out in another context - another dimension to T.H. Marshall's classic analysis of the three (civil, political and social) basic aspects of citizenship. Communication rights must be seen as an indispensable extension of social rights; in this view, democracy is not complete unless citizens have real opportunities of joining in the social discourse and using mechanisms for user feedback and participation in the media. To classify Solidarity's approach in terms of the three ideal types of communicative democracy distinguished above, it might be said therefore that this concept of the Self-Governing Commonwealth was intended to involve society-wide representative participatory communicative democracy, ensured by structural guarantees of social feedback, access to, and participation in, media activities and direct media accountability to society.[30]

Let us put aside the question of how practicable the concept of society-wide representative participatory communicative democracy really is. Let us also disregard for the moment the fundamental change of perspective on social communication once the former opposition movements took over power. This concept and ideal must be treated as a reference point and a criterion by which to judge the media policies of the Central and Eastern European governments which arose out of the opposition movements of the communist era.

Having said that, we must also - treating Solidarity as a case study of those opposition movements - make a distinction between its idealistic, but vague, long-

---

[30] There was even a suggestion at one point that to ensure direct social input into the process, members of Polish Radio and Television's governing body should be elected in a national election.

range plans and its tactics in promoting political change under what it assumed
would be a long period of continued communist rule. Writing about Solidarity's
goals in Poland in 1980-1981,[31] Goldfarb makes the following telling point:
"Solidarity ... sought to expand a zone of independence from totalitarian definitions
of control, to detotalize parts of the social order ... Polish society sought to get
official recognition for the *coexistence* of pluralism and totalitarianism". Solidarity
did not see any chance to overthrow the communist system soon; rather, it strived
to create civil society, understood as a free social space for the self-organization of
society against the totalitarian or authoritarian state[32] - and then successively to
expand that space and fill it with more and more types of alternative institutions in
the hope that one day they could take over from the institutions of the communist
state. In adopting a "long-march" strategy, opposition movements in Poland and
elsewhere in Central and Eastern Europe saw civil society as a sphere distinct form,
independent of, and opposed to the sphere of state action. As a social reality, civil
society was initially conceived of as creating "parallel structures", independent
public spheres and an alternative culture. As social action it primarily meant gradual
and self-limited (re)construction of social reality "from below", legalistic and non-
revolutionary in principle.[33]

Underground media and an independent public sphere, comprising not only
periodicals and publishing houses, but also alternative artistic events, "flying
universities", etc. were seen as a major component of civil society in this sense.[34]
Accordingly, Solidarity's platform in the media sphere in 1980-81 and later was
based on the assumption that the communist state would continue in existence for a
long time to come. So, in addition to whatever one could do in the underground,

---

[31]   J.C. Goldfarb, *Beyond Glasnost: The Post-Totalitarian Mind*, Chicago and London,
       The University of Chicago Press, 22 (1989).

[32]   Cf. A. Arato, *Civil Society vs. the State: Poland 1980- 81*, Telos, No. 47 (Spring
       1981).

[33]   T. Mastnak, *The Powerless in Power: Political Identity in Post-Communist Eastern
       Europe*, 13(3) Media Cult. & Soc. (1991), 399 402; cf. S. Splichal, *Media Beyond
       Socialism: The 'Civil Society' Paradox and the Media in Post Socialist Countries*
       (Univ of Llubjana 1992), mimeograph.

[34]   H. Fedorowicz, *Civil Society as a Communication Project: The Polish Laboratory
       for Democratization in East Central Europe*, *in* Democratization and the Media,
       supra note 30.

media reform should be pursued by bringing pressure to bear on the authorities. As a result, Solidarity's battle for the democratization of mass communications aimed primarily at obtaining concession from the state and the passage of new laws so as to restructure existing media institutions. During the Round Table conference in 1989, Solidarity accepted - however unwillingly and under protest - continued government and party control of broadcasting. Even after the election of June 1989, it assumed that communists would remain in power for quite a few years yet and viewed its strategy in exactly the terms of expanding civil society as a zone of independence from the state. It had done very little work on defining the principles on which a new system of democratic mass communications would be based and gave no consideration to the effects of introducing the free market into the media field. Accordingly, it had no blueprint for action when it finally took over power in September 1989.

III.   After the Revolution: Groping in the Dark

As the situation in East Germany, Hungary and Poland has shown, Solidarity's approach to the underlying principles and values of social communication found continuation in efforts to define the new legal and institutional structures of the media once the opportunity to do that arose.

In East Germany, a most interesting debate on the shape of the new media order took place during the transition period between the collapse of communist Party control and the run-up to reunificaion and assimilation of East Germany into the West German system. During that debate, "the classic liberal notion of the marketplace of ideas was rejected out of hand"[35] and an effort was made to design a media order along the lines of the antipolitics ideal espoused by the grass-roots democratic forces which were in the forefront of the movement. They "wished to fashion citizen politics ... these antipolitics politicians attempted to work out a new kind of public sphere infrastructure to ensure the vitality and involvement of citizen movements",[36] by institutionalizing possibilities for citizen-to-citizen dialogue,

---

[35]   M. Boyle, *The Revolt of the Communist Journalist in the German Democratic Republic*, 17 (1989-90), mimeograph.

[36]   Id. at 4.

subjecting the media to direct social control and opening the government to public inspection.

In Hungary and in Poland, a somewhat more realistic approach was adopted, accepting the existence of commercially-driven media, but with great emphasis being placed by reformers (especially in Hungary) on designing a media system serving primarily the civil society. That was to be achieved by creating socially-representative governing bodies of public broadcast media, but most of all by providing for the emergence of a "third sector" of the broadcast media: non-profit private stations representing a wide variety of opinions, orientations and beliefs. In Poland, the Broadcasting Reform Commission appointed in 1989 named this the "civic sector" of broadcasting,[37] comprising, as its chairman has explained, socially-motivated privately or collectively owned stations, mostly local and community ones, speaking for, on behalf of, or to various groups, parties, organizations, movements, minorities, territorial groups and communities (at this time of fast social and political change in post-communist countries, there is an unusually high level of need for opportunities for active communication, especially in the field of political communication).[38]

This concept, which has been recognized as one of a whole range of solutions practiced or proposed in many countries in order to combine collectivist and market approaches in a synthesis that incorporates the strength of both, is clearly oriented towards ensuring equality in mass communications. Its stated goal of lowering barriers to market entry for new communicators and ensuring the emergence and survival of this sector, required, it was assumed, considerable support in terms of public policy and potentially also public funds.

Meanwhile, when the new democratic governments finally assumed power and could translate these ideas into practice, they largely adopted a different track. They were reluctant to regulate strictly the media for fear of repeating the mistakes of the past. This was true especially in the field of the printed press. Except for dismantling the old system of controls they were unable and unwilling to develop any policy stance of their own on what form the press scene should take and what rules should govern it, with the exception of a clear desire in many countries that

---

[37]   *Glowne zalozenia reformy radiofonii i telewizji*, Przekazy i Opinie 1. 7-61, (1991).

[38]   K. Jakubowicz, *Solidarity and Media Reform in Poland*, 5(23) Eur. J. Comm. 333-354 (1990).

major new political parties should receive, be allotted or allowed to buy some newspapers in order to develop a pluralistic press system. Since then, however, they have been left to swim or sink depending on their sales, and many have indeed gone under. In general, the print media were left to the operation of the free market, with all the limitations of access to possibilities of communicating that this entails. Processes of media concentrations and penetration by foreign capital[39] have already been set in motion and will further curtail access to the print media.

In broadcasting, the situation has been quite different. While the need to re-regulate broadcasting was widely recognized, the process of developing new laws has been politically contentious and therefore protracted. Part of the problem is that "there is a lack of a historical legal tradition concerning free and independent media in a democratic society".[40] There is also a strong distrust, inherited from the past and compounded by recent experience, of intense politisation of public authorities, of public regulation of social life. This has complicated the process of drafting new laws. There are also genuine constitutional issues in that the institutional arrangements for regulating and overseeing public and private broadcasting usually reflect a country's system of government - and this is far from finally settled in post-communist countries. Areas of competence and division of power between the various state authorities and branches of the government are still being agreed upon. As shown, for example, by the Hungarian conflict between the Prime Minister and the President over the nomination of top executives for Hungarian Radio and Hungarian Television,[41] or political battles over control of Slovak Television[42] this poses major difficulties as far as developing the new system of broadcasting is concerned. Most importantly, however, the beleaguered and insecure new

---

[39]   K. Jakubowicz, *Media Concentrations and Foreign Media Presence in Central and Eastern Europe*, Report commissioned by the Council of Europe, Strasbourg (forthcoming); M. Galik & F. Dénes, From Command Media to Media Market; The Role of Foreign Capital in the Transition of the Hungarian Media, Budapest University of Economics, Budapest (1992).

[40]   W. Kleinwächter, *Old Problems in a New Environment: Broadcasting Legislation in Eastern Europe and the Republics of the Former Soviet Union*, 1 (1992) mimeograph.

[41]   J. Pataki, *Political Battle in Hungary over Broadcasting Dismissals*, 1(30) RFE/RL Research Report 26-30 (1992).

[42]   A. Kalniczk, *Slovak Television: Back to State Control?*, 1(45) REF/RL Research Report 64-68 (1992).

governments, which in many cases do not have a stable parliamentary majority or a secure power base in society, have been reluctant to give up control of broadcasting.

In part this is because of the rough treatment they received from the print media - a stunning experience for the new administrations which perceived themselves to be victors of a popular revolution and liberators of their peoples from communist oppression. As one commentator noted in the Hungarian context "in the post-revolutionary euphoria all the parties did seriously believe in the sanctity of the principle of the freedom of the press. (They were yet to discover) how annoying the practice of this freedom (would) soon become to many of them".[43] The press in many cases adopted a highly critical and aggressive attitude towards them in order to gain or maintain credibility. The old guard of journalists, known to have kowtowed to the communist government, now sought to atone for its past behavior by adopting an uncompromising attitude to the new one. The new guard, people once involved in the opposition movement and otherwise highly supportive of the new system, still felt uncomfortable about working for quasi-official media and tried to retain credibility by an equally critical stance towards it. Stung by such partly undeserved treatment, the new governments could perhaps be forgiven for feeling that they needed support from some media and were not happy about the prospect of losing those they could rely on, i.e. broadcasting.

Nevertheless, new laws and institutional structures of radio and television organizations are slowly emerging. The analysis below should offer some indication, the concept of access, which underlies current thinking and practice in this area.

If we look at these developments in terms of the whole concept of civil society and media freedom, it will become clear that while great progress on the way to democracy has of course been made, civil society as a social space for self-organization of society to counteract the expansionist policy of the state has lost much ground. Its former leaders have moved into positions of importance in the power structure and in the political establishment, taking their organizations and media with them, and leaving behind a void which will not easily be filled. Among the reasons for this are the following:

---

[43]   E. Hankiss, *The Hungarian Media War of Independence,* Budapest, Centre for Social Studies (1993).

- a deliberate policy pursued by governments in some countries of discouraging social participation in public and political life, i.e. of mobilizing the population for the purpose of elections or other short-lived campaign, and dampening their enthusiasm at other times;

- a feeling of anti-climax among the population, following the inevitable disappointment of hope that abolition of communism would help solve other problems easily;

- disillusionment with the new governments in consequence of their adoption of tough liberal economic policies;

- disappointment with the media because of the sometimes stridently propagandistic tone of both broadcasting and the new advocacy press, their inability to cover developments so as to make sense of developments unfolding in the country (competent, unbiased, impartial reporting and analysis of public life area hard to find) and their inadequacy in performing the watch-dog function.

Splichal notes that the revitalization of civil society is again blocked because:

> "[h]aving overthrown the old undemocratic regimes, (civil society) lost its own autonomy ... Decisions of public consequence are, as they were in the former system, removed from the public and the citizens lose their ability to participate in political processes. The access of both oppositional parties and particularly autonomous groups from civil society to national broadcast media and mainstream print media is being limited ... parliamentary mechanisms of party pluralism and formal democracy are considered as the only legitimate way to articulate the interests and opinions of "society", while non-institutional arrangements of civil society are ignored".[44]

In addition to the expansion of the state, civil society is in retreat also because the population has largely opted out of public life, discouraged by lack of progress in solving the particular countries' problems and by what it perceives to be the interminable power struggle of politicians concentrating on issues without relevance to the everyday life of the people. Yet another reason is the expansion of capital,

---

[44] Splichal, supra note 33, at 36.

itself a factor limiting press freedom, which is gaining control of many areas of public life. In East Germany, journalists were complaining that they were as powerless against their new publishers as they were against the Communist Party.

IV.   New Broadcasting Laws

We will analyze new broadcasting laws and drafts[45] of such laws, where available, in order to establish to what extent the ideals of communicative democracy in general and participatory representative communicative democracy in particular, served as a guide to developing the institutional structures and procedures in the new broadcasting systems. Naturally, in addition to licensing procedures and criteria for awarding licenses to private broadcasters (which might for example provide for special treatment of non-commercial private stations), it is primarily the new public service broadcasting systems that can be treated as a test case in this latter regard, in terms for example of any system of public accountability or mechanisms of access and participation built into them by law.

In analyzing these laws and drafts, it must be remembered that they represent three distinctive "generations" of law-making. Some, like the 1990 Decree of the President of the USSR on Democratization and Development of TV and Radio Broadcasting are an expression of *glasnost*, with its mixture of carefully calibrated liberalization and continued government control and supervision of broadcasting.[46] Others, like the 1991 Law on the Statue of Albanian Radio and Television, whose almost sole purpose is to guard against politisation, and political control of the state

---

[45]   These are: the Polish Broadcasting Act of Dec. 29, 1992; the Romanian Law on Radio and Television Broadcasting of May 1992; the Law on the Statute of Albanian Radio and Television of April 1991; the Czechoslovak Law on the Operation of Radio and Television Broadcasts of October 1991; the Slovak National Council Act on Slovak Radio of May 1991: Hungarian Television's "proposal on the concept of the draft bill on radio and television" of February 1991 and the Draft of the Hungarian Law on Radio and Television of Summer 1992; General Principles of Temporary Statute of Bulgarian Television and Bulgarian Radio of December 1990; the Latvian Law on Radio and Television of May 1992; Decree of the President of the USSR on Democratization and Development of TV and Radio Broadcasting of July 1990; Draft Law of the Russian Federation on TV and Radio Broadcasting of January 1992; the Draft of Slovenian Law on Public Media. Drafts, while obviously inconclusive and subject to many changes, do offer some insight into the thinking underlying the development of the new broadcasting systems. We will also use information on other broadcasting systems where it is available. See Kleinwächter, supra note 40.

[46]   Cf. Jakubowicz, supra note 38.

154

broadcasting system (with no provision for turning it into a public system, or its demonopolization and licensing private stations), come from the first impatient impulse of creating a new system primarily by negating the old one, with little appreciation of the fact that guarding against the mistakes of the past is no guarantee of creating a truly new system and indeed provides little understanding of the dilemmas involved. And finally, laws like the Polish Broadcasting Act, represent the first relatively mature effort to design a complete new broadcasting system. It is, for example, the only new law in force which in addition to creating a regulatory body and laying out a procedure for licensing private stations, defines the legal form, general structure, and permit of public service broadcasters. However, even this "third-generation" act will need to be amended and expanded quite soon into a "fourth generation" law to do justice to the real complexities of contemporary broadcasting driven by the market and new technologies.

Thus, the laws and draft under consideration here are not fully comparable. Nevertheless, together they do provide evidence of the general direction of change in this area.

The first issue facing political elites and legislators was which public or state authority or branch of government would be responsible for regulating and overseeing public and private broadcasting. Given the constitutional difficulties referred to above (concerning the division of power and competence between various state authorities), the solutions adopted were indicative of the general balance of power in the new system of government. They are summed up below in a table which shows which authorities appoint (or would appoint if draft laws were in force) how many members[47] of the regulatory body in the countries where they have been set up or proposed.

---

[47] The numerical ratios are not without importance. In Poland, the first draft, written in early 1990, when General Jaruzelski was still President of Poland and the newly emergent Solidarity-led government was still very popular, the government, the Diet, and the Senate were to appoint 3 members of the Council each, and the President was to appoint 1 member (3:3:3:1). This was subsequently changed to a formula in which the government would not appoint anybody, while both Houses of Parliament and the President would appoint 3 people each (3:3:3). That formula was accepted for a long time and changed for the one now written into the law and adopted at the last moment in the Diet (4:2:3) which subsequently rejected a Senate amendment restoring the 3:3:3 formula. At one point, it was also suggested during the debate in the Diet that since it was more important than the Senate, it should be able to appoint six members of the National Council, i.e. twice as many as the Senate (6:3:3). One of the governments at one point proposed that it would appoint an additional group of 3 members (3:3:3:3) and that it should also appoint three Council's Secretary (the Chairman is be appointed by the President), who would hold all the executive power. Thus, the matter was clearly the object of a prolonged power struggle.

Members of Broadcasting Regulatory Bodies Appointed by Particular State Authorities (Table 1.)

	Parl't		Gov't	President	Const'l. Court	Active politicians barred from membership
	Lower House	Upper House				
Poland	4	2		3		no
Romania	3	3	3	2		yes
Slovak Republik		9				yes
Czech Republic		9				yes
Russia[a]	2	2		5[b]	3	yes
Latvia		1 (chairman)				

[a] This represents the provisions of the 1992 Draft of the Russian Federation on TV and Radio Broadcasting. According to an earlier version, the Commission was to consist of 12 members: 3 to be appointed by the President, 3 by each of the two Houses of Parliament and 3 by the Constitutional Court. *See* Kleinwächter, *supra* note 40.

[b] According to the 1992 Draft Law of the Russian Federation on TV and Radio Broadcasting, the President would appoint 2 members of the Federal Commission on Mass Communication "from among the ranks of representatives culture and art" and 3 more "from among qualified specialists in the sphere of social psychology, TV and radio broadcasting, journalism, philology, law and representatives of culture and art".

Czechoslovakia, as a federal country was a special case. Its Federal Council for Radio and Television Broadcasting was a creation of the Federal Assembly (which elected 3 members) and Czech and Slovak National Councils (3 members each). Another special case was Hungary where an attempt was made to circumvent political conflicts between different state authorities by involving all, or most of them in decision-making concerning broadcasting. The 1991 draft of the Hungarian broadcasting law provided for the existence of a one-man regulatory authority (Radio and Television Office) whose president was to be nominated by the Prime Minister and then appointed by Parliament by a two-third majority vote, following a hearing in a parliamentary committee.

Yet another solution has been adopted in Latvia. There, the regulatory body, the Council of Radio and Television of Latvia, is composed of the following persons: "the chief of the Council of Radio and Television of Latvia Republic, the representative of Latvia Writers Union, the member of Composers Union of Latvia Republic, the member of Cinematographist Society of Latvia Republic, the member of Theater Society of Latvia Republic, the member of Journalists Society of Latvia Republic, the member of Cultural Found of Latvia Republic, three deputies of the Supreme Soviet of Latvia Republic, the member of Social Consultative Soviet of Nationalities of the Supreme of Latvia Republic, the member of religious of the Consultative Soviet of the Supreme Soviet of Latvia Republic, the member of the Ministry of Culture of Latvia Republic, the member of the state enterprise of Latvia Radio, the member of the state enterprise of Latvia Television, the members of two other societies of radio and television, the members of state inspection, the members of the center of radio and television of Latvia Republic, the members of the Sociologists Association of Latvia Republic, the members of three municipal societies of radio and television". While the translation[48] does not make every detail clear, this solution (while perhaps patterned to some extent on the composition of the councils of Western German public service broadcasting organizations) seems characteristic of the spirit of "first" or "second generation" broadcasting laws. In the first case, communist governments created, as evidence of their democratic independence, "representative" executive or advisory bodies, giving them little or no real power. In the second, in an effort to ensure that every relevant social group, organization and institution is involved in running the media procedure, large bodies

---

[48]   Published in Kleinwächter, supra note 40.

were created which incorporated their representatives. If we assume that we have to do here with the second case, then this is the only instance of the ideal of participatory representative communicative democracy applied in creating regulatory bodies in the countries under consideration. This is all the more so that council members are delegated and recalled by the organizations and bodies they represent - and since there is no fixed term of office, they can presumably be recalled at will, giving their mother organizations considerable power over their activities on the council.

In redesigning the broadcasting system, a decision had to be made on who would appoint the top management of state/public radio or television. The present situation is shown in Table 2 below.

Organ which Appoints Top Management of Public Broadcasting Stations (Table 2.)

Country	Gov't	Parl't	President	Regulatory body
Poland				x[a]
Romania			x	
Bulgaria		-----		
Albania		-----		
Czech Republic		x		
Slovak Republic		x		
Hungary	--------------------------------------			
Russia			x	
Ukraine	----------------------			
Belarus	x			
Latvia		x		
Estonia		x		
Lithuania		x		
Slovenia		x		

----   means that one body nominates (e.g. a parliamentary committee), and another (e.g. the full House) appoints, broadcasting personnel or approves the appointment.

a   The regulatory body appoints the Supervisory Boards of public radio and television, which in turn appoint and dismiss the boards of management.

Hungary is again a special case, inasmuch as the system proposed in the 1991 draft was to involve in the decision making just about everyone among the top authorities of the country (potentially creating a deadlock in the case of a conflict among them, which in fact happened, making public broadcasters pawns in, and victims of, a running political feud between the Prime Minister and the President.

This situation, and others like it in other countries, contradict what has been a clear and unequivocal desire to insulate broadcasting from political influence. Expressions of this desire can be found in many of the legal instruments under consideration here. Already the 1990 Decree of the President of the USSR on Democratization and Development of TV and Radio Broadcasting stated that: "Monopolization of broadcasting by any party or political grouping, as well as using the State TV and Radio channels for promotion of the staff's personal political ideas is regarded as inadmissible". The 1991 Law on the Statue of Albanian Radio and TV actually bans membership in a party as well as the conduct of political activity by the directors and employees of Albanian Radio and TV. The 1992 Draft Law of the Russian Federation on TV and Radio Broadcasting would, if adopted, prevent political parties from being able to found radio or television stations.

However, all these hopes and intentions notwithstanding, insulating broadcasting from political influence proved more difficult than expected. For

Sources of Public Broadcasting Stations' Financing (Table 3.)

Country	Gov't or state budget	Licence fees	Advertising	Other
Albania	x		x	x
Bulgaria	x		x	x
Poland		x	x	x
Czech Republic		x	x	x
Slovak Republic		x	x	x
Romania		x	x	x
Russia	x		x	x
Hungary	x	x	x	x
Ukraine	x		x	x
Belarus	x		x	x
Latvia	x			x
Estonia	x		x	x

example, in most communist countries, state broadcasting was financed out of the state budget, which created an obvious situation of dependence on the government. Not much has changed since then (Table 3).

Let us note that even where license fees account for the bulk of the broadcasting organization's income, they are usually paid by the public into the state treasury. State authorities then allot this money to the broadcasting organization in what is unavoidably a politicized process of decision-making. Thus Hungarian TV was "punished" for its behavior by the withdrawal of most of its budget, and ultimately the governing majority in Parliament passed a law incorporating the budgets of Hungarian Radio and Hungarian Television into that of the Prime Minister's Office, giving the government direct financial control over them.[49]

A clear test of new broadcasting policies (and of whether they are oriented towards freedom or equality as a main value of public communication) is the question of demonopolization. First generation regulations allowed for it, if at all, on a very limited scale, as shown by the 1990 Decree of the President of the USSR on Democratization and Development of TV and Radio Broadcasting which gave the "right to establish new TV and Radio centers" to "the Soviets of People's Deputies, public organizations and parties". Later laws demonopolize broadcasting by creating a private sector open to all comers, but contain few provisions ensuring anything like equal access to opportunities to communicate by easing entry for smaller and poorer groups, minorities and communities.

The Romanian Law on Radio and Television Broadcasting says in Article 12 that "the criteria for deciding between [applications for licenses] must ensure the pluralism of opinions, equality of the participants treatment, the quality and diversification of programs ...The access of social and cultural organizations, political, religious, and of other applicant's to audio-visual programs shall be allowed ...". This however, is a general guideline, not accompanied by any operative clauses laying down precise procedures and criteria for ensuring equality of access. Similarly vague provisions are written into most new laws or draft laws.

The Polish Broadcasting Act says in Article 40 that the fee charged for granting of a broadcasting license is to be determined "taking into account the nature of particular broadcasting establishments and their programming". This is an indication that the fee may potentially be lowered for non-commercial private broadcasters, but there is no certainty that it will be.

The 1991 Czechoslovak Law on the Operation of the Radio and Television Broadcasts says in Article 20 that fines imposed for offenses under the law "shall be purposefully used for the support of the broadcasting of license holders [i.e.

private broadcasters - K.J.], with priority being given to the needs of local broadcasts". The 1992 Draft Law of the Russian Federation on TV and Radio Broadcasting proposes that non-commercial broadcasters may receive government subsidies and suggests the establishment of privileged tax status for stations "which are distributing programs for children, educational programs, cultural enlightenment programs for the hearing-impaired". The Czechoslovak Law puts cable operators under an obligation to reserve free of charge one channel for the needs of the local community. The 1991 Hungarian Television proposal for a draft broadcasting bill goes furthest in actually spelling out a rationale for an interventionist policy: it is "a matter of general public interest that [local public broadcasting and community broadcasting services] operate in the largest possible numbers. To this end, it is worth considering that [they] be *guaranteed* access to certain additional equipment, to be financed from state resources.[50] To this end, the document proposed the establishment of a National Broadcasting Fund (1-2 per cent of new state revenues from broadcasting and frequency fees).

The status of the Russian and Hungarian proposals is of course uncertain, given that they were formulated in draft bills which have not been given parliamentary approval. An interesting light on broadcasting policies is thrown by the extent of demonopolization and privatization of state broadcasting. In the Czech and Slovak Republics, for example, the policy is to leave public television with one channel alone. In the Russian debates on the shape of television to come, the view is sometimes forcefully expressed that no public television is needed at all, and the state should connect itself with the legal possibility of buying time for its programming from commercial broadcasters. This policy, if implemented, would create more space for the corporate voice and would reduce the size of the public sector - duty-bound to provide at least internal pluralism in its programming and at least recognize the need for social access and participation.

Another form of easing entry into the market for new domestic communicators would of course be a policy of limiting foreign capital participation in broadcasting establishments. The following table illustrates policies pursued in various countries (Table 4).

A policy of lowering barriers to entry for new communicators would naturally need to involve limiting media concentrations so as to prevent large media conglomerates from forming and controlling the media scene. Policies actually pursued in particular countries, provided they have been adopted at all, are summed up below (Table 5).

---

[50]   *Proposal on the Concept of the Draft Bill on Radio and Television*, Hungarian Television, Budapest (1991).

Cap on Foreign Capital Involvement in Broadcasting Establishments, if Any (Table 4.)

Poland	33 per cent
Bulgaria	25 per cent
Latvia	49 per cent
Lithuania	0 per cent
Romania	none
Slovak Republic	none (but gov't unwilling to let foreign capital in)
Czech Republic	none
Albania	0 per cent
Slovenia	0 per cent[a] (49 per cent proposed)

[a]   In Slovenia, the old (federal) Law on Foreign Investments is still in force. It expressly bans foreign ownership of companies in the field of the media and telecommunications. Similarly, the law on telecommunications does not permit the allocation of broadcasting frequencies to foreign natural or legal persons.

Legal Limits on Media Concentrations (Table 5.)

Bulgaria	"dominant position" in media inadmissible
Poland	n.a.
Latvia	n.a.
Romania	no-one can be majority shareholder in one audio-visual communication company and have more than 20 per cent of the stock in another
Slovak Republic	"dominant position" in media inadmissible
Russia	n.a.[a]
Slovenia	n.a.

[a]   The 1992 Draft law of the Russian Federation on TV and Radio Broadcasting says that no person or corporate entity, with the exception of the Russian Federation or its member states, may "Act as an owner, partner or participant in more than four organizations; own more than 60 per cent of the total values of stocks or votes in the administrative organs of any one organization; own more than 30 per cent of the total value of stocks or votes in the administrative organs of one organization if it is an owner or more than 15 percent of the total value of stocks or votes in the administrative organs of another organization". "No organization may receive more than three licences for radio broadcasting and two licences for TV broadcasting by means of air distribution with fully or partially overlapping zones of realistic reception".

And finally, let us look at yet another set of provisions which might be used to favor access by domestic communicators and producers to air time: the domestic production quota (Table 6).

Domestic Production Quota (Table 6.)

Poland	at least 30 per cent
Bulgaria	n.a.
Latvia	none
Lithuania	
Romania	none
Slovak Republic	none
Czech Republic	none
Russia	n.a.
Slovenia	n.a.

Poland is the only country to have introduced in its broadcasting law a quota of independent production (of at least 10 per cent of air time) - which might have been still another way of promoting access.

IV.   Access, Yes, but for Whom?

As it happens, some broadcasting laws and draft laws do incorporate specific provisions guaranteeing access - but to governments and other state authorities and politicians. The 1992 Draft Law of the Russian Federation on TV and Radio Broadcasting says that "The Russian Federation or its member state has the right to broadcast, in this name ... TV or Radio broadcasting on the channel which has been licensed to a non- governmental organization... an organization is obligated to provide a government enterprise a channel of distribution and [air] time ... for pay" (it may not exceed one-tenth of the organization's air time). Article 4 of the General

Principles of Temporary Statue of Bulgarian Television and Bulgarian Radio lays down the principle that: "The President of the Republic, the Chairman of the Great National Assembly, the Prime Minister and state officials authorized by them are entitled to program time, which is given immediately on demand. The Chairman of the Committee for Radio and Television is also entitled to program time within the sphere of activities of the Committee. Spokesmen of political parties within the National Assembly have the right to demand program time no longer than five minutes". Similarly, Estonian Radio and Estonian Television are obliged to give broadcasting time for the broadcasting of announcements and officials statements of the Estonian Parliament and of the government. The Statue of Lithuanian Radio and Television says in Article 5 that deputies of the Supreme Council (Parliament), the leaders of the state institutions responsible to the Supreme Council and members of the government have a priority to use Lithuanian Radio and Television to discuss the questions within their competence. There is a special program, "Position of the Head of State", as there is in Poland, where the weekly show "Straight from the Belvedere" deals with the activities and policies of the President, reported on and explained by his closest aides.

These provisions, seen in the entire political context in which broadcasting in post-communist countries operates, must clearly be seen as signifying that the goal of participatory representative communicative democracy still remains in force - but has been redefined. What it seems to mean in practice today is not access, representation and participation in the operation of the media by society as a whole, but by the political class, the power elite which seeks direct involvement in, and influence upon, broadcasting policy and particularly the state/public broadcast media. While the situation is changing and gradual improvement is noticeable, it will take some time yet before the consequences of the immediate post-revolutionary period - when in most countries governments and the power structure considered broadcasting as their exclusive domain - are superseded by a different approach. However, because the main stress is on freedom rather than equality as the underlying value of public communication, access will largely be governed by market mechanisms.

THE DEVELOPMENT OF RIGHTS OF ACCESS TO BROADCASTING IN THE CZECH REPUBLIC AFTER 1989

by Milan Jakobec

The first important condition of the development of rights of access to broadcasting in post-communist countries is the transformation of the communist system of centralized monopolistic broadcaster to an open society system with media consisting of a plurality of independent broadcasters. The second condition is a society composed of active subjects who are able to express themselves in the media and who are equipped with suitable and necessary facilities for free expression.

I.   Transformation of the Public Media

The transformation of the communist broadcasting system started in post-communist countries with the transformation of monopolist totalitarian broadcasters. The broadcasters of the former communist propaganda, confronting the changed conditions of a post-totalitarian society had to be reshaped with the introduction of ideas of public access and public service.

Under the former regime, employees of the state broadcasting agency, together with communist party leaders were the only persons who were able to use the rights of access to broadcasting. For most of these individuals, this means more the abuse rather than the use of their rights.

The basic idea behind the Laws on Czech Television and the one on Czech Radio (the "Broadcasting Laws") passed by the Federal Parliament of Czechoslovakia in 1991 was the ideological transformation of institutions run by the state and entirely financed by the state budget into independent public institutions under public control by an independent council. The broadcast institutions would also be accountable to Parliament, financed through subscriber license fees and a variety of other diversified sources of revenue including commercial activity not at variance with the purpose of public broadcasting.

Under the 1991 Laws, the activity of public broadcasters is controlled by two independent councils - the Council of Czech Radio and the Council of Czech Television. Each council has 9 members elected by the Czech Parliament to be representatives of important regional, social, political and cultural streams. The term

165

A. Sajó (ed.), *Rights of Access to the Media*, 165-175.
© 1996 *Kluwer Law International. Printed in the Netherlands.*

of office is five years. Membership in either Council is incompatible with being the President, a member of Parliament, a member of the Government generally, or the head of a State administrative body. Furthermore, the council members must not be active members of a political party or act to the advantage of a political party. Additionally, council members may not be representatives of a broadcasting organization or represent commercial interests, that may influence the impartiality and objectivity of their decisions. Similarly, neither the council member nor his relatives may have a financial interest in any type of broadcasting entity.

As a matter of fact, the members of the contemporary broadcasting Councils in the Czech Republic were elected according to non-political principles influenced by President Havel's ideas of apolitical politics. Now that the political arena has become more politicized again, the idea of apolitical councils has been reconsidered in Parliament. This issue has arisen during the Parliamentary debates about the Councils' annual reports. The Councils are responsible to Parliament and may be dissolved by Parliament if Parliament issues more than one statement in a period of six months that the Czech Television or the Czech Radio is not fulfilling its legal mission.

According to the Broadcasting Laws, the mission of the public broadcaster is to service the citizens of the Czech Republic through the transmission of programs whose subject matter reflected the entire territory and population of the Republic. The Radio and Television Councils' own missions are to provide objective, verified, impartial and balanced information that allows for the free formation of opinions and permits the development of the cultural identity of the Czech nation and of the national and ethnic minorities living in the Czech Republic. They also aim to provide the public with ecological information, to foster the educational and moral development of children and minors, and to provide entertainment for the viewers and listeners.

The Councils have the legal authority or competence to appoint the directors of Czech Radio and Television, to approve the budget for both entities, to establish regional studios, and to decide about complaints which criticize the director of either public broadcaster.

The independent Councils as controlling mechanisms of the public are important tools of ensuring and implementing rights of public access to public broadcasting. From the beginning of their activities, they have tried to break the fortress of self indulgence and self satisfaction that existed among former state broadcasting agencies.

The threat to the proper functioning of the Councils as the tools of public access is political pressure from politicians who seek broadcasting access for themselves and their political parties, in the name of the public. This is a cheap and easy substitute for true public access.

II.   The Building of Media Pluralism After November 1989

The fundamental task faced by the State administration after November 1989 was the abolition of censorship and of the censor's office for mass media, known as the Federal Press and Information Office ("FUTI"), and securing pluralism of information in the mass media.

The simplest task was the abolition of FUTI by the Federal Minister of Information during the first weeks after the changes in November of 1989. But a legislative framework in the form of a law on mass media had first to be created to ensure pluralism of information and of the mass media. A new team at the Federal Ministry of Information and later the department of State Information Policy at the ČSFR government was entrusted to prepare the law. In view of the protracted legislation process it was evident that if the plurality of radio and television broadcasting was to be translated into political life as soon as possible essential steps would have to be taken prior to the adoption of the law on mass media.

The ČSFR government took these steps with its decision of June 11, 1990, setting up an inter-departmental commission for the selection of applicants for non-state radio and television broadcasting. The commission was headed by the deputy prime minster responsible for mass media.

II.1   Radio broadcasting

The decision of the ČSFR Prime Minister's Office of June 14, 1990, authorized nationwide medium-wave frequencies for Radio Free Europe. The decision of the

ČSFR government of October 18, 1990 permitted the technical facilities of the telecommunications system to be used by the BBC and Radio Free Europe.[1]

In an attempt to introduce the plurality of radio broadcasts as quickly as possible, the ČSFR government thereby gave its consent to the broadcasting of non-commercial news radio stations which in the days of totalitarianism used to have programs beamed to Czechoslovak territory from abroad, partly in Czech and partly in Slovak.

The inter-departmental commission of the ČSFR government, in agreement with the pertinent Czech government officials, set out to establish a dual broadcasting model by granting licenses to private radio stations. Prior to the license procedure the frequency possibilities for private broadcasting had to be mapped out in collaboration with the Federal Telecommunications Ministry and the radio communications administration. The Federal Telecommunications Ministry agreed to the utilization of the secondary frequency network for private broadcasting. These were frequencies with an output of 1 kW in the FM II band, which until then had been waiting for efficient utilization. These frequencies were suitable for local broadcasting with the prerequisite of successful international coordination.[2]

When Law No. 36/1991 on the dividing of jurisdiction in matters of the press and other information media came into force, the right to issue broadcast licenses in the Czech Republic was transferred in mid-April 1991 to the relevant governmental body of the Czech Republic. Radio broadcasting in the Republic continued to be de-monopolized by the inter-departmental commission of the Ministry of Culture, appointed and run by the Minister of Culture. The technical

---

[1] The BBC began to broadcast in the FM II band in 1990 and 1991 in Prague, Brno, Bratislava, České, Budějovice, Plzeň, Pardubice, Košice and Bánská Bystrica. The RFE/CTK radio station under the name of Radio Plus broadcasts on the FM 11 band in Prague alone.

[2] The easiest frequencies to coordinate were those for Prague, where, in view of the geographic position of the city, there was the least likelihood of interfering with frequencies used by neighbouring states. That is why on March 22, 1991, the inter-departmental commission was able to take the historic decision of issuing the first licenses for private broadcasting in Prague and its environs.

Licenses were awarded to the following radio stations: HALLO WORLD, RADIO I, BONTON, VOX, EUROPA 2, COLLEGIUM/INDEPENDENT AND RIO. The radio stations were required to respect 14 conditions in their experimental broadcasts, most of which coincided with the stipulations of the planned law on broadcasting. The program requirements and the restrictions on the broadcasting of commercials were based on the provisions of the European Convention on Transfrontier Television.

broadcasting conditions and the conditions for licenses awarded prior to the validity of the law on broadcasting remained the same as those who applied for licenses awarded by the new federal commission.[3]

Law No. 468/1991 on radio and television broadcasting which came into force in November 1991, created the regulatory framework for broadcasts by licensed radio stations, originally limited to 1992, was extended to the end of 1995.[4] The law also established the Federal Radio and Television Broadcasting Council as an independent body consisting of nine members elected by the Federal Assembly; it is similar to the British Independent Broadcasting Authority of the French *Conseil Superieur de l'Audiovisuel*.

In February 1992, the Czech National Council adopted Law No. 103/1992 on the establishment of a Radio and Television Broadcasting Council for the Czech Republic. When this law came into force the responsibility for all radio and television broadcasting matters was given to the Council which was entrusted to act as the state administration in this area and indirectly responsible to Parliament through its annual report to Parliament.

After the difficulties involved in establishing the Council and creating conditions for its activities, the Council continued to issue licenses for local radio stations realizing that the network of these stations created the backbone of modern plurality of a democratic mass media.

The goal of building a dual radio broadcasting system was accomplished when a license for nationwide radio broadcasting in the FM II band was given to the stations RADIO ALFA owned by the Kaskol company and the RG FREKVENCE I projected as a so-called family radio station. The successful Prague stations EUROPA I and RADIO GOLEM are the main shareholders of the latter station.

The legislative conditions for nationwide licensing were set out in Law No. 36/1993 on certain measures in radio and television broadcasting. This law divided

---

[3]   In the course of 1991, and in the first two months of 1992, the inter-departmental commission of the Ministry of Culture granted a further five licenses for broadcasting in Prague. The licenses were awarded to the following radio stations: GOLEM, INTERPRAGUE, BOHEMIA, KOBRA, AND HIFI-KLUB-VOA

[4]   In mid-1992, 42 operators altogether held radio broadcasting licenses in Czechoslovakia, of these 35 in the Czech Republic and 7 in the Slovak Republic. Two public broadcasting companies - the Czech Radio and the Czech Television - established by a law of the Czech National Council in November 1991 - existed at that time and as of March 1993 still existed in the Czech Republic.

the nationwide frequency networks among broadcasters in accordance with international agreements.

The Council issued licenses pursuant to the 1993 law in March 1993 and set forth license conditions that would prevent mutually destructive competition between the two private nationwide stations as well as prevent abuse of their dominant market position vis-a-vis local radio stations. Both private nationwide stations accepted these conditions which marked the beginning of the 180-day legal deadline for the commencement of their broadcasting (after receipt of a license).

After this, the Council continued to implement the dual pluralist broadcasting system by issuing further local and regional radio licenses and also planned to start dealing with the problem of cable broadcasting in March 1993.

When issuing licenses under the terms of the 1993 law, the Council takes into account the proportion of the applicant's own programs as part of its overall broadcasting, the share of Czech programing and, last but not least, the amount of the applicant's domestic and foreign capital. The grant commission of the Ministry of Culture used the same criteria when in 1992 it offered financial grants to radio stations with no foreign capital participation.

II.2   Television Broadcasting

With regard to creating a dual system of television broadcasting, the de-monopolization of television transmission was an incomparably more complicated task than breaking the monopoly in radio broadcasting. The expenses and investment associated with the inauguration of television broadcasting, and the size and long-term returns in television, made it impossible to start issuing television transmission licenses on the basis of a short-term experimental regime, as in the case of radio broadcasting.

Only a law that stipulated a binding framework can provide guarantees for television business enterprise. The law on radio and television broadcasting set out this regulatory framework and reserved the third television channel for license holders. This channel, however, reached only 30 percent of the population, but the Regional Administrative Radio Conferences' system sets forth the frequency capacities for allowing the channel to reach viewers nationwide.

The Federal Radio and Television Council attempted to grant a license to the two Republics (i.e, the Czech and the Slovak Republics) linked in a federation.

But this attempt was thwarted at the very outset by constitutional developments of devolution and the negative attitude of the representatives of the Slovak Republic to a joint private television channel. This may be one of the reasons for the very prompt issuance of a license for television broadcasting on channel T3 (analogous to the OK3 channel in the Czech Republic) to the M5 and the Ister companies in Slovakia during 1992.

The task to de-monopolize television broadcasting in the Czech Republic therefore fell to the Radio and Television Broadcasting Council, which shortly after its establishment, began to prepare licensing procedures, license conditions and the criteria to be applied to the projects of private television stations.

First, before the end of 1992, the Council issued a license to the PREMIERA TV company.[5] The issuance of this first television license in the Czech Republic had virtually no public response although from a commercial standpoint it covered an extremely attractive urban conglomeration. For the private regional station to have obtained this license was functionally equivalent to the nationwide license held by the public broadcasting system which, by law, reaches every corner of the land.

The competition for the third nationwide television channel set forth the following requirements for the applicants: screen high quality news programs during peak viewing time, support domestic production, ensure regional programs and reliable financial backing of the project.[6]

The breakup of the Federation of the Czech and Slovak Republics at the end of 1992 seriously affected the license procedure on the third television channel. The Law on Certain Measures in Radio and Television broadcasting, passed by the Czech National Council on December 22, 1992, decided that Czech Television should be the operator of a public channel, one of the two nationwide television channels to be named by the Radio and Television Broadcasting Council, and the

---

[5] The station had renowned film director Jiří Menzel as one of the leading owners. PREMIERA TV would broadcast throghout the Prague and Central Bohemian regions, reaching an audience of approximately 2.5 million. The company started broadcasting on Channel 24 in mid-1993.

[6] The competition was announced in November 1992 and also set forth criteria with regard to the technical capacities of the channel. December 3, 1992 was set as the deadline for submitting projects. By that date, 22 companies had submitted their projects.

third channel had to be allocated by 1995. License holders would be given the second nationwide channel.

During the television-licensing procedure, prior to the public hearing, the license procedure had to be reassessed to ensure its conformity with the law. All license applicants had to be informed that the competition was no longer for the third but for the *second* channel. New opportunities had to be created for those license applicants who did not intend to take part in the bid for the third channel, arguing that they were waiting for the privatization of the nationwide federal channel. The majority of the original 22 applicants confirmed their intention to take part in the competition for the second channel; a number of additional companies joined the competition, bringing the total number of applicants to 26.

The public hearing for the applicants took place between January 25-30, 1993 and the CET 21 television station (Central European Television for the 21st Century), was awarded a license for 12 years.[7] The victorious company accepted 31 license conditions concerning, above all, support for domestic television production and conformity with the Czech Constitution, the charter of fundamental rights and freedoms, legislation of the Republic and the standards of the Council of Europe and the European Community. The company must start its broadcasting in February 1994.

The license issuing procedure demonstrated that one single vacant nationwide channel can become a political issue in a society only beginning to discover the mechanisms of democracy. Political attacks against the Council and against the holders of the license questioned the legitimacy of the Council's decision and even of individual Council members who had been properly elected by the Czech Parliament. The independent Council used its independence during the license granting process and did not ensure the consent of the various political parties to its decision. After the issuance of the national television license to CET 21, the independence of the Council was reconsidered during Parliamentary debates and the withdrawal of the Council was expected during the May session of Parliament on the basis of the second rejection of its annual report by Parliament.

---

[7]   CET 21 is a company financed 70 percent by the Central European Development Company, an American-Canadian firm, and thirty percent by the Czech Savings Bank.

The campaign against the independent Council for Broadcasting presents additional proof of the tendency of post-communist states to prefer political party access to broadcasting to public access to the media, and the interests of the viewers.

The programing of the CET 21 private television channel is based on the idea of public access to broadcasting, with an emphasis on the news, current affairs programming, regular windows for sociological research, and direct access of viewers to broadcasting. The obligation of providing one hour in a month to public access programming is one of the 31 conditions imposed by Council on the license holder.

In spite of the private nature of CET 21's TV station project, it nonetheless fulfills the public service mission of television in democratic society in a manner comparable to public television. The standard of programs offered, the flexible reaction to the needs of the public. support for domestic programming, and the development of a market for programs made by independent producers were the main reasons for the success of CET 21 during the open tender for the license. Unfortunately, critical political parties and the majority of journalists are not interested in the quality of the project and the public service offered by private television. Instead, they are interested only in the question of who is behind it and who will be influencing the minds of television viewers for 12 years.

The first grant of a national television license to a private broadcaster in a post-communist country only stressed the vulnerability and fragile position of newly independent regulatory bodies and the necessity of such bodies' independence for the protection of the rights of public access to broadcasting.

The tendency to criticize the Council for its important decisions is expected to be the same in all post-communist countries. The criticism that leads to the rejection of the very idea of the independent, apolitical, regulatory body is very dangerous for future media space in post-totalitarian states. The concentration of the power to license private broadcasters in the hands of the government or a ministry once again is a step backward and away from democratic mechanisms in the field of media and it may lead to the total politicization of broadcasting. This would be contrary to the interests of viewers and listeners. The success of the idea of independent regulatory bodies in post-communist states is very important for further development of an open society and of public access to broadcasting.

III.   Public Access in Cable Networks

Broadcasting reform in post-communist countries is mostly based on a dual system of broadcasting composed of the public and the private broadcasters.

The third sector of broadcasting - university or community stations - has only a slight chance of being developed at present. People who could start this type of broadcasting usually have little financial resources and cannot afford to pay post and telephone and telegraph (i.e., "PTT") fees, copyright fees, and purchase expensive technical facilities, etc., in the way that private broadcasters can. New broadcasting laws hardly differentiate between a communal and a private station. Moreover, the possibilities to acquire financial support from a private foundation, a "town hall" or from other sources are very limited.

The chance for the development of the third sector of broadcasting is hidden within the licensing policy of the regulatory bodies who license multi-channel cable operators. The conditions imposed on cable operators may include a duty to develop communal channels for public access programming. Other conditions may include an obligation to provide a local community channel as well as an obligation to equip a studio to be at the disposal of the community. The cable operator might also have to pay for the staff needed to operate a studio, and the training of the public in use of the necessary broadcast equipment. The contribution to public access may be used as obligatory compensation for an exclusive area license issued to a cable operator. These conditions are known as "Robin Hood practices" because they force the cable operator to provide and finance community access to broadcasting facilities as a precondition to receiving an operating license.

The broadcasting laws valid in the Czech Republic took a first step toward to development of public access cable by stating that the operator of a cable distribution network shall reserve one channel for the meeds of a given geographic area (limited in scope) serviced by the cable network.

IV.   Conclusion

The right of access of the media as a legal provision is a necessary instrument of a democratic reform of broadcasting in post-communist countries, but it will remain only a nice-sounding sentence if the conditions for access are not created.

Such conditions involve:

1. The transformation of the public broadcasting sector to serve the public and to become an open institution of access;

2. The building of the private broadcasting sector on the basis of the idea of public service. Conditions or obligations of providing public access should be conditions of the granting of a license; and

3. The training of the public in how to use their rights of access and in how to use modern technical facilities. This can be accomplished through the use of Robin Hood taxes imposed on prosperous private broadcasters.

CHAPTER III

JUDICIAL REVIEW OF ACCESS TO THE MEDIA/NEW TRENDS IN ACCESS TO THE MEDIA

BEYOND THE VOICE AND INTENDED VIEW CONCEPTION OF SPEECH: EXPANDING THE FIRST AMENDMENT GOAL OF RICH PUBLIC DEBATE TO PROTECT A MULTIPLICITY OF DISCOURSES

by Ethan Klingsberg

I.   Introduction

The Supreme Court has adopted First Amendment aspirations that include related concepts like "widespread dissemination of information" and "rich public debate". The Court often subordinates such goals by openly pursuing the goal of protecting an individual's right to self-fulfillment through communication.[1] However, deference to the individual's right to self-fulfillment is not solely responsible for stunting the Court's development of "rich public debate". The Court's current, self-limiting articulation of "rich public debate" related goals is also responsible. This Paper examines how the Court can further develop the conception of how to attain an informative public debate.

The Court's perception of "rich public debate" is almost exclusively shaped by reference to two factors: the "source", "voice" or speaker and the "idea" or "view" that is trying to be said or signified.

The first Amendment ... was designed to "secure the widest possible dissemination of information from diverse and antagonistic sources" and "to assure unfettered interchange of *ideas* ..."[2]

---

[1]   See Fiss, *Free Speech and Social Structure*, 71 Iowa L. Rev. 1405 (1986).

[2]   *Buckley v. Valeo* 424 U.S. 1, 49 (1976) (per curiam) quoting from *New York Times Co. v. Sullivan* 376 U.S. 254, 266, 269 (1964) quoting from *Associated Press v. U.S.* 326 U.S. 1, 20 (1945) and *Roth v. U.S.* 354 U.S. 476, 484 (1957).

A. Sajó (ed.), Rights of Access to the Media, 177-203.
© 1996 Kluwer Law International. Printed in the Netherlands.

However, more than a speaker and an intended idea constitute a speech's "message", i.e., the informative contribution speech makes to debate. The messages of speech are intertwined with the discourse or the structural discipline by which the speech is communicated. A voice and the intended view are only two components of the discipline that shapes a communication. Other components of communicative discipline can be identified by examining the set of factors that make up the structure of the medium and content. For instance, the contribution of the speech of Mayor Ed Koch to public debate is a result of not only the ideas he intends to voice, but also the speaker's identity, the rhythm of the speech, and the metaphors utilized by the speaker. If all speakers were required to rely upon the same predominant metaphors, rhythmic patterns and other elements "that designate such matters as relevance, propriety, regularity, [and] conviction[3] as Mayor Koch then the spectrum of messages would be severely restricted even though all speakers could still intend to convey any viewpoint.

An example of the way a discourse can dominate intended ideas can be found in Professor Edward Said's analysis of the ways in which the imposition of the discourse of Western scholarship upon the cultures of the East severely restrained the informative contribution that Eastern culture could make to academia in West. Even though the Western scholars had access to primary sources in their study of the Orient, by running the intended ideas of the East through the filter of Western discourse, only Western "canons of truth" ended up being voiced.[4]

Communicative disciplines or discourses are able to define the message because they play a strategic role: a discipline tailored (often unintentionally or only subconsciously) so that certain messages can be effective. The strategies of many communicative disciplines overlap primarily in the necessity of certain minimum amounts of money. A conception of "rich public debate" limited by concentrating merely on protecting a spectrum of views trying to be signified by voices, has enabled the Court to avoid including in its First Amendment jurisprudence, the protection of other strategic factors that are essential to disciplines of communication.

The Court's limited "rich public debate" analysis leaves the definition of debate too simplistic, thereby result in a debate that is unnecessarily narrow. Under

---

[3]   E. Said, *The World, The Text, The Critic*, 216 (1983).

[4]   Id.; See also Said, *Orientalism*, (1978).

the current "voice and view" conception of "rich public debate", the Court is able to consider a speaker already to be within the debate without ever determining whether the speaker has access to many resources strategic to his message's communicative discipline. Thus, only a multiplicity of speakers and intended ideas - rather than a multiplicity of communicative disciplines or discourses - are protected.

This Paper lays out a framework for a First Amendment goal of "rich public debate" that is not so considered. Part II explains the significant difference between the worldly or information conveying potential of a debate characterized by a multiplicity of discourses. Then Part II assesses how to pursue the goal of a multiplicity of discourses and settles on a balancing test. In light of this balancing test, Part III critiques the way the Court has recently pursued rich public debate in holdings on rights of access. Part III dismisses the Court's embracement of the fairness doctrine in *Red Lion Broadcasting v. FCC* as inadequate for worldly public debate purposes. Then Part III reveals that more recent opinions on interference with corporate speech contain roots for a comprehensive outlook upon what makes a contribution meaningful to public debate. Finally, Part III explains how the future courts can utilize these roots to expand right of access jurisprudence. In Part IV, the potential future embracement of the realizations of Parts II and III on how to pursue the First Amendment goal of an informative public debate are shown to be endangered by recent developments in time, place and manner scrutiny. These developments are critiqued to reveal their incongruity with the protection of rich public debate. In addition, Part IV proposes ways for modifying these developments in time, place and manner scrutiny so that debate characterized by a multiplicity of discourses still has a chance of thriving.

II.   Towards Heterotopian First Amendment Goals

Expression within the American legal system - among lawyers in their professional capacities - is essentially a "utopian" enterprise with occasional "heterotopian" elements. Expression within the law is conducted in a relation to a common locus - i.e., all expression is incorporated into only one discourse, only one discipline. The result is a very comforting environment, because theoretically the discipline of communication within the legal system is able to recognize all the circumstantial or empirical knowledge that is necessary for the law to operate. The following passage from *Tar Baby* is an appropriate description of a debate with only one discourse:

> "He was satisfied with what he did know. Knowing more was inconvenient and frightening. Like a bucket of water with no bottom. If you know how to tread, bottomlessness need not concern you".[5]

Nevertheless, "in human history", as in *Tar Baby*,

> "There is always something beyond the reach of dominating systems, no matter how deeply they saturate ... and this is obviously what makes change possible, limits power ... and hobbles the theory of that power".[6]

Hence, realizations will seep into the law from other disciplines. For example, a judge will read an unratified, international bill of human rights or hear from a mother about the plights of large, poor, single parent families and will realize that something "curious" is happening in our legal system which confidently does not include adequate food and shelter within the concept "fundamental Rights"..[7] But in many instances our legal discourse is willing to settle for itself - its "utopian" or "no-place" characteristic - because turning towards certain discourses (including for many judges the discourse of unratified international human rights bills or the discourse of a poor, single, mother)[8] is just not considered "legitimate", even though these "illegitimate" modes of communication with their distinct disciplines might lead to an empirical or worldly realization that the American legal discourse has not perceived or does not reveal.

Often good reasons exist for this limit, upon the degree of heterotopianism ("of other places"), and hence circumstantiality, possible within juridical discourse. The most prominent justification is the burden society places upon the Law to be efficient and constructive. Without strict disciplining rules that enable lawyers to filter out certain discourses as illegitimate, the law could be overwhelmed with revelations of "curious" discontinuities within its discourse.

---

[5]   T. Morrison, *Tar Baby*, 242 (1981).

[6]   Said, supra note 3 at 246-47 (describing Foucault's sense of power through disciplines or discourses as a reason to believe in the possibility of change).

[7]   See *Dandridge v. Williams* 397 U.S. 471, 520, n.14 (1970) (Marshall, J. dissenting) (Through references to Universal Declaration of Human Rights and reality of Mrs. Williams's situation as mother of large, poor family, Justice Marshall questions the "curious" validity of majority's holding that no fundamental right is at stake in challenge to welfare grant limitation).

[8]   Id.

But the Law also has shown a tendency to extend this underlying "fear of ... the mass of spoken things, of everything that could possibly be violent, discontinuous, querulous, disordered even and perilous in ... discourse"[9] to the delineation of First Amendment goals. "Free speech" has historically been limited by fears of the potential babel that the protection of a multitude of discourses carries with it. John Milton's aspirations of "free speech" in pursuit of uncovering the "truth" did not let into the debate those discourses supposedly unworthy of divine truths.[10] And the more contemporary goal of "rich public debate" does not protect access to components of a discourse other than a source or speaker and the intention of signifying an idea.

Hence a "rich public debate" can take place under current First Amendment theory even though many positions strategic to certain discourses remain inaccessible to those discourses. For instance, in *Associated Press v. U.S.*, the Court claimed to be fulfilling the goal of the widest possible dissemination of information merely by assuring the participation of a large quantity of voices.[11] Even a monastery seeks a large quantity of voices. By analogy, if the informative potential of debate in a university is to be enriched, more than affirmative action admissions and hiring programs are needed; issues like textbook canon and rules of class discussion, teacher presentation, student writing and grading must be addressed.[12] Since the extreme pressures that justify restraining the potential heterotopianism of expression in jurisprudence (and perhaps in other government functions like the legislative process, to some extent the educational process[13] and maybe even the election

---

[9]   Foucault, The Discourse on Language in *The Archeology of Knowledge*, 229 (1972).

[10]   See Cole, *Agon at Agora: Creative Misreadings in the First Amendment Tradition*, 95 Yale L. J. 857, 876-77 (1986).

[11]   326 U.S. 1, 20 & n. (1945).

[12]   See forthcoming Note in Yale Law Journal by J. O'Brien or removing "orthodoxy" from schools.

[13]   See the debate on literary canon reform between literary critics like E.D. Hirsch, who insist upon maximizing the amount of information conveyed to students, and educators like Robert Scholes, who insist that the goal of dispensing information conflicts with the goal of teaching effectively, in *Salmagundi* (Fall, 1986). See infra on "purpose of forum" factor.

process[14]) are absent in routine public debate, the conception of rich public debate should be expanded to protect a multiplicity of discourses, rather than just a multiplicity of voices and views. As Circuit Judge Skelly Wright observed in his attempt to include attention to the significance of "what issues are to be discussed by whom and when" in assessing "discrimination against controversial speech" on television[15], the only result of having a variety of discourses emanating from the TV set, as opposed to just a variety of voiced views, would be to "unsettle" the continuity cherished by the apathetic viewer.[16]

The worldly revelation on the inherent discontinuity of a discourse which the authority of legal discourse often represses in the realm of jurisprudence, should be a goal of First Amendment theory in the realm of public debate. The First Amendment pursuit of the value of an informed society should aspire to a public debate that replicates experiences like that of the lawyer who realizes a discontinuity in the legal discourse upon immersing himself in an extra-legal discipline. This proposed First Amendment goal bears no relation to John Milton's designs to find a unified truth via public debate.[17] This Paper's First Amendment goal is to undercut the will to a unified truth respectively embodied by all discourse. Along with the appearance of discourses' discontinuities when distinct discourses can

---

[14]   In a recent address to Professor Fiss's "Free Speech" class, an expert on the West German political system referred to efforts by the Green Party to use an alternative discipline - no "foundations" - in expressing their message in the election process. The expert dismissed the efforts of the Green as counterproductive. Perhaps the political process could be changed to accommodate the discipline of the Greens. But the expert seemed to think that when in a well-defined and limited process like the West German elections, the Greens' desire to exercise their ideal discipline of a communication was silly. The counter argument to this sentiment is that no process is really "efficient" from a worldly perspective if certain discourses are intrinsically rendered counterproductive. See infra on "purpose of forum" factor.

[15]   See *CBS v. DNC*, 412 U.S. 94, 130 (1973) reversing 450 F.2d 642, 658; infra Part II-A.

[16]   *Business Executives Move For Peace v. FCC* 450 F.2d 642, 665-66; See also Marcuse, *Representative Tolerance* in A Critique of Pure Tolerance 98 (1969) (on how so-called "objectivity" of speaker can control message, e.g. by voicing news of murder in same tone as stock market report a distinct, unified message is conveyed despite "objective" treatment of different intended ideas).

[17]   See supra note 10.

flourish in the same community, there arises the affirmative prospect of new realizations by listeners who are exposed to different discourse.[18]

The pursuit of a debate characterized by a multiplicity of discourses requires involvement in the difficult task of assessing what composes a discourse in order to assure that a distinct discourse is able to flourish. The crux of such an assessment would be the identification of the resources strategic to the communicative discipline - i.e., what Michel Foucault calls "strategic positions".[19] Foucault compares communicative discipline to a military exercise: depending upon the nature of the military campaign (or discourse), certain unique and certain common positions are strategic.[20] Explaining the importance of Foucault's observations regarding the connections between discourse, access to strategic positions and messages ultimately conveyed, Professor Said writes:

> "Foucault's theories move criticism from a consideration of the signifier to a description of the signifier's place, a place rarely innocent, dismensionless, or without the affirmative authority of discursive discipline. ... Its (Foucault's 'strategic position' outlook) greatest value is that it awakens criticism to the recognition that a signifier is occupying a place, signifying in a place, is - rather than represents - an act of will with ascertainable political and intellectual consequences, and an act fulfilling a strategic desire to administer and comprehend a vast detailed field of material".[21]

Many factors control a discourse: the message is constituted not by just what idea is trying to be said (merely the declaration of war), but also the components of how the speech is conveyed (what weapons are fired, where and when). Moreover, the strategicness of these factors changes as the characteristics of listeners change with time and locale. If we lived in an ideal world, then the best way to pursue a heterotopian public debate would be to avoid having a third party structure what a

---

[18] As Paul de Man once wrote, the American view of modernism has always stressed the dark confused side of its nihilism - neglecting the aspect of Nietzsche's nihilism, for instance which was a revitalized sense of rational learning and a radically constitutive sense of human sciences.

[19] Said, supra note 3 at 221. See, e.g., Foucault's study of the strategic positions that make the discourse of punishment in the penal system able to work. Foucault, Discipline and Punish (1977).

[20] Foucault, *Questions on Geography*, (1976 interview) in Power/Knowledge 77 (1980).

[21] Said, supra note 3 at 220.

speaker needs for his discourse. Absolute protection of each speaker's autonomy would be the best way to assure that each speaker is able to contribute a unique discourse[22] to enlarge public debate's potential worldly revelations. The problem with this approach is that many disciplines share strategic resources that are scarce.

When two discourses (A & B) both require a limited resource (strategic position C), the resolution should be based upon the following balancing test: how strategic position C is to the discipline of Discourse A in comparison to any alternative positions strategic to Discourse A which infringe less upon other discourses' disciplines balanced against how strategic Position C is to Discourse B in comparison to any alternative positions strategic to Discourse B which infringe less upon other discourses' disciplines. Among the alternative positions that should be evaluated is the possibility of some short of sharing of position C so that both A and B can carry our their communicative disciplines.

A factor that should temper this balancing test would be consideration of the purpose of the debate. If the debate is merely to inform the public of general knowledge than a multiplicity of discourses should be pursued fully. But if the purpose of the forum is one in which efficient, constructive results are deemed necessary (such as a first grade classroom) then the degree of government interface to protect the potential multiplicity of discourses should be limited. Some judges might, however, perceive public debate to have a constructive purpose that requires as much protection as the legal profession from the potential Tower of Babel atmosphere fostered by a multiplicity of discourses. Such a conclusion would require an extremely conservative interpretation of the statement that public debate has "a structural role to play in securing and fostering our republican system of government.[23] The implementation of this "purpose" factor would be analogous to the Court's less than full-fledged pursuit of procedural due process standards in

---

[22]   "Liberty of the press is in peril as soon as the government tries to compel what is to go into a newspaper. A journal does not merely print observed facts the way a cow is photographed through a plateglass window. As soon as the facts are set in their context, you have interpretation and you have selection, and editorial selection opens the way to editorial suppression. Then how can the state force abstention from discrimination without dictating selection?"
Miami Herald Publishing Co. v. Tornillio, 418 U.S. 241, n. 24 (quoting from Chafee, Government and Mass Communications 633 (1947).

[23]   *Finzer v. Barry* 798 F.2d 1450, 1492 (Wald, C.J., dissentingt) (D.C. Cir. 1986) cert. granted 107 S.Ct. 1282 (1987) (challenge to statute prohibiting hostile demonstrations within 500 feet of an embassy).

deference to overriding pressure to fulfill a purpose like education[24] or giving out welfare money.[25]

The measurements necessary for the balancing test present dangerous possibilities for the First Amendment to be exploited to help some speakers and not others. To prevent the balancing test evaluation from being reified into the product of one discourse, its criteria will have to be frequently updated and its results subject to change. This problem could be potentially significant because, as Part II explains, the Law only perceives circumstantiality via a limited debate. To recognize the strategicness of position to various discourses, the Legal system will have to step outside of its own favored way of assessing strategicness. The law cannot evaluate what is strategic to a speaker's discourse with legal disciplining rules as a guide to what empowers speech.[26] Hence, this Paper's proposal presents a challenge to not only First Amendment theories of rich public debate but also the notion of law as a system which can act only upon the perceptions of one, severely limited discourse.

Perhaps the most prudent, if not the most courageous, route would be to advocate a ban on government interference; then at least certain discourses would be able to be conveyed in an uninhibited manner.[27] Part III shows, however, that the Court's recent rich public debate analysis demonstrates the confidence to undertake in a sophisticated manner the empirical examinations of communicative disciplines necessary for the proposed balancing test.

---

[24] *Goss v. Lopez* 419 U.S. 565 (1975) (purpose of education preserved in resolving what procedures are required by due process in school setting).

[25] *Mathews v. Eldridge* 424 U.S. 319 (1976) (even if procedural due process balancing test had come out in favor of extensive safeguards, these should not be implemented if they will cost so much that the purpose of the procedure - putting money in the hands of the poor - will be hindered).

[26] In addition to critiquing the Court's various analyses of what is necessary for speakers to contribute to informing public debate (See infra Part III), it would also be interesting to access what Courts consider necessary for a distinct voice to be heard in a courtroom: how the series of rights related to and restraints upon expression in a courtroom operate to protect and to restrict distinct discourses and messages.

[27] See supra note 22 quoting Chafee from *Miami Herald*.

III.   Implementing the Goal of Worldliness Through an Expansion of the
         Conception of Rich Public Debate.

A.   The *Red Lion - CBS v. DNC* Model of Rich Public Debate: Access to a
         Voice and Intended View

Red Lion Broadcasting v. FCC embodies the Supreme Court's limited vision of rich
public debate. Ironically this case which deserves praise for subordinating speaker
autonomy values to the goal of expanding public debate,[28] evidences the Court's
rejection of more recent efforts to expand further public debate's informative
potential. In *Red Lion* the Supreme Court "unhealed" the fairness doctrine because
"multiplying the voices and views presented to the public"[29] over the airwaves
would enhance the informative value of television. The conclusion reached by *Red
Lion* is faulty because it assumes (1) that access to the airwaves would be strategic
for the alternative speech and (2) that all that is needed to enrich the debate on
television is to grant an alternative point of view access to a voice.

        If access television time is not strategic to an alternative discourse then the
access will not enable that discourse to enrich debate. Granting an unnecessary or
highly inefficient right of access can only hinder the information conveying potential
of other discourses for which the use of the television airwaves is strategic. And if
television is a strategic resource for the alternative speech covered by the fairness
doctrine, then *Red Lion* fails to realize that access to more than just a voice might
be necessary if the fairness doctrine is truly to enrich debate and not just reinforce
the dominance of certain discourses on TV. Herbert Marcuse points out, for
example, that if the broadcasted alternative viewpoint is surrounded by particular
types of commercials, then the message of the alternative discourse becomes that of
the commercials.[30] Thus, the pursuit of "fairness" should include consideration of
contextual factors in addition to voice and view.

        The Court could have avoided the first fault by determining that for certain
discourses access to a segment of television time is absolutely essential and that little

---

28   See Fiss, supra note 1.

29   395 U.S. 367, 401 n.28.

30   Marcuse, supra note 16. Cf. Chafee, supra note 22.

interference with the ability of the broadcaster (*Red Lion*) to communicate is caused by granting this right of access. This exercise would have involved using the balancing test advocated in Part II. Instead, the Court appears to have upheld interference with a broadcaster's exclusive control of the airwaves merely because the idea of a "monopoly" by one speaker over a limited resource is repugnant per se. Actually, a monopoly by a speaker over a resource can benefit the goal of an informative public debate if the resource is only strategic to that autonomous speaker's discourse.[31]

The Court could have avoided the second fault by examining whether it takes more than access to voice and a view to remove the dominance over the airwaves of one discourse. In *CBS v. DNC*, the Court had an opportunity to remedy the second fault of *Red Lion*. *CBS v. DNC* presented the question of whether the First Amendment goal of an informed public debate leads to a requirement that broadcasters air the "special and separate mode of expression"[32] contained in editorial advertisements in addition to the *Red Lion*-fairness doctrine "all you need is a voice espousing a view" requirement for rich public debate. The *CBS v. DNC* Court answered the question by following the *Red Lion* view that as long as broadcaster "is required to present representative community views and voices",[33] the public debate is kept well-informed.

B.   How to Make Access Meaningful: The *PG&E* Analysis - Halfway There

In addition to the irony of *Red Lion* playing, in part, the role of the "obstacle" to worldly public debate, is the irony that a line of cases protecting the autonomy of corporate speech from government interference might end up serving as the precedent for a more expansive model of worldly public debate. After *CBS v. DNC*, the Court had a chance to further examine the protection of the societal interest in receiving information via public debate. This opportunity arose in rulings on challenges to the regulation of corporate and other types of speech to which no

---

[31]   See Part II-B.

[32]   412 U.S. at 130.

[33]   412 U.S. at 131.

individual speaker's right to self-fulfillment attaches. The Court's analysis in these cases can serve as an initial step towards a jurisprudence that recognizes the informational value of speech as the product of more than just a source and the intended idea.

If every aspect of a communication is viewed as an element of the discipline that shapes speech or its informational value to the public, then the best way to assure that the potential of a discourse's worldly insights will reach the public would be to permit one to speak without any forces restricting the possibilities of disciplines that one can employ. The Supreme Court's corporate speech holdings lean towards this connection between the potential for uninhibited conveyance of information to the public and the protection of speaker autonomy. Recent decisions, like *First National Bank of Boston v. Belloti*,[34] *Con Ed v. Public Service Comm'n of N.Y.*[35] and *Pacific Gas & Electric v. PUB of California*,[36] aspire to preserve the informational value of corporate speech to society by invalidating State regulations that might inhibit corporate speech.

Buckley v. Valeo is a seminal predecessor of these holdings that protect corporate speech's autonomy in adherence to the goal of enlarging the amount of information available to the public. *Buckley* invalidated a limitation upon campaign expenditures because the restrictions upon the use of money severely skewed the wealthy, politically active individual's communicative discipline. The determination that access to more than $1,000 was strategic to the discourse of the wealthy, political actor was a simple determination. Over the next decade the Court, in pursuit of protecting the informational value of public debate, further developed its confidence in analyzing how much regulations interference with a discourse.

These analyses of the effect of a regulation upon a corporation's speech are commendable because they recognize that whether the public will have access to the unique informational value of a corporation's discourse depends upon factors having to do with the means by which the speech is conveyed. The recognition that the informational value of a letter writer's discourse can be affected by an insert in the mailing envelope is a great step from the statement in *CBS v. DNC* that the

---

[34]   435 U.S. 765 (1978).

[35]   447 U.S. 530 (1980).

[36]   106 S. Ct. 903 (1986).

informational value of speech delivered over the airwaves depends only upon the chance to present "representative views and voices", regardless of contextual circumstances.

The most recent of these holdings, *PG&E*, is particularly praiseworthy because it is not just a *per se* holding that any regulation interferences with a corporation's discourse. The plurality and the dissenting Chief Justice deliver extensive critiques in pursuit of answering the "empirical question"[37] of how much interference with the information conveying potential of PG&E's discourse is caused by a third party's use of "extra space" in their billing envelopes. If the Court in *CBS v. DNC* had used the type of exhaustive analyses conducted in regard to the effects of the insert on *PG&E*'s speech, then the *CBS v. DNC* court would have found that the informational value of television speech depends on who speaks, when he or she speaks, what commercials surround the predestination and other circumstances essential to whether access to TV is strategic to discourse.

The problem with the Court's efforts to protect a well-informed public debate in the *Buckley* line of cases is that the empirical scrutiny of a regulation's effect upon a discourse's access to strategic positions is only applied to one discourse. A public debate that informs must consist of a multiplicity of effective discourses - a goal which requires balancing if there are mutual and scarce positions. In *Buckley* and its progeny, the Court merely assumes in footnotes that the regulations have no unique, strategic role for the communicative disciplines of the poor political speaker (in *Buckley*) and *TURN* - a private advocacy group - (in *PG&E*).[38]

The lack of fully developed discourse analyses of the speech of the poor political actor and *TURN* is due to the Court's decision to use *Red Lion - CBS v. DNC* "voice and view" analysis to test if these speakers are precluded from using a resource to contribute to the informational value of public debate. Thus, the positions at stake for the poor political speaker and *TURN* in *Buckley* and *PG&E*, respectively, were held to be insignificant to the information conveying potential of

---

[37]   106 S.Ct. at 919 (Rehnquist, C.J., dissenting).

[38]   106 S.Ct. 903,907 n.4, 908 n.6; 424 U.S. 1, 49-50 N.55.

public debate simply because the poor political speaker of *Buckley* could still speak, write or publish and *TURN* could still mail a letter.[39]

If interference with one speaker's communicative discipline (the wealthy political speaker or *PG&E*) fails to provide another discourse (that of the poor political actor or *TURN*) with a position strategic to the latter's communicative discipline which is unavailable through more isolated measures (i.e., measures that do not interfere with the purity of other discourses), then the regulation detracts from the goal of creating a more well-informed public. But after establishing that the $1,000 limitation statute has a severe effect upon the wealthy speaker's discourse, it is hypocritical for the Court to hold summarily that with or without the $1,000 limitation the poor speaker's ability to contribute to public debate is the same. Buckley attempts to make it appear as if the poor political speaker's discourse only depends upon being able to put forward a voice and a view the rich political speaker's discourse depends upon the additional factor of how much money can be spent on political speech. Similarly, the Court determines that *PG&E*'s speech is forwarded by a voice and a view remains uninhibited; yet, the *PG&E* Court simply assumes that *TURN*'s other opportunities to present voice and view via the mail are sufficient for *TURN*'s discourse to make a contribution to informing the public. The brief *Red Lion -CBS v. DNC* analysis of *TURN*'s discourse contains no analysis of the strategicness of the insert to *TURN*'s communicative discipline. The Chief Justice's dissent in *PG&E* is just as limited as the plurality opinion, because he also fails to analyze the importance of the insert to *TURN* and public debate. Without a two sided analysis followed by a comprehensive balancing, Rehnquist's conclusion that granting the right of access will enlarge public debate's informative potential is empty.[40]

There is no justification for assessing a regulation's effect upon the speech of *TURN* and speech of *PG&E* in different ways as neither speaker is of a category with inherent constitutional rights to self-fulfillment[41] and the effectiveness of both

---

[39]   106 S.Ct. 903,907 n.4, 908 n.6; 424 U.S. 1, 49-50 N.55.

[40]   106 S.Ct. at 921 (Rhenquist, C.J. dissenting).

[41]   This paper does not specify how the overcome cases like *Miami Herald* in which the Court's extreme deference to the autonomy of the regulated speaker is based not solely on the goal of informing the public, but also on an inherent right of a particular individual speaker to autonomy - i.e., a right to self-fulfillment. See also *CBS v. DNC*, 422 U.S. at 117-118 (noting that there is a significant distinction

discourses are equally important to the goal of a constructive and informative public debate. Updating *Red Lion - CBS v. DNC* analysis of speech's potential to inform debate to the perceptions of the analysis of *PG&E*'s discourse could be viewed as merely a scientific update by the Court and not a totally new First Amendment goal. The Part II balancing test already underlines the *Buckley* line. In *PG&E*, the Court analyzes the effect of the regulation on the information conveying potential of the speech for both *PG&E* and *TURN*. The only problem is that a different level of scrutiny is applied in assessing the weight of each side. Since the critique of PG&E's information conveying potential is more advanced, it should replace the use of the *Red Lion - CBS v. DNC* voice and view analysis to determine whether the First Amendment goal of an informative public debate requires some protection of what *TURN* and the poor speaker have at stake in *PG&E* and *Buckley*, respectively, as well as what both the broadcasters and the alternative speakers have at stake in *Red Lion* and *CBS v. DNC*.

C. Using *Wooley - Barnette* Sentiments to Temper the Expansion of the *Red Lion - CBS v. DNC* Analysis so that It Does Not Become a *PG&E* Analysis Is Like a Rabbi Applying Kashruth to the Main Course After Permitting Shrimp Cocktail as an Appetizer

One rationale for only applying a *Red Lion* "voice and view" analysis to test whether public debate is adequately informed by *DNC* and *TURN* is regarded for the First Amendment interest in not making a speaker serve as an instrument for alien speech. This value, enunciated in *West Virginia v. Barnette* and *Wooley v. Maynard*, is distinct from the right of an individual speaker to self-fulfillment. In *PG&E*, the Court explicitly recognized that no individual right to autonomy existed for a corporation - only listeners' rights to a robust debate were at stake; but, over the dissent of the Chief Justice, the plurality held that even a speaker without an

---

between First Amendment freedom of a newspaper editor and that of a broadcast licensee); *Red Lion*, 395 U.S. at 389-90 (same). Bringing about the demise of decisions based only on one's right to be free from government interface with one's quest for self-fulfillment through speech is left to Professor Owen Fiss. See Fiss, 71 Iowa L. Rev. at 1417 (arguing that government interference should be viewed as a way of preserving neglected speaker's autonomy or fulfillment right). This paper is merely intended to inform the Court's analysis when it is explicitly pursuing rich public debate.

inherent right to autonomous speech could be the beneficiary of protection from having to bear the burden of alien speech. Apparently, in deference to this *Wooley - Barnette* value, the Court decided to temper any trend towards expanding approval of rights of access by only sanctioning access where access to a voice and intended view was absent. Both *CBS v. DNC* and *PG&E* refer to sentiments embodied in *Wooley* and *Barnette* to support the decision not to find a right to access beyond the voice and view provided for in *Red Lion*.[42]

The problem with sticking to the *Red Lion* "bare bones" access approach via the *Wooley - Barnette* doctrine is that *Wooley* and *Barnette* indicate no tolerance for even the "voice and intended view" access requirement of *Red Lion*. *Barnette* contains no indication that, even though forcing the student to utter the pledge of allegiance is constitutionally repugnant, the government could still have required the student to facilitate a view merely representative of the pledge of allegiance. Similarly, under *Wooley* the New Hampshire driver was not permitted to remove the bold phrase, "Live free or die", from his license plate only still to be vulnerable to the possibility of being required to convey a view representative of the sentiments of the State motto. *Red Lion* strays dramatically from *Wooley* and *Barnette*, basing its holding on the premise, "There is no sanctuary in the First Amendment for unlimited private censorship".[43] This language sounds more like the Rehnquist dissent *Wooley*.

Red Lion is so different from *Wooley* and *Barnette* because of the presence in *Red Lion* of an informative public debate as a primary goal: in *Wooley* and *Barnette* this aspiration was not a factor.[44] Thus, the Court in *Red Lion* abandoned the *Wooley-Barnette* value of protecting a speaker from facilitating alien speech because the value of rich public debate was present. This was the only way that *Red Lion* could be decided because the two types of holdings are in direct conflict.

---

[42] The *CBS v. DNC* sentiments foreshadowed the Court's updated approval of *Barnette* which occurred a few years later in *Wooley*. In *CBS v. DNC*, a basic flaw the Supreme Court found in the Court of Appeals opinion was that the lower court "did not ... order that either BEM's or DNC's proposed announcements must be accepted by the broadcasters". 412 U.S. at 100. Thus, the Supreme Court held that the lower court decision would result in another party controlling the broadcaster's "journalistic judgment of priorities". 412 U.S. at 118-120.

[43] 395 U.S. at 392.

[44] See *Barnette* at 631 (utterance in question is solely a pledge of belief and not imparting knowledge). See also *Wooley* at 717 & n.14 (same).

The Court, however, has chosen to ignore this key aspect of the *Red Lion* holding. In *CBS v. DNC* and *PG&E,* both of which have rich public debate as the primary value at stake, the Court uses *Wooley-Barnette* interests as a basis for not expanding *Red Lion* and recognizing the possible legitimacy of a right of access to more than a voice and a view. If *Wooley* and *Barnette* are applicable, then even a voice and view access of *Red Lion* cannot be upheld. The Court's adherence to the limited "voice and view" analysis of an adequate contribution to public debate justified by deference to *Wooley* and *Barnette* is like a rabbi eating a shrimp cocktail appetizer but not a pork main course because of Kashruth. Perhaps, if the rabbi is started on a ship with only non-kosher food then his decision to eat the shrimp cocktail could be justified by pursuit of the value of health. However, the rabbi will soon realize that he or she must exempt more than the appetizer from Kashruth if he or she is to be healthy. Similarly, the Court should realize that to pursue effectively rich public debate, the *Wooley-Barnette* concerns must be cast aside in regard to more than the appetizer access of *Red Lion.*

The Court's willingness to leave open to *TURN*[45] and DNC the limited *Red Lion* voice and view access is incompatible with any recognition of the applicability of *Wooley-Barnette* interests to the Court's pursuit of rich public debate. Thus, *Wooley-Barnette* sentiments should not serve as a basis for failing to expand the *Red Lion* vision of what type of access is needed for an informative public debate unless the Court intends to abandon even *Red Lion.*[46] If *TURN* and *DNC* had been found to be in a need of *Red Lion* type access, it is difficult to see how the interference with *PG&E* and *CBS,* respectively, could have been tolerated with the sentiments of *Wooley* and *Barnette* being applied.

IV.   Reforming Developments in Time, Place and Manner Scrutiny which Threaten the Possibility of a Debate Characterized by a Multiplicity of Discourses

In addition to causing inconsistency in the Court's scrutiny of the effect of rights of access on public debate, the Court's application of the limited voice and view

---

[45]   106 S. Ct. 908 n.6.

[46]   See *Syracuse Peace Council.*

analysis of speech results in a dangerously deferential scrutiny of time, place and manner restrictions. Even if First Amendment jurisprudence recognized the legitimacy of private actions for rights of access to "strategic positions" based upon the balancing test proposed in Part I, the potential expansion of public debate could be hindered by deference to time, place and manner ordinances. Hence, it is important to also update the Court's time, place and manner jurisprudence so that worldly public debate goals are protected.

First Amendment precedent requires examination of three issues in accessing the legitimacy of time, place and manner rules: (1) Is a legitimate government interest being pursued? (2) Is the regulation content neutral? (3) Are adequate alternatives for expression still available? The neglect of the importance of a multiplicity of discourses to the informative potential of public debate manifested in the Court's recent examination of these factors could lead to a First Amendment that overlooks significant government imposed restraints upon the richness of public debate.

A.   **Government Interest: Aesthetic Aspects of Speech: From a Protected Component of Rich Public Debate to a Legitimate Government Interest. The Need for Re-instituting First Amendment Goals into the Assessment of the Legitimacy of Government Interests in Aesthetic Regulation**

Traditionally, the government interest prong of time, place and manner scrutiny could only be satisfied by what Justice Brennan calls "objective grounds"' like health, safety and national security.[47] In *Taxpayers for Vincent v. City of Los Angeles*, a majority of the Court for the first time announced that a restriction upon speech could legitimately be based solely upon the government interest in "proscribing intrusive and unpleasant formats of expression".[48] Earlier cases had found aesthetic values to be sufficient to invoke the police power,[49] but the First Amendment had only sanctioned regulations in pursuit of aesthetic concerns when

---

[47]   *Taxpayers for Vincent* 104 S. Ct 2118,2138 & n. 3 (Brennan, J. dissenting).

[48]   104 S. Ct at 2130.

[49]   *Berman v. Parker*, 348 U.S. 26, 32-33 (1954) (removal of blighted housing upheld).

the listener or viewer was a captive: "left practically helpless to escape" the intrusion of speech upon one's privacy.[50]

In 1971, the captive audience test was still whether the listener or viewer could avoid the offensive speech "simply by turning his eyes".[51] Thus, anywhere outside the home and the classroom seemed to be limits for aesthetically motivated restrictions upon speech. The First Amendment successfully eliminated any government interest in imposing an ordinance aimed exclusively at suppressing "verbal tumult, discord or even offensive utterance".[52] The Court justified his limitation upon government interests:

> "[W]e think it is largely because government officials cannot make principled distinctions in this area that the Constitution leaves matters of taste and style so largely to the individual".[53]

Furthermore, this outlook, articulated in *Cohen v. California*, is harmonious with the idea that discontinuity brought out by a multitude of discourses increases the worldliness of debate. "That the air may be filled with verbal cacophony" wrote the Court, "is not a sign of weakness but of strength"[54] *Cohen* was a great opinion for public debate goals; its reasoning includes recognition of the connection between the richness of public debate and aspects of the speech other then access to voice and an untended viewpoint.

However, *Cohen's* vision of a First Amendment that de-legitimizes government interests in intruding upon aspects of communication other than access to a voice and intended content was short-lived. It probably was *Cohen's* reference to preserving "*verbal* cacophony" that enabled the development of First Amendment scrutiny of government interests to skip over the realizations of *Cohen* and start

---

[50]   *Kovacs v. Cooper*, 336 U.S. 77 (1949).

[51]   *Cohen v. California* 403 U.S. 15,21 Cf. *Heffron v. Int'l Society for Krishna Consciousness*, 452 U.S. 640, 657 n.1 (1981) (not a captive audience if can say no upon being approached) (citing *Martin v. Struthers*, 319 U.S. 141, 143-44 (1943) (voiding ordinance prohibiting door to door distribution of advertisements).

[52]   *Cohen*, 403 U.S. at 24-5.

[53]   *Cohen*, 403 U.S. at 25.

[54]   *Cohen*, 403 U.S. at 24-5.

finding legitimate government interests in restricting the medium of expressing the message that has the adverse impact on the landscape".[55] The post-*Cohen*, aesthetic interest precedent appears to be based upon an expansion of captive audience doctrine reasoning. The Court's rationale in *Taxpayers for Vincent* is that one cannot just "reject it or accept it"[56] when looking at a small, temporary poster display. This is a substantial expansion of the earlier "captive" standard in *Cohen* which was based on one's prerogative to "avert the eyes".[57] The premise of *Cohen* that "we are often 'captives' outside the sanctuary of the home and subject to objectionable speech",[58] has been transposed into an argument in favor of expanding the captive audience doctrine and consequently the scope of legitimate government interests in aesthetic regulation of speech. Even a "verbal"-aesthetic regulation, like the one struck down in *Cohen*, would appear to be an exercise of a legitimate government interest under the First Amendment reasoning of *Vincent*.

The Court's expansion of the captive audience doctrine beyond one's home and classroom needs to be limited by a standard other than aesthetic taste. The same inherent difficulty that the Court found to exist in evaluating distinctions of "taste and style" in verbal usage in *Cohen*, also pertains to assessments of the "taste and style" of all components of expression. All speech is intrusive;[59] whether the intrusion is pleasant depends upon a listener's preferred discourse or appetite for exposure to other discourses.

A way to restrict an aesthetically based, captive audience doctrine is important because the value of a worldly public debate is at stake in *Taxpayers for Vincent*, as it was in *Cohen*. Professor Costonis describes the government interest

---

[55]   *Taxpayers for Vincent; Metromedia*, (plurality opinion) (billboards).

[56]   *Taxpayers for Vincent*, at 2131 (distinguishing *Schneider v. State*, 308 U.S. 147, 162 (no captive audience when a pamphlet being offered on street)).

[57]   But see, *Packer Corp. v. Utah*, 285 U.S. 105, 110 (1932) (Brandeis, J.) (on unavoidable thrust of a billboard display) (cited in *Erzoznik v. City of Jacksonville*, 422 U.S. 205,221,223 (Burger, C.J. dissenting)).

[58]   *Cohen*, 403 U.S. at 21 (citing *Rowan*, 397 U.S. 728 (1970) (upholding addressee's statutory right to stop one from mailing him offensive materials)).

[59]   See, e.g., *Erzoznik v. Jacksonville*, 422 U.S. 205, 218 (Douglas, J. concurring) (a puritan movie is likely to be just as intrusive on one's privacy as a movie with nudity).

in regulating outdoor aesthetics as an effort to protect "cultural stability - identity" values through the preservation of specific, "cherished associations".[60] Such a government interest can be direct conflict with the aspiration of enlarging the informative aspect of public debate. Although the preservation a cherished discourse is important to public debate, worldliness also springs from alternative discourses which reveal discontinuities in the stable vision by the "cherished associations" of a dominant discourse.

The Court explains that aesthetic regulations are a means of pursuing psychological and economic benefits[61]. But can the advancement of psychological serenity and economic stability for the adherents of certain discourses be an appropriate goal in First Amendment scrutiny of restrictions upon the public debate? The elevation of certain associations to a sacred, untouchable level, through limitations upon the range of expressive disciplines available, preserves the utopian[62] aspects of debate and restricts the development of alternative discourses.

The value of an informative public debate should play a more well-developed role in First Amendment analyses of the legitimacy of government interests in promulgating aesthetic regulations of speech. The "captive audience" evaluation of the legitimacy of the government interest in implementing aesthetic rules should reflect the balancing test of Part II. Courts should uphold aesthetic rules not in blind deference to the stylistic preferences of majorities, but in order to protect certain discourses from being drowned out or rendered unable to function. Shades of this use of the captive audience doctrine can be found in Justice Jackson's concurrence in *Kovacs v. Cooper,* an early explanation of the captive audience rationale in the context of upholding an ordinance on the operation of loud soundtracks. While the majority focuses on the need for the First Amendment to be sensitive "to claims by citizens to comfort and convenience",[63] Jackson asserts, that "freedom of speech for Kovacs [the owner of the sound truck] does not in my view

---

[60]   Costonis, *Law and Aesthetics: A Critique and Reformation of the Dilemma*, 80 Mich. L. Rev. 355,446 (cited in *Taxpayers for Vincent*, 104 S.Ct. at 2138 n.4. (Brennan, J. dissenting).

[61]   104 S.Ct at 2135-36.

[62]   See, Part II.

[63]   336 U.S. 77, 88.

include freedom to ... drown out the natural speech of others".[64] Under the balancing test of Part II, an aesthetic regulation against loudspeakers could be held valid because (1) the volume drowns out the opportunity for other discourses to function and (2) the volume is not strategic to any discourse or at least is a strategic element that can be replaced with less intrusive, equally strategic, available resources. Conversely, if the aesthetic regulation only presents an obstacle for certain discourses without protecting any discourse from being drowned out - i.e., the regulation only protects a cherished discourse from having to compete in a rich public debate - then a legitimate government interest is absent. Protecting a discourse from being drowned out or from being unable to function is different from protecting a discourse from being exposed as discontinuous in the presence of a multiplicity of discourses. Through the suggested assessment, the Court could synthesize the worldly public debate value embraced by the Court in its recognition of the affirmative quality of "cacophony" in *Cohen*, and the interest in preserving traditional discourses from being drowned out, aspired to by the advocates of aesthetic rules. The result would be that legitimate, aesthetic interests would be restricted to those that function to enhance the multiplicity of discourses in public debate.

B.   Content Neutrality: The Secondary Effect Doctrine and Rich Public Debate

The recent time, place and manner assessment by the Supreme Court in *City of Renton v. Playtime Theaters, Inc.* shows that the examination of the issue of content neutrality is also moving away from a regard for the aspiration of public debate characterized by a multiplicity of discourses. The municipal ordinance under scrutiny restricted the locations available to all theaters showing movies with certain content. The Court held that the regulation was content neutral because it was motivated by the "secondary effects" of the expression upon the "quality" of urban life.[65]

---

[64]   366 U.S. at 97 (Jackson, J. concurring).

[65]   106 S. Ct. 925, 929.

The Court failed to distinguish clearly a "secondary effect" from any other communicative effect that expression might have. In response to *Renton*, Circuit Judge Wald recently pondered whether any listener impact is a secondary effect?[66] What the *Renton* decision posits is that the effect of speech is not its content. But from the comprehensive content of the societal interest in an informative public debate, the content of speech is not just the ideas trying to be conveyed but the speech's ability to function as a discourse that can affect listeners.

Ironically, in the opinion preceding *Renton* the Court held that the placement of an insert into a PG&E billing envelope is an act directed at the content of the PG&E speech. This is a more perceptive assessment of what constitutes content. Even though the regulation was only aimed at the "effect" of presenting PG&E's speech without the speech of TURN, the Court realized that the content of PG&E's speech is tied to any rule that modifies PG&E's communicative discipline and consequently the speech's communicative impact or effect.[67]

What is most disturbing about the expansive "secondary effect" doctrine of Renton is that in the near future the Court will probably try to distinguish further a "secondary effect" of speech from content. The Court will strain to explain that a "secondary effect" doctrine is not anathema to the information conveying potential of speech, because the "secondary effect" doctrine is not aimed at what the listener learns or perceives from an expression. Rather, this doctrine is aimed only at what happens next. Efforts to regulate deviance from traditional lifestyle, which is essentially the asserted "secondary effect" of the adult films in *Renton*, would seem more worthy of heightened content scrutiny[68] than a regulation aimed solely at the information that the film is conveying. After all, if the revelations of an expression are so powerful that they result in not only new realizations, but also marked

---

[66]   *Finzer v. Barry*, 798 F.2d 1450,

[67]   But this was the only half the story in *PG&E*. See supra Part III for how the Court managed to ignore this realization in its analysis of the regulation's effect upon other discourses, thereby leaving the connection between the holding and the pursuit of rich public debate not fully established.Even though an ordinance is content based, if it can be justified under the Part II balancing test then it should be permissible. Thus, in *Renton* a court would plug into the test the discourse of the adult theaters and the discourses supposedly threatened by the presence of the theaters.

[68]   For an explanation of the dramatic difference in results of content neutral scrutiny see Stone, Content-Neutral Restrictions 54 U.Chic. L. Rev. 46 (1987).

200

changes in adult lifestyles, then it is in the interest of an informed society to have this speech expressed unless the effects are dangerous, clear and present.

C.   Adequate Alternatives: Another Unnecessarily Limited Analysis

The Court's critiques of whether time, place and manner regulations leave open adequate alternatives for expression also fail to attempt to protect a multiplicity of discourses. A full analysis to determine whether a distinct communicative discipline will be able to function after the enforcement of a time, place and manner regulation can be difficult. Hence, an insistence by the Court that an adequate alternative simply consists of an opportunity for the speaker to voice his intended ideas might seem reasonable.

Yet, often the facts of whether an alternative is adequate in terms of discourse analysis, rather then voice and view analysis, are so obvious and within the Court's reach that the route of ignorance chosen by The Court cannot be justified. In *City of Renton v. Playtime Theaters, Inc.*, the district court found and the appellate court affirmed that in general there are no commercially viable adult theater sites within the 520 acres left open [to adult theaters] by the Renton ordinance.[69] But the Court chose to ignore "commercial viability" as a factor worth considering in its adequate alternative critique, because it reasoned that the economics of real estate problems do not pertain to any First Amendment concerns.[70] Certainly if a theater cannot be "commercially viable" in the alternative sites left open, the communicative discipline will not be able to function.

Moreover, if the City of Renton were required to subsidize the Playtime Theaters so that it could survive economically in a more remote location, then the discourse of Playtime still might not be able to function. A proper discourse analysis should extend beyond an analysis of the economic effect on the speaker of a mandated change in a component of his discourse. Only by evaluating the strategicness of the new position in communicative discipline terms can the adequacy of the alternative for the listeners or public debate be determined. Thus, the "commercial viability" finding should be used as an indication that Playtime is no

[69]   106 S.Ct. at 932.

[70]   106 S.Ct. at 932.

longer able to speak from a "strategic position" not only in economic terms but more importantly in discourse analysis terms.

The Court also overlooked easy facts pertinent to the adequacy of alternatives in *Clark v. Community for Creative Non-Violence*. The disputed regulation in *Clark* prohibited sleeping in the park across from the White House. In the Court of Appeals, Circuit Judge Edwards explained in his concurrence:

> "The appellants have stated, numerous times, that sleeping is necessary to attract demonstrators and capture media attention. But there is more to it than that, for in this case sleeping itself may express the message that these persons are homeless and so have nowhere else to go".[71]

In short, access to sleeping in the park was a strategic aspect of the discourse of the Community for Creative Non-Violence. But the Supreme Court, as well as Circuit Judge Edwards, never apply this realization to the adequacy of alternatives critique. For Edwards, this factor is only important in establishing at the outset of the opinion that the act of sleeping is speech. But if Edwards perceives sleeping as an important component of the Community's speech, how can the absence of this component not be an important factor in assessing the adequacy of alternatives?

The Supreme Court avoids blatantly assessing the speech of the Community in two inconsistent modes by conveniently assuming *arguendo* that sleeping is speech. The Court thereby avoids any elaboration in the beginning of the opinion upon the strategic position that sleeping occupies in the Community's discourse. Then when it comes time for the adequacy of alternatives issue, the Court observes that with or without access to sleep, the Community can still, in some manner, voice their intended view; hence, for the Supreme Court, the regulation presents no "barrier to delivering to the media or to the public by other means, the intended message concerning the plight of the homeless".[72] When knowledge of the effect of time, place and manner restrictions, upon a discourse's strategic position is available, the Court should consider this knowledge in its evaluation of the adequacy of the alternative positions.

---

[71]   703 F.2d 586, 601 (D.C.Cir. 1983) (Edwards, J. concurring); See also 468 U.S. 288 (Marshall, J. dissenting).

[72]   468 U.S. at 295.

V.   Conclusion

A First Amendment goal of materiality or worldliness is in many ways pessimistic. This Paper's goal is premised upon the theoretical impossibility of any single discourse or set of discourses ever bringing debate to a final Truth. After accepting that all discourses are to some extent discontinuous (because all disciplining rules of expression are violence committed upon the things of the world), then affirmative steps can be taken towards what Foucaoult calls "exteriority": avoidance of permitting debate to become burrowed within one core discourse by looking instead to the limits of each discourse.[73] A debate can only reveal these limits if a multiplicity of discourses flourishes. For many listeners it is much more rewarding to be in a "will to truth" debate in which the worldly revelations of all speech can be easily classified as "in error" or "correct"; but only by enabling the "monsters" of speech - the voices that one discourse labels as neither right nor wrong because they are operating within a different discourse - have a chance will the debate be potentially informative in a more authentic sense.

If this Paper's model of rich public debate is ever to have a chance of endorsement by the Courts, then the Courts must be willing to subordinate values of speaker autonomy to the societal interest in receiving information. As the Court in the *Buckley* line of cases realizes, there is a place for autonomy in promotion of the value of an informed society. It is time for the Court to build upon the sophisticated discourse analysis that enables one to realize the potential place for autonomy in the pursuit of informative public debate goals. The same reasoning that reveals the importance of speaker autonomy to rich public debate can also reveal the importance to the rich public debate of granting rights of access in certain situations. The implementation of a balancing test based upon evaluations of degrees of interference with discourses' strategic position is necessary to identify those situations in which rights of access will enrich public debate. If the proposed balancing test is to serve as an instrument for enhancing the multiplicity of discourses able to thrive in public debate then the assessments of strategicness by the courts must extend beyond the perceptions of a single, legally favoured, "legitimate" discourse. Furthermore, the realization that a discipline, rather than a voice and

---

[73]   Foucault, supra note 9 at 229.

intended view, composes speech's informative contribution should signal the Court to modify recent trends in time, place and manner scrutiny so that a multiplicity of discourses can be protected.

THE NEW TYPES OF MEDIA AND THE STATE
OR THE END OF LIBERALISM

by Gábor Halmai

I.   Introduction

The expression of opinion and thought has existed as long as mankind has existed. But, because of the lack of the means of dissemination, different opinions and thoughts have not been able to reach their possible public, the *Öffentlichkeit* (the public sphere). Indisputably, the first important step towards the emergence of publicity was the invention of book printing at the beginning of the new age. This was the beginning of differentiation within the communicative media, which greatly facilitated the circulation the information within society.

The next important milestone was the emergence of political publicity starting in the middle of 18th century, a process mainly characterized by the growing importance of the press (print media). In this period the main concern of legislative activity with respect to freedom of expression was not the freedom of individual expression but the freedom of the press. This meant that the freedom of expression was represented by those who participated in the process of forming political opinion and were endowed with the necessary cultural assets, and who were willing and able to conduct political discussions. The determinative ideology of the era itself, liberalism, was not disposed to the opening of discussion for the whole public.

However, approximately in the middle of our century, the era that was dominated by the press (print media) came to an end, due to the spread of the of electronic media. This resulted in the almost unlimited extension of publicity. From this time on, publicity has not been the domain of just a relatively small group of educated and socially active people. The involvement of the masses in the public sphere by the means of the media brought about two important consequences.

On the one hand, the circle of the people participating in, or, at least, witnessing the political process was significantly extended. Ongoing politics became observed by whole nations or sometimes by the whole world. We can recall the events of the 1989 Romanian revolution, of the 1990 Gulf war, or of the August Putsch in Moscow in 1993, which television brought into our homes. Another main change initiated by the appearance of new types of the media is that publicity lost its almost exclusively political character and became a domain of the arts, sciences

A. Sajó (ed.), *Rights of Access to the Media*, 205-223.
© 1996 *Kluwer Law International. Printed in the Netherlands.*

etc., a means of the expression of the existing opinions and thoughts in these fields. As a result of this change which has been brought about by the appearance of new types of the media, new examples of constitutional regulation extend beyond conventional freedom of the press and include the subjective elements of individual self expression, and the objective elements of freedom of the radio and television broadcasting as well. Of course, the American and European legal systems have been affected differently by the emergence of new types of the media.

II.   The First Amendment and the Jurisprudence of the United States Supreme Court

II.1   Freedom of press versus freedom of individuals

In the legal system of the United States these changes can be detected as modifications in the jurisprudence of the courts instead of changes in the stable and very laconic regulation at the constitutional level. At this point a question arises whether the seemingly specific legal status of the print and electronic media in comparison with the individual freedom of speech stems from the public functions of the former. There is another question closely related to this. Namely, to what extent is government obliged (and able) to provide for the optimal functioning of John Stuart Mill's "market place of ideas" - using legal and institutional means in order to ensure the equal opportunity of expression of different opinions and thoughts in the media, and thus guaranteeing balanced information for the public. To put this dilemma another way: can the privileged position of institutions of mass information be justified or not?

The decisions of the United States Supreme Court (the "Supreme Court") to date have presupposed the equivalence of individual and institutional rights concerning the First Amendment of the United States Constitution. According to this, the rights of journalists or broadcasters in the field of the print and electronic media do not exceed the freedoms of private persons. According to a 1972 decision of the Supreme Court, "[t]he First Amendment does not provide for the press the constitutional right of any specific access to information which is not accessible to the public generally".[1]

---

[1]   *Branzburg vs. Hayes*, 408 U.S. 665, 684 (1972).

In general, this direction was followed in the decisions of the Supreme Court in the later period. For example in 1978, the Court declared that neither the public nor the press have the right to visit prison. Nevertheless, the Supreme Court concluded, if legislation had provided this right, such legislation should not differentiate between private persons and the press. According to this decision: "neither the First Amendment nor the Fourteenth guarantee the access to that governmental information or sources of information which are under the control of the government" because the Constitution, "does not compel the government to provide the media on their request with information or to provide the access to the information".[2]

Two justices of the Supreme Court, however, forcefully defended the so called structural, institutional interpretation of the "free speech" proviso of the First Amendment. These minority opinions have not left the jurisprudence of the Supreme Court unaffected. According to Justice Potter Stewart, a member of the Supreme Court between 1958 and 1981:

> "[T]he guarantee of the free press is a structural prescription of the Constitution. The most of the other provisions of the Bill of Rights protect the specific freedoms and rights of the individual. The proviso of freedom of the speech has its protective effect on an institution. The reason for giving constitutional guarantee to the free press was the establishment of the fourth institution which is an additional check on the three branches of power. The proper metaphor is the fourth power. So the First Amendment is protecting the institutional autonomy of the press".[3]

A similar opinion was expressed by Justice Brennan who for three decades, until the beginning of the 1990's, was the decisive liberal personality of the Court. Justice Brennan stated: "There are two specific models of the press in our society... The traditional 'free speech' model referring to the First Amendment excludes any interference with the freedom of the expression of the opinion. The second model is of structural character. This follows from the communicative function of the press. . . The 'structural' model significantly extends the constitutional protection

---

[2]   *Houchins v. KQED*, 438 U.S. 1, 9ff. (1978).

[3]   See Justice Potter Stewart, 26 Hast. L J. 631, 633 ff. (1975). It is a matter of course that the concept of the fourth branch of power cannot be interpreted as a constitutional category, because the press in the contrary to the three branches of Montesquieu is not an institution of public power, so its function in the structure of power can be interpreted within the system of the categories of the political science.

of the press. The press deserves protection not only when it is stating something, but when it performs those tasks which are important concerning the collection and circulation of the news." If somebody prefers this structural, institutional model of the freedom of the press, Brennan continues, "the range of extension of the protection is unlimited. Every kind of restriction affects in some extent the capability of the press to fulfill its protected duties."[4] Brennan clearly points to the consequence of this model, i.e, that in this structural-institutional model of the freedom of the press in the last resort the public is regarded as a subject of the guarantee of the dissemination of information.

Thus, for Justices Brennan and Stewart the objective function of freedom of the press is more important than the right of an individual against the state. However, the mingling of these two models of the freedom of the press has been criticized several times, even by the camp of liberal legal philosophers who otherwise highly regard the achievements of Justice Brennan. Ronald Dworkin in his book, *A Matter of Principle*, which appeared in 1985, regards the simultaneous use of these two models as a threat to the traditional conception of freedom as a basic right.[5] Dworkin in an article published in 1992, repeated his criticism in connection with Brennan. Brennan wrote the majority opinion in the case of *New York Times v. Sullivan*. According to a critique offered by Dworkin, Justice Brennan, almost exclusively, emphasizes the instrumental character of freedom of speech, and bases its justification on the advantageous social consequences of freedom of expression. Doworkin also states that Brennan almost completely fails to discuss the moral right of the individual to say what he wants.[6]

In spite of that fact that it is not uniform, American legal jurisprudence tends not to establish a privileged position for the press. The Supreme Court in a 1937 decision did not detect a threat to the freedom of the press when regulations concerning collective labor contracts were applied to press companies, saying: "a publisher of a paper has no exemption from the general application of the law. He has no privilege entitling him to offend other people's rights and freedoms. He is

---

[4]   Justice Brennan, 32 Rutgers L. Rev. 175-177 (1979).

[5]   See Ronald Dworkin, *Is the Press Losing the First Amendment?*, 381, *in* A Matter of Principle (1985).

[6]   See Ronald Dworkin, *The Coming Battles over Free Speech*, N.Y. Rev. of Books, June 11, 1992, at 57.

responsible for the slander...".[7] In the case of *Branzburg v. Hayes*, the Supreme Court held that journalists had no constitutionally guaranteed right in a criminal proceeding in front of the jury to refuse to give testimony in order to protect their information and sources of information, provided that the information sought by the jury is relevant to the proceeding itself. At the same time, the Supreme Court left open the possibility that states could proceed further in the regulation of this issue. By 1983, 25 states gave journalists the right to refuse to testify in order to protect their confidential sources of information. Under a 1978 decision, courts have the power, within the confines of the Fourth Amendment, to order the search of a media organization's offices, and to order the seizure evidence.[8]

With regard to the issue of publicity of criminal proceedings, The Supreme Court, in a 1979 decision, *Gannett v. DePasquale*, held that the public and the press may be excluded from a preliminary court procedure if this step is necessary to ensure the right of a defendant to the due process guaranteed under the Sixth Amendment.[9] Nevertheless, seven years later, in *Press Enterprises v. Superior Court*, the Court permitted normal publicity during the preliminary phases of a case without explicitly reversing their previous decision.[10] Finally, in a third decision handed down between the two mentioned above it is very difficult to interpret the position of the justices. In *Richmond Newspapers v. Virginia* the Court held that both the public and the press have a right (are entitled) to publicize a trial (so there is no privilege for the press), and this right can be restricted only in extraordinary cases because the press functions as a "representative of the public" implying that there is a privilege.[11]

---

[7]   *Associated Press v. N.L.R.B.*, 301 U.S. 103, 132 (1937).

[8]   *Zurcher v. Stanford Daily*, 436 U.S. 547 (1978).

[9]   *Gannet Co. v. De Pasquale*, 443 U.S. 368(1979).

[10]   *Press-Enterprise Co. v. Superior Court*, 106 S.Ct. 2735 (1986).

[11]   *Richmond Newspapers. Inc. v. Virginia*, 448 U.S. 555 (1980).

II.2   Legal regulation of mass media

The issue of the privileged (or not privileged) position of the press is closely related to the question of the extent government can proceed in the legal regulation of mass media, and to what extent this legal regulation can differ from the rules applied with regard to individual expression of opinion. In relation to the general rules of the freedom of speech, the precedents of the Supreme Court on this issue declare every kind of discrimination as running contrary to the spirit of the First Amendment.

At best, only some positive discrimination in favor of socially and economically weak groups is admissible, but the infringement of the rights of economically strong people is not allowed.[12] At the same time, a legislator can take into consideration and can ensure to some extent the equality of the opportunities of the different strata in the society. The Justices of the Supreme Court explain this by referring to the fact that the freedom of the mass media is not an original right included in the First Amendment but only derived from it, and this circumstance leaves some room for the legislator to factor in specific considerations.

Such specific considerations have been taken into account in the area of the commercial radio broadcasting, which was commenced after the First World War, first by the Radio Act of 1927, then by the 1934 Communications Act (which is in force now) mainly by establishing the Federal Communications Commission (the "FCC"). The Supreme Court legitimized the distribution of the frequencies (first of radio then of television) by the FCC in which the FCC unavoidably takes into consideration the motives of the television or radio report saying: "this regulation is of vital necessity as the control of the traffic because of the development of the cars".[13] At the same time, the justices left no doubt that in the field of the press a licensing system similar to this would be unconstitutional.[14]

However, the number of the radio stations in the United States is considerably higher than the number of daily papers, so it seems that scarcity of the frequencies is technically resolvable. Thus, the relevant differences between the electronic and print media from the point of view of state regulation now seems to

---

[12]   *Buckley vs. Valeo*, 424 U.S. 1 (1976).

[13]   *National Broadcasting Co. v. U.S.*, 319 U.S.190, 213 (1943).

[14]   Cf. *Near v. Minnesota*, 283 U.S. 697 (1931); *New York Times Co. v. U.S.*, 403 U.S.713 (1971).

be fading. Nevertheless, the Justices of the Supreme Court still adhere to the position that the right of the individual to have acces to radio and television broadcasting should be deducted from the original right of the public to balanced and fair information in public matters: "the right of a listener or a viewer has priority, not the right of the broadcasting company".[15] This privileged right of the public includes receiving information on social, political, aesthetic, moral and other opinions. Because of this, the Court argues, the state cannot tolerate the monopolization of the broadcasting market by the government or by a private licensed broadcaster.[16]

This argument can justify the application of some content criteria in the process of the awarding broadcasting licenses.[17] The most well-known of these criteria is the so called *fairness-doctrine*, which on one hand prescribes the dedication of some portion of broadcasting time to public purposes and on the other hand prescribes fairness regarding public debates. This means giving the opportunity for each side to publicize its opinion. The side which has not been treated fairly has the right to respond, similarly to an election candidate who has been turned away by a broadcasting company in favor of other candidates. At the same time, the Supreme Court declared a regulation concerning the printed media unconstitutional which prescribed a right of a political candidate who has been criticized to respond (this is also known as a right of reply).[18] Similarly, according to the Communications Act, if a radio station provides broadcasting time for a candidate, it should proceed similarly concerning the other candidates. An additional rule for the electronic media is that the restriction of obscene and indelicate programming in electronic media is easier than in print media.[19] The provision that a broadcaster must dedicate at least one hour of broadcasting time for the presentation of local issues is also one of the preconditions for receiving a broadcasting license.

---

[15]   *Red Lion Broadcasting Co. v. F.C.C.*, 395 U.S. 367, 386 (1969) (emphasis supplied).

[16]   Id. at 390.

[17]   Licenses are valid for a radio station for five years, for a TV station seven years and can be prolonged.

[18]   *Miami Herald Publishing Co. v. Tornillo*, 418 U.S. 241 (1975).

[19]   *F.C.C. v. Pacifica Foundation*, 438 U.S. 726 (1978).

It is a very interesting fact that while the technical progress did not affect the opinion of the Supreme Court, the FCC itself initiated the abandonment of the fairness-doctrine, arguing that market competition would reliably ensure the exchange of thoughts and opinions.[20] Nevertheless, the Supreme Court insists on the importance of differentiating between print and electronic media: The daily papers have the right to inform the public one-sidedly or to limit themselves to non-political issues only, but a radio or a television station should at the same time endeavor "to find a balance between the way it would act as a private enterprise and it would act as a representative of the public".[21] One further argument in favor of the special requirements for radio and television stations is their characteristic of being "unstoppable", which similarly to the "captive audience" of the traditional freedom of the speech argument, legitimates a more strong state intervention.[22]

To summarize and to a certain extent simplify American Constitutional jurisprudence concerning the new types of media, one can say that it the Supreme Court has attempted to use legal methods in order to enforce the requirements of enlarged social publicity (*Öffentlichkeit*). However, concerning the rights due to the new forms of media, generally the media has been denied a privileged status.

III.   The *Grundegesetz* and the Jurisprudence of Karlsruhe

In European legal systems not only the changing legal stance of the constitutional courts but the constitutional provisions themselves indicate the presence of new media. The first new constitution containing new elements of freedom of the expression was the 1949 Bonn *Grundgesetz* of the Federal Republic of Germany which put an end to its national-socialist past. The fifth article of this document regulates the traditional freedom of opinion, the freedom of information, of press,

---

[20]   Cf. *General Fairness Doctrine Obligation of Broadcast Licensees*, 102 F.C.C.2d. 143 (1985).

[21]   *Columbia Broadcasting System, Inc. v. Democratic National Committee*, 412 U.S. 94, 117 (1973). We should note that this distinction was made not between private- and state-owned radio and television stations, since the last category in the United States is nonexistent.

[22]   *F.C.C. v. Pacifica Foundation*, 438 U.S. 726, 748 (1978).

of art, of science of research, and of teaching. This article also deals with the possibilities of restricting some forms of the expression of opinion.

The first observations on the *Grundgesetz* were made from the traditional liberal point of view interpreting these rights exclusively as fundamental rights of an individual who is entitled to free development of his or her personality.[23] In this respect, these comments do not differ from the comments made about Article 118 of the Constitution of the Weimar Republic.[24] However, in legal literature, the emphasis on the institutional elements of freedom of expression soon appeared, encompassing the areas of both the print and electronic media. Some constitutional legal experts interpret the Fifth Article of the Grundgesetz as an institutional guarantee, others emphasize the mingling of individual and institutional elements.[25]

The legal opinions of the Federal Constitutional Court from the second half of the 1950's onward, connected the freedom of expression with the free democratic order put down in the *Grundgesetz*. The famous *Lüth* decision declared freedom of expression, following the 1789 French Declaration, as one of the basic human rights which is necessary "for the free democratic order of the state as an explicitly constitutive element because only this will make possible the permanent intellectual debate, the free struggle of opinions essential for the free democratic order".[26] Three years later, a decision of the German Constitutional Court (the "Constitutional Court") identified print media, radio and television as the main means of open discussion on public affairs and of the emerging publicity, resulting from this. The decision deduced from this premise the special protection of freedom of the press as *a basic right*.[27] This opinion has been embodied in the jurisprudence of the Constitutional Court as several decisions of the Court demonstrate. However, this

---

[23]   See, e.g,. H V. Mangoldt & Fr. Klein, *Das Bonner Grundegetz*, Bd./ 1, 1. Aufl. (Berlin/Frankfurt 1957), 60.

[24]   Gerhard Anschutz, *Die Verfassung die Deutschen Reiches*, 14 Aufl, (Berlin 1933), 550.

[25]   An example of the former conception is H. Ridder, *Meinungsfreihet*, in: Fr. L. Neumann, H.C. Nipperdey, & U. Scheuner, *Die Grundrechte*, Bd. 2 (Berlin 1954); an example for the latter is Roman Herzog, *Artikel 5 Abs. I-II, in* Th. Maunz & Th. Durig, *Grundegesetz Kommentar*. 5. Aufl. (Munich 1983), 7-8.

[26]   BVerfGE 7, 198, (208).

[27]   BVerfGE 12, 113, (125).

does not mean that the importance of the freedom of opinion in the free development of the personality has not been emphasized in the decisions of the United States Supreme Court.

The Constitutional Court also interprets freedom of opinion and the freedom of the press as the right of an individual to have his or her voice (*sich-hören-lassen*). In this case, contrary to the issue of freedom to access to the media, the main point is not the right of the "receiver" to listen to an opinion but of the "sender" not to be separated by the state from the "receivers".[28] At the same time, this does not mean a right to be listened to (von anderen angehört zu werden), or the right to have an audience provided by the state. The promotion of the expression of opinion does not imply a right to the access to the means of mass communication. What is more, the Constitutional Court did not recognize the right of political parties to have broadcasting time, only to have equal opportunity in the event that parties have been provided with broadcasting time at all.[29]

In respect to the print media according to the opinion of the German Constitutional Court, the traditional concept of the right of an individual to protection should apply. This means entitlement to an absence of state intervention, but does not imply an entitlement of promotion of press activity by the state. In other words, the institutions of the press have no enforceable basic rights in front of the courts against the organs of the state. This does not exclude a legislator from formulating such a right but this right means only "voluntary service (rendering)".[30]

In the Federal Republic of Germany, the legal status of television and radio, similar to the case of the print media, is determined by the constitutional concept of freedom from state intervention, meaning freedom from the intervention of the current government and the actual parliamentary majority ("*Staatsfreiheit*"). This applies both to private and to public television and radio stations. However, even the first decision of the Constitutional Court on television issues (the *1. Fernsehurteil*) argues that while in the case of print media the balanced character of the supply and demand comes about by itself, in the case of television and radio stations (which exist in much less number due to technical and financial constraints), the

---

[28]   Cf. BVerfGE 27, 71, (81).

[29]   Cf. especially BVerfGE 14, 121 (131).

[30]   Cf. BVerfGE 20, 162,(176).

guaranteeing of freedom of broadcasting and balanced supply and demand requires "specific measures".[31]

One of these measures could be, according to the opinion of the judges of the Constitutional Court, the organizational structure of the broadcasting companies itself. For the purpose of broadcasting, it is legally possible to form public law personalities (i.e. public broadcasting stations) which are exempt from the influence of the state (and which remain under limited legal control). The governing bodies of such broadcast stations must include in a defined proportion, representatives of all political, ideological and social groups. According to the decision of the Constitutional Court, it is not unconstitutional that broadcasting institutions which function under public law are in a monopolistic position at the *Land* level.

At the same time, the German Constitution does not require that broadcasting institutions function under public law. But the organizational structure of a private broadcasting company should provide some guarantee for the appropriate representation of all socially relevant groups. According to a later decision of the Karlsruhe Court this independence in program production should include "the selection of the materials to be reported of and also the option for a special type of presentation inclusive of the particular form of a program".[32]

The third Television Decision of the Constitutional Court (*3. Fernsehurteil*) again confirmed the necessity of legal regulation of private radio stations, with measures that would ensure the freedom of radio broadcasting. "This necessity remains notwithstanding that the special character of the radio broadcasting caused by the scarcity of the frequencies and the high costs in the result of recent developments ceases to exist."[33] This means that the legislator should ensure that the whole range of domestic programs reflect the diversified character of the existing opinions and conforms with the requirement of a balanced and professional reporting. To achieve this goal, the decision of the Constitutional Court offers two kinds of regulation for the *Land* legislators.

The first is the "inner pluralist" model, which up to this point had been the dominant model. This model requires a balanced offering of programs from each

---

[31]   BVerfGE 12, 205, 261).

[32]   See the so called *Lebach* decision, BVerfGE 35, 202.

[33]   BVerfGE 57, 295, (323).

broadcasting company. The other model requires "external pluralist" diversity (*"aussenplurastische Vielfalt"*) of programs which preciously was a characteristic feature only of print media and film production. According to this model, democratic and balanced programming should be achieved through the programs offered.

In this externalist model, directors and commentators are required to provide information in a professional, realistic and comprehensive way, but they are not required to take into consideration the balanced quality of the whole program. In the field of print media and film production, mutually balancing influences are present without any intervention. In the case of television and radio, legislators should affirmatively monitor the situation and determine the need for balanced programming. When necessary, the legislator should change regulations to ensure a balanced presentation of opinions.

The Fourth Television Decision (*4. Fernsehurteil*) confirms the constitutional necessity of guaranteeing the access of characteristic opinions, to the media and of preventing the dominance of one opinion through the use financial, organizational and procedural rules. Such access serves as a precondition to a diversity of opinions in private radio broadcasting. At the same time this decision states that in Germany, given the dual structure of public and private radio and television companies, the "basic provision" of information is the task of the institutions functioning under public law. These broadcast institutions can reach almost the whole population with their comprehesive programming. So to some extent in contradiction with its decision of 1981, the German Constitutional Court reached the conclusion that "until and in so far as the fulfillment of these duties is guaranteed by the public radio companies it is reasonable not to require such high standards from the private stations."[34]

However, the Constitutional Court added a new twist to this issue in February of 1991, in a case regarding the constitutional validity of the radio law of North Rhein Westfalia.[35] Petitioners objected to the very strict requirements of the law towards the private radio stations, arguing that those excessive requirements for private stations were almost equal to the requirements imposed on public stations and that they harmed the autonomy of the stations. Petitioners further argued that the

---

[34]   BVerfGE 73, 118, (153).

[35]   Europäische Grundrechte Zeitschrift (EuGRZ) 1991, Heft 3/4.

principle of "model consistency" was deducible neither from the Constitution nor from the previous decisions of the Constitutional Court on media issues. The Court also stated that the legal requirements for private stations should be more lenient than towards public stations. According to the reasoning of the Constitutional Court, only those requirements, which contravene the provisions of the *Grundgesetz* concerning freedoms in the field of the television and radio broadcasting make it impossible or almost impossible to launch new television and radio stations.

The jurisprudence of the German Constitutional Court does not seem to be very liberal concerning radio and television issues. This runs contrary to the reasoning of the Court on issues concerning traditional freedom of opinion. However, that fact that the decisions of the Court consistently reject the principle of "the division of power in the area of publicity" slightly contradicts this. According to the opinion of the judges of the Constitutional Court, it does not contradict the principles of the Constitution for companies interested in the print media also to be involved in private radio and television stations.[36] Only the emergence of "dominant opinion" should be prevented. This practice of the Constitutional Court corresponds to the reasoning of the Court on the issue of the concentration of the print media. The essence of this reasoning is that the liberal point of view disregards the organizational structure of the press and accepts regulations against the broadcasting companies capable of controlling the media market only in cases of serious violations of the democratic principles of the Constitution.

The legal reasoning of the Constitutional Court concerning private and public television and radio stations does not affect the film industry which is organized exclusively on a private basis. In this area a limited system of licensing by an authority remains in force instead of a system of continuous supervision and organization prescribed by legislation. The non-governmental type of organization that performs the duty of voluntary self-control of the film industry (*Freiwillige Selbskontrolle der Filmwirtschaft*) can impose a ban on films (e.g., because of their pornographic content), and can prescribe age limitations for viewers, based on the German Law on Youth.

---

[36]   BVerfGE 73, 118, (175).

IV. The Hungarian Constitution and the Custom of the Constitutional Court

The appearance of new types of media had no effect on the Constitution of the People's Republic of Hungary (Law number XX. of 1949) which was adopted almost at the same time as the German *Grundgesetz*. The lower level of technical development in Hungary's media could explain this fact. However, the overall reform of the Hungarian Constitution in 1972 did not change this situation, notwithstanding that at that time almost every household possessed a radio and a considerable percentage of families also had a television set. The first law on media (press) appeared in 1986 and remained in force in almost unchanged form through 1995. It was no more that a set of provisions on media wrapped in certain political declarations.[37]

The so called "Trilateral Roundtable Discussions" held from June till September of 1989 with the participation of the State-party, various social organizations, and the democratic opposition, set for itself the objective of preparing a new draft legal regulation on print and electronic media as a part of the so called "basic laws" of the democratic transition. However, the special subcommission of experts designed to perform this task failed to reach any consensus regarding the content of this regulation, presumably because of the foreseen decisive power character of the media in the coming elections.[38] As a result, freedom of expression in the legal regulation that determined the transition to a new political system, were dealt with only in Article 61 of the thoroughly modified Hungarian Constitution, which came into force on 23rd of October, 1989.

The new element of this article was that the reference to socialism and the interest of the people, as a necessary condition for exercising the basic right,

---

[37] See the detailed critique of this law in a study written in 1987 by the request of the editors of the *Turning point and Reform*: M. Gálik, G. Halmai, R. Hirschler, & G. Lázár, *A Proposal for the Reform of the Media Öffentlichkeit*. Kritika, 1988/10.

[38] The protocols of the proceedings of these political roundtable discussions which had a crucial decisive role in the constitutional change in Hungary have not been published yet because some participants did not permitted the publication of the materials. Following from this, the content of the discussions of the expert subcommissions is difficult to reconstruct. First of all, I tried to retrace of the debate on constitutional issues using those few documents which were available to me. These documents were given at my disposal generously by constitutional lawyer Péter Szalay. See G. Halmai, *From the People's Republic to Republic*. Társadalomtudományi Közlemények, 1991. 1-2. szám.

disappeared. Freedom of speech was replaced by the reference to the more broad concept of freedom of expression, (which included communication rights), and the right to be acquainted with and to circulate information of public interest, i.e., freedom of information was added. This right had been part of the German *Grundgesetz* since 1949. As a result of the so called "Pact", which was an agreement between the largest governing party and the largest opposition party, the new parliament has added to Article 61 of the Constitution the following: "the adoption of the Act concerning the supervision and appointment of the heads of the public service radio and television company, and news agency, the licensing commercial television and radio companies, and further the prevention of a monopoly in the field of the information requires the votes of two-third of the members of Parliament present."

However, until this law on media was passed by the Parliament, freedom of communication in the field of radio and television broadcasting was suspended. The awarding of broadcast licenses was denied through an intra-governmental decree. This is not a normative act and the decree also created a moratorium on frequencies. Although the new Parliament required the government to submit a draft bill on the moratorium on frequencies in order to legalize the moratorium, this draft never was submitted to the Parliament. This meant that the illegal moratorium on frequencies remained in force. This prevented the emergence of new radio and television stations.[39]

The legal regulation, or rather the absence of it, made the emergence of new radio and television broadcasting stations impossible (except for Hungarian Radio and Television). It also made freedom of expression by new media impossible. At the same time, the 1986 Press Law barely addressed the legal status of the national public television and radio company which was in a monopolistic position. Also, a 1974 government decree on Hungarian Television and Radio remained in force. The sixth article of this decree prescribed the state supervision of these institutions.

---

[39] In this absurd situation anybody who tried to launch a radio or television broadcasting according to his or her constitutional right could not get permission to do so. At the same time, a criminal proceeding was started against Tilos Rádió, a radio company that broadcasted without permission since 1991. The Nyilvánosság Klub (Öffentlichkeit Club), awarded the Civil Kurázsi Award (Civil Courage Award) to Tilos Rádió.

The Hungarian Constitutional Court (the "Constitutional Court") ruled this decree unconstitutional, but postponed its nullification until the new media law was passed. The Court used the very doubtful argument that it is better to have unconstitutional governmental supervision than to not have any supervision at all.[40] At the same time, the reasoning of the decision contains very important statements concerning the desirability for the electronic media to have a balanced character and to be independent from the state. The Constitutional Court of Germany has repeatedly mentioned this conceptual goal.

The justices of the Hungarian Constitutional Court, in several steps, deduced from the "maternal" right of freedom of expression, freedom of television and radio broadcasting in several steps. The first step was freedom of the press, of which freedom of expression was already a part. This meant that the freedom of the press should be guaranteed by the state taking into consideration that the press is an extraordinarily important means of gathering the information necessary for the formation, expression and shaping of opinion. The task of guaranteeing the freedom of expression of opinion and the freedom of gathering information required additional measures with respect to television and radio as compared to freedom of the press.

The reason behind this was, according to the Constitutional Court, that the exercise of the fundamental right in this case should be reconciled with the "scarcity" of the technical resources for exercising this right (i.e., with the limited number of the available frequencies). According to the decision of the Court, this scarcity of electronic media was not likely to change within a reasonable period of time. Contrary to the print media, it did permit the unrestricted founding of television and radio companies. However, even in the area of the television and radio broadcasting, special measures would be reasonable with respect to national public television and radio companies which were for the time being in a monopolistic position. Regarding public broadcasting, the Court stated that media legislation should guarantee objective, comprehensive and balanced information through the use of financial, procedural and organizational prescriptions.

Similar to their colleagues in Karlsruhe, the Hungarian Justices of the Constitutional Court did not bind the specific guarantees of the freedom of television and radio broadcasting to any particular or concrete manner of organization or to any particular legal form. The constitutional or unconstitutional character of the

---

[40]   Decision of the Constitutional Court No. 37/1992 (June 10).

organizational structures, which are to be created by the legislature freely, shall be determined by

(1) their capacity to guarantee in principle the comprehensive, balanced and objective expression of all opinions existing in the whole society and

(2) to provide the public with information of public interest.

The fulfillment of these conditions, by a new media law, would mean that national and regional public broadcasting and commercial broadcasting would be treated the same. The distribution of the allocation burden between national public television and radio on the one side and local and commercial broadcasting from another, was to be established by the legislature (within constitutional confines). Such a balance is needed in order to achieve the objective, comprehensive and balanced supply of information. Thus, the Hungarian Constitutional Court applied the so called "inner pluralistic" model recommended by the Third German *Fernsehurteil* to the national public media, and the so called "external" pluralistic model to the entire electronic media.

An additional requirement of public radio and television companies, which has also been outlined in the German Constitutional Court decisions, is freedom from the state. To this requirement, the Hungarian decision added the requirement of freedom for various social groups. The concrete method of regulation to be chosen by the legislature: "should exclude the possibility that the organs of the state, or any other group of the society have influence on the content of the programs resulting in the injury to the comprehensive, balanced and proportional and objective way of presentation of the existing opinions in the society,....". According to the justices of the Constitutional Court the "freedom from the state organs" implies freedom not only from the government which is mentioned in the decree of 1974, but also freedom from the legislature. The unprecedented delay of the passage of the media law by the Hungarian Parliament resulted in a situation where the principal requirements established by the Constitutional Court concerning the 1974 governmental decree did not speed up the political decision-making but at least helped the legislators opt for constitutional methods of regulation.[41]

---

[41]   Since the parliamentary parties were not able to reach an agreement on the content of the media law we cannot determine on what extent the coming legal regulation will fulfill the requirements of the Constitutional Court.

V.   How to Proceed?

The appearance of new types of media even in democratic rule-of-law states has compelled legislators and courts to abandon traditional liberal methods of regulation of the freedom of expression, at least concerning the electronic media. The common feature of laws and constitutional decisions regarding electronic media is that they prescribe positive rules in order to ensure the balanced character of television and radio companies and also to ensure their freedom form state intervention. This rather well-spread constitutional practice permits, or even more, requires the legal intervention of the state into the private realm of opinion formation. This is justified by a limited number of available frequencies, which makes regulation necessary. However, it remains an open question at the current level of technological advancement, as the division of frequencies becomes more and more feasible, and the use of satellite and cable programming expands, whether state regulation should not retreat into the area of public media and regulate exclusively in this field. In the remaining area of television and radio broadcasting, free rein would be given to the free market of thoughts and opinions. It seems, at least on first sight, that the organization of the electronic media along private-market lines can achieve one of the goals of state regulation, independence from the state. The question to be answered is whether in television and radio broadcasting, which is much more effective than the print media, the objective supply of information can be safely entrusted to the market (i.e., it is enough to apply the same aposteriori regulation as in the area of the print media).

Undoubtedly, institutional guarantees may be justified based on the fact that the modern media is an incomparably effective and powerful tool for dissemination of information to the public. It can reach everybody through the push of a button. Thus, freedom of television and radio broadcasting contains the traditional right of protection against the interference by the state, but also contains a right to state regulation to some extent. In this respect, I propose to make a distinction between public and commercial electronic media.

It is obvious that public radio and television stations were established to provide information, entertainment, and cultural programs for the public, i.e., for the tax payers (which often means also subscription fee payers). On the grounds of this goal, the public is entitled to expect that the media perform their task professionally and in a balanced manner. This requires the fulfillment of the diversified expectations of listeners and viewers, and also implies ideological and political neutrality. In order to attain these requirements, institutional, procedural guarantees worked out by legislation are needed. In certain cases, these guarantees may restrict the freedom of expression.

The situation is entirely different in the case of the commercial television and radio companies. Given the extended technical possibilities of electronic communication, it is not justifiable to influence the content of programs in order to attain either the "inner plurality" of a given station or the "external plurality" concerning the whole of the commercial station. The imbalance caused by commercial stations may be corrected by the state only through the regulation applied to the public stations. So the acceptable level of state regulation concerning electronic public media is equivalent to the level of justifiable regulation in the area of print media. This cannot be more than anti-monopolistic regulation because if the state does not guarantee freedom of competition, freedom of expression could be endangered. In the area of print and electronic media any other regulation should not exceed what is legally permissible concerning freedom of expression.

THE HUNGARIAN CONSTITUTIONAL COURT IN THE MEDIA WAR: INTERPRETATIONS OF SEPARATION OF POWERS AND MODELS OF DEMOCRACY

by Andrew Arato

I. Introduction: The Politics of Court Decisions in the Media War

This paper attempts to evaluate the five decisions of the Hungarian Constitutional Court that stemmed from the Hungarian Media War of 1991-1993. While I will briefly discuss the immediate political meaning as well as the legal character of the decisions, I will in particular focus on three theoretical issues: 1. The court's interest in maintaining legal continuity and security in the context of the Hungarian transition; 2. the Court's apparent weakening of elements of consensus (or pluralistic) democracy in the Hungarian political system; and 3. the Court's continued interpretive activism in the context of a relatively "soft" constitutional background.

In my view, (aside from numerous earlier skirmishes) the Media War began in the summer of 1991 when the Hungarian Government and the leadership of the MDF (Hungarian Democratic Forum - the senior party in the governing coalition) first adopted the arguments of the right wing of this party, according to which there was a need to assert greater majoritarian control over the electronic media. Up till this point, bound by agreements made with the leading Opposition party that were subsequently enshrined in Article 61(4) of the Hungarian Constitution and in the Media Appointments Law of 1990 (the "Appointments Law")[1] as well as in the actual choice of media presidents in Messrs. Elemér Hankiss and Csaba Gombár. Through these actions, the Government repeatedly reaffirmed its acceptance of television and radio free of party interference.[2]

---

[1] Act LIV of 1990.

[2] I am accepting Elemér Hankiss's chronology of events during the Media War. See Telehir, March 1993, at 150 and 159.; One might say he was in good position to know when the Media War began. On the other hand it seems perfectly legitimate to date the beginning, as does János Kenedi, with Member of Parliament, István Csurka's first demands after the national elections of 1990, for a media controlled by the electoral winners, coupled with his broadsides against the supposedly communist holdovers in Hungarian Television and Radio. See Kenedi, *A*

A. Sajó (ed.), *Rights of Access to the Media*, 225-241.
© 1996 *Kluwer Law International. Printed in the Netherlands.*

The strategy of the Government involved several important elements. First, there was a repeated attempt (using governmental recommendations, parliamentary hearings and discussions, and appeals to the Constitutional Court) to displace or replace the Hungarian Media Presidents with new vice presidents. Second, there was an attempt to assert direct governmental control over the media by insisting on the validity of a 1974 governmental decree, Directive 1047/1974 (Directive 1047). Point 6 of this Directive provided for governmental supervision of the media. The current Government interpreted this provision as *operative* control over the media. Third, the governmental majority, on two occasions, deprived Hungarian Radio and Television of the budgetary resources for independent operation. Fourth, with the failure of the Government's initial strategy to replace the Media Presidents, the Government tried to remove the President of Hungarian Television, Elemer Hankiss, through a disciplinary procedure, coupled with criminal procedures against his two closest co-workers. Fifth, the governmental majority made every effort to convert the requirement, that a new media law be passed by 2/3 majority into a requirement that the law be passed by simple majority. Finally, throughout the period many members of the ruling coalition participated in extra-parliamentary mobilization against the Presidents of Hungarian Radio and Television as well as the President of the Hungarian Republic who protected them.

Opposition to the Government's actions took place on many levels as well. First, under the Appointments Law, President Árpád Göncz refused to sign the recommended removal of the Media Presidents and initially, the appointment of new vice presidents. Second, the parliamentary Opposition appealed to the Constitutional Court to rule Directive 1047 unconstitutional. Third, in December of 1992 the Opposition, through parliamentary maneuvering, was able to defeat the coalition's attempt to pass its own media law on the bases of a simple majority. Fourth, many members of opposition parties participated in civic activities and extra-parliamentary mobilization to support President Göncz and, in their view, the freedom of the media.

As the list of strategies and counter-strategies indicate, the governmental side had more powerful resources and alternatives throughout the conflict. And indeed, as in most countries of the region, the Government in Hungary in the end

---

médiaháború füstje és lángja, Magyar Hirlap, June 12, 1992. The difference between the two views is not just a terminological one ("war" vs. "skirmish"), but has to do with the evaluation of how close Csurka's and Prime Minister Antall's media strategies were before the summer of 1991.

succeeded in asserting (or, given the past, reasserting) its direct control of the electronic media. Media Presidents were forced to resign and vice presidents were put in charge to assert Government control.

While the country has gone through an important learning experience, the ruling parties have gained vantage points they desired by the eve of the next election. Of course, they were not able to fully exploit these, due to their internal tensions, their amateurish handling of media-programming, and the well-learned skepticism of the population toward what they heard on radio and television.

It should be noted, that since the decline of support for the Hungarian ruling parties from 1990-1992 was not due to the hostility of the media and the press, as many imagined, it can also not be reversed by asserting state control over the most important organs of public communication. Nevertheless, through the Media War, some extremely troubling precedents for governmental action have been established. It will take great efforts in the future to reverse these and to create a genuine public-service media.

Evidently, appeals to the Hungarian Constitutional Court have played an important role in the Media War both for the Government and the parliamentary Opposition. Five decisions in all were made by the Constitutional Court - three on the ability of the President of the Republic of Hungary (hereinafter: the President) to refuse to sign government recommendations for appointment and removal of officials,[3] and two on the constitutional and legal status of Directive 1047,[4] which the coalition tried to use to justify its efforts to exert direct control over the media. In general it is easy to characterize these decisions. The first group progressively narrowed the ability of the President to refuse to sign appointments or removals, except in cases of formal procedural irregularity, or for substantive reasons, when, the president can argue "on solid grounds" that signing would "gravely disturb the democratic operation of the organization of the state".[5]

This last requirement was itself further narrowed from one decision to the next: the danger to the democratic operation of the state must lie specifically in the person to be appointed (or who will succeed after a removal) and must relate to the

---

[3]   Those cases were: Numbers 48/1991 (IX.26); 8/1992 (I.30); and 765/G/1992/3 (VI.8).

[4]   Those cases were: Numbers 431/B/1992/3 (VI.8) and 431/B/1992/5 (III.16,1993).

[5]   Magyar Közlöny, September 26, 1991, No. 103, at 2120.

operation only of the specific institution to which the appointment would be made.[6] Moreover, the Court insisted that the president sign orders of appointment or removals within a reasonable time, to avoid a kind of "pocket" veto of the appointment or demission.[7]

The Court did not take away, however, the president's power to subjectively consider and weigh whether he should sign, and in one respect expanded his possible reasons for doing so by agreeing with him (and not with the prime minister) that the violation of a fundamental right implies grave danger to democratic functioning.[8] Above all, the Court claimed lack of competence to adjudicate the concrete controversy between the president and the prime minister, in effect ratifying, that unless the ruling coalition had the necessary 2/3 vote to impeach President Göncz, his ability to resist would survive.[9]

Finally, we should note that this group of decisions were internally controversial within the Court. Three out of ten justices, Justices Schmidt, Vörös, and Kilényi, disagreed with the narrowness of limits drawn around presidential action, with the Courts rejection of the need of consensus between the president and the prime minister, and with the very ability of the Court to draw these conclusions through interpretation given the silence of the constitutional text on the issue.

In the second group of (two) decisions, the Court affirmed that the disputed Point 6 of Directive 1047 was indeed unconstitutional. The point was unconstitutional because it did not provide any guarantees against the Government converting its right to regulate the media into a one-sided influence over the media, thereby potentially damaging the freedoms of speech, freedoms of the press and the free emergence of public opinion.[10] The Court moreover chided Parliament for "the violation of the constitution through omission", through not creating the media law.

In the absence of such a new media law, however, the first Court decision refused to immediately set aside the governmental decree judged unconstitutional.

---

[6]   Case No. 765/G/1992/3 (mimeographic version), supra note 3, at 7-10.

[7]   Magyar Közlöny, No. 11 (1992).

[8]   Case No. 765/G/1992/3, supra note 3, at 2-3 and 8.

[9]   Id. at 4. This was also confirmed by Justice Sólyom in a private letter to Prime Minister Antall.

[10]   Case No. 431/B/1992/3, supra note 4, at 3.

Instead, Parliament was given a deadline of November 30, 1992, to establish the new media law. The Court threatened to reopen the case if Parliament failed to do its constitutional duty, and to "determine the time of the elimination of the governmental order".

The second decision, without setting any new deadlines, once again did not set aside Directive 1047. Instead, the Court tied the directive's elimination to the parliamentary creation of a new media law, irrespective of the time when this would happen. This shift from a temporal deadline to a future political event, (i.e., the eventful enactment of a law) in determining the elimination of an unconstitutional regulation, brought about the vigorous dissenting opinion of Justice Vörös. And indeed, the decision provided for a legal sanction of the continued governmental control of the media, even though such control and the regulation on which it was based were both judged unconstitutional.

One might argue that the two sets of decisions neatly complemented one another, in terms of a balanced handling of the politics of the media war. The appointment decisions weakened the constitutional case of the President, but left him the power to resist government mandates. The regulation decisions removed the constitutional case for governmental control of the media, but left the Government the right to control the media until it got a media law fully to its liking. Thus, one might say, the status quo was maintained by the Court.

Nevertheless, such a state of affairs in itself could be interpreted as a reinforcement of the stronger, in this case the governmental side. However, that side won not by relying on either of the Court's opinions, but by utilizing its budgetary powers as well its ability to initiate disciplinary and criminal proceedings that would cripple the Media Presidents, even though each case was legally very weak.[11] At the same time, however, the content and timing of the Court's decisions seriously effected some of the actual conflicts that were taking place. The Court's dramatic restriction of the Hungarian president's ability to deny to sign (or to make) appointments and demissions, as well as its repeated denial that consensus is necessary in these cases, turned the opposition parties (as well as Hankiss) against

---

[11] The criminal case of Gábor Bányai was dismissed after a few days, in December, 1992. In the case of László Nagy, the police authorities eventually, in May, 1993 sent the case to the Public Prosecutor without actually recommending that charges be raised. Any study of the protocols of the Hankiss disciplinary procedure (which was discontinued before a verdict, upon his resignation) would show the extreme weakness of the Government's charges. Those charges depended, in part, on the charges against Hankiss' subordinates. See generally Telehir, March, 1993.

the previously approved part of the media law, the Appointments Law.[12] As a result, it became much harder to actually pass a media law. The Opposition could not easily agree on an overall regulation that contained this more limited element (relating to the power of appointment), and the Government had less of an incentive to agree to any compromise since it already had an appointment law it liked. Similarly, the second decision of the Court concerning regulation, which kept the 1974 governmental decree in effect, indefinitely removed whatever incentive the Government could still have to produce a media law.[13]

The two decisions taken together in fact meant that if there was no consensus achieved on the coalition's terms, the Government could potentially control the media under the reinterpreted appointments law and the 1974 governmental directive, and could do so indefinitely. Such seems to be the political balance sheet resulting from the Court's several decisions, even though the Court gave both sides many points to rejoice about.[14]

Did this outcome actually matter? With Hankiss and Gombár out of the way, the Government could control even formally the independent media through the power of the vice-presidents who were their men all along, and who were eventually placed fully in charge. Thus, by the time the Court made its second decision on the regulation of the media, there were arguably no political stakes involved. By confirming the legality of the (unconstitutional) regulation used by the Government, the Court only gave procedural legitimacy to already accomplished

---

[12]   See the protocols on the six party parliamentary deliberations on the media law, in Telehir, November, 1992 at 61-62 and 76. For Hankiss's view see Telehir, August, 1992 at 43 and 48.

[13]   The correct expectation by Messrs. Elek and Kulin, members of the MDF liberal wing, that the Court would do as it finally did and remove any deadline, already weakened their incentive to produce a media law before the Court's actual decision. See the protocols on the Cultural Committee of Parliament's hearings on the "suitability" of Hankiss as Television President in May-June, 1992 in Telehir, August, 1992 at 133 and 139-140.

[14]   Thus, Miklós Haraszti, perhaps the most determined and knowledgeable advocate on the side of the opposition, was not wrong when he claimed that the Court's last decision on appointments established a kind of first amendment for Hungary. See Beszélő, December 19, 1992, at 6-7. The Court did this both in the decision about Directive 1047, and in the last appointments decision. Unfortunately, the application of this was postponed in the former case, though not in the latter one according to which the President may deny appointments on the basis of possible injury to the freedoms of press and speech.

actions. Nevertheless, the earlier decisions also influenced the actual method chosen by the Government to deal with Hankiss.

At least, initially, the Government based its disciplinary proceedings, both formally and in terms of the content of the charges against him on the disputed Directive 1047. The same was true for the case of the governmental coalition against Hankiss during the Parliamentary hearings of May and June 1992, and the MDF deputies who were very relieved to get the Court's decision before the last session when they had to pass judgement on Hankiss.[15]

In short, at both times, the major part of the coalition's case against Hankiss was that he carried out organizational changes, without the initiative or the approval of the Government. This, if true, they argued, (Hankiss cogently argued it was not) was a violation of the letter (and indeed the spirit) of Directive 1047. Against the Court's decision it counted for little that Hankiss could claim that he acted against an unconstitutional law, in the spirit of the constitution.[16] Whether or not the Government had reason to think that its administrative action against Hankiss, based on the most negative interpretation of the meaning and application of Directive 1047, would stand up in all the Courts (perhaps eventually in the Supreme or Constitutional Courts themselves), the mere continued existence of the regulation gave it some reasonable presumption to initiate the disciplinary procedure.

II.　　Legal Problems of the Media-Related Decisions of the Constitutional Court

How strong were the Court's media-related decisions from a legal point of view? Not wishing to anticipate the work of legal analysts, and constitutional historians, several points seem nevertheless striking:

1. In the case of the two decisions on the validity of Directive 1047, the Court omitted to define or even to discuss what government "supervision" of the media meant in this particular instance. In the case of the original communist rule,

---

[15]　　Telehir, August, 1992 at 133 et. seq.

[16]　　It made little difference that oppositional deputies could argue that the particular and most explicitly statist interpretation of Directive 1047, on which Hankiss would be condemned, was unconstitutional, since the court provided, unfortunately, no interpretation at all of the regulation.

created at the time of the rollback of the 1968 economic reforms, the term evidently meant nothing and everything. The government in fact was not the organ of supervision of the media; this role was played by the relevant official of the politburo. But the supervision that existed included normative, hierarchical and operative controls. Which of these was to be still pertinent? The original text of Point 6 of the 1974 directive mentions "approval of organizational rules", "naming the vice presidents" and "carrying out other tasks determined by other rules".[17] The second of these functions became obsolete, given the Appointments Law passed in 1990, and the third referred to nothing given the absence of a new media law.

This left the first, and on the bases of this Hankiss and his lawyers repeatedly argued that only "legal supervision" (or supervision of legality) remained pertinent. At the same time, the Government and its lawyers repeatedly argued that the directive gave them operative control, though to my knowledge they never outlined the content of this. In reality, of course, they sought to influence the internal hierarchy, appointments, and organizational rules of Hungarian Radio and Television. But only in one case mentioned by Miklós Haraszti of SzDSz and confirmed by Hankiss did top government officials use Directive 1047 as the legal foundation of their interference.

Prime Minister Antall, in a March 1992 letter to Hankiss indicated that he would approve the new organizational rules of Hungarian Television (his prerogative under Directive 1047) only if the vice-president took over all major functions of the president, especially control of news programs.[18] As objectionable as this form of pressure was, it was, as Hankiss recognized, only the formally possible misuse of "supervision" in the legal sense as explicitly referred to by the text of Directive 1047. The problem is that Hankiss believed that he had the legal right to resist such misuse, and the Government believed he did not. This ambiguity should have been resolved by the Constitutional Court.

In its one vaguely relevant remark the Court indicated its fear (in case of the immediate annihilation of Directive 1047) of a legal vacuum and its rejection of a situation in which the Media Presidents would not be responsible to any

---

[17]   Magyar Hirlap, July 9, 1992.

[18]   See Telehir, August, 1992 at 40 and 124.

authority.[19] These two dangers are treated as one. Yet, they are not. One seems to refer to a legal supervision, one that makes sure that the practices and internal rules of the media live up to the demands of the legal system, even short of violations of the criminal law. The second refers to undisclosed types of political control themselves, circumscribed by the law.

But, it is just such limiting boundaries that do not exist, at present, and that is what makes the rule in question unconstitutional according to the Court. In spite of this state of affairs, the Court's language could be interpreted as stating that it wished to maintain political rather than merely legal supervision. This is the textual basis (however vague and ambiguous) of the governmental interpretation of the Court's decision.

Ferenc Kulin, (during the Parliament's cultural committee hearing of Hankiss), stated that the very fact that the Court declared the unconstitutionality of the directive means that the Court must have had in mind the right of full, operative government interference in "every aspect of the life of television". Otherwise, he reasoned, why they declare the directive unconstitutional; certainly mere supervision of legality would not be unconstitutional. Thus, the fact of the Court's peculiar double decision (stating that the Directive 1047 was unconstitutional but for the moment legal) is used even by the liberals of MDF to affirm the legality in principle at least of continuing the communist-statist direction of the "life" of the media.

To the benefit of the Court's reputation however it must be said that Kulin's interpretation of its decision is false. The Court considered Directive 1047 unconstitutional not because it was openly statist, but because it was ambivalent about what the state can do, not because it *permits* statist controls but because it *does not eliminate* such a possibility. The Court ended its decision by pointing out that the Government can use its right of supervision to promote as well as to frustrate the freedom of press. But since it is the constitutional responsibility of the Government, according to the Court, to defend the constitutional order and the rights of the citizens, it was implicitly obvious that the Government had a duty to forego the unconstitutional options which the directive *per se* did not eliminate.

Thus, the Court had in mind (without explicitly saying so) two forms of unconstitutionality: (i) the existence of the directive itself without guarantees against

---

[19]   "Public service radio and television would leave any legal supervision, or [*illetve* = either "respectively" or "rather"] the sphere of legally operating relations of political responsibility'. Case No. 431/B/1992/3, supra note 4, at 6.

misuse (i.e. the unconstitutionality of the legal rule itself) and (ii) government actions exploiting the ambiguity of the directive to the detriment of the freedom of the press (i.e., unconstitutional actions by the executive). The Court reluctantly and temporarily prolonged the first form of unconstitutionality, but made no concessions to the second. Unfortunately, however, by not discussing the meaning of supervision, or the types of actions permissible as part of supervision, the Court itself gave rise to a form of ambivalence, that could be exploited, as Kulin's remarks show, on behalf of unconstitutional actions (or threats) by the executive, or the governing majority.

This omission is all the more serious, since the Court had to know of the alternative interpretations advanced by the various sides in the conflict. Indeed, the fact that the second decision concerning the validity of Directive 1047 continued to avoid interpreting the meaning of supervision, was even more serious. It was serious given the prevalence of its statist-interpretation within the ruling coalition, its open articulation at various governmental fora (as in the aforementioned case of Kulin), and indeed its embodiment in the resolutions of both Parliament's Constitutional and Cultural Committees concerning Hankiss.[20]

The first of these resolutions adopted by the Constitutional Committee sought to establish the point that Hankiss was a state official, thus, he could be directed as such. The second resolution adopted by the Cultural Committee, specifically referred to its (statist) interpretation of the Court's decision (that came between the two resolutions) as confirming this very claim. Finally, the utilization of the same interpretation was an important legal basis of the disciplinary process against Hankiss. It was an ostrich-like tactic for the Court to simply disregard these interpretations of its first decision as it was about to make the second one on the fate of the same regulation (Directive 1047).

2. The Court's discussion of what would happen if it immediately annihilated directive 1047 is surprisingly tendentious. It is not true, first of all, that the Hungarian criminal law or libel law would represent the only legal protection against actions of the media or its leadership; labor law, and contract law, for example, apply to the media that are not under governmental supervision. Thus, one cannot speak of an absence of legal supervision in the full sense, but rather the shift of supervision from government to the Courts.

---

[20]   The resolutions were adopted on May 18 and June 17, 1992. See Telehir, August, 1992 at 7 and 132.

More disturbingly, the Court claimed that "the media would be completely at the mercy of party conflicts, or the power conflicts of groups operating within the media. This situation would definitely be to the detriment of free expression of opinion".[21] One cannot of course exclude this possibility. But it is only a worst case scenario, or rather the depiction of the actual state of affairs only from the point of view of the MDF radicals. This is a position the Court undoubtedly did not wish to, or had the right to take for granted. It should have at least considered the possibility, that with an end to the possibility of governmental interference, the Media Presidents, under internationally-approved internal rules, would quell internal conflicts, and guarantee the operation of a genuine public-service media.

After all, this is what the Media Presidents were working on before they were confronted with a variety of external pressures. Of course, it is also not the Court's duty (or right even) to believe that this second scenario would have been either actual or likely. But for what reason did the Court present the first, negative scenario as the only one possible? In the case of the continuation of Government supervision under Directive 1047, the Court told us that we have no right to believe in the unavoidability of negative consequences for the freedom of the press: "One cannot start out either from the premise that the Government will not defend the freedom of the press, or from the assumption that it will limit it". Perhaps inadvertently, the Court here did not actually mention two possibilities that we should not assume, but only two versions of the same one. But even if it wanted to also say that "we should not assume that the government will *not* limit the freedom of the press" this possible negative scenario was neither fleshed out, nor considered particularly likely.

Given the efforts of the coalition for about a year, and of its right wing for two and a half years, this omission was rather strange. After all, Hankiss and Gombar certainly did not aim at the chaos warned against by the Court, while Istvan Csurka and his friends admittedly aimed at governmental domination of the electronic media. Again, the Court did not have to share this assessment. They could have believed that Csurka would fail[22] and that whatever Mr. Hankiss' and Mr.

---

[21]   Case No. 431/B/1992/3, supra note 4, at 6.

[22]   And by the time they made their second decision on Directive 1047, they knew that he did fail. Antall's first complete rejection of Csurka and his politics was published in Pesti Hirlap on exactly the same day, March 16, that the Court announced this decision.

Gombar's intentions were, they were not able to bring the Media War to an end. By presenting one option - media independence from government supervision - only in terms of its most negative outcome possible, and the other option - government supervision over the media - in terms of ambivalence at best, and by leaning toward a best case scenario at worst, the Court came very dangerously close to adjudicating the concrete case of contention between the Media Presidents and the Government, a case that was not even brought to the Court for judgement.

3. The two decisions concerning the constitutionality and validity of Directive 1047 are inconsistent. This point was made by Justice Vörös, whose dissent in the second case is about twice as long as the incredibly skimpy argument from the majority written by Justice Sólyom. Justice Vörös stressed, quite cogently, the absurdity of moving from a temporal deadline, that would lead to the definite annihilation of Directive 1047, to the use of an uncertain event as the new deadline. The first decision actually promised that a second one, if necessary because of Parliament's failure to produce a media law, would actually determine *the point in time* of the annihilation of the governmental directive. The second decision did no such a thing, and extended the directive's validity indefinitely.

I would only add that thereby the whole logical status of the two decisions changes. The first, backed up by the threat of annihilation of the unconstitutional regulation, still contained a strong incentive for the governing parties to produce a media law. For the Opposition it had an incentive as well, because the Court did not name the time period when the regulation would be definitively destroyed. Thus, the Opposition had reason to fear that the Government may have the regulation at its disposal throughout the all important-electoral period, or at least until the Media Presidents were finally replaced by more pliant successors. The second decision, though increasing the incentive for the minority to come to terms, no longer contained any incentive whatsoever for the majority, the governmental parties. These parties no longer had any reason to produce a media law, since they could continue to utilize (for an indefinite time) the 1974 directive that favored them. Thus, the event or the condition to which the Court now tied future annihilation was not only uncertain, as Justice Vörös stated, but became unlikely, in part because of the very decision that proposed this condition. Finally, Justice Vörös was also right to point out that the toleration of an unconstitutional condition indefinitely endangered the very legal security the Court wished to protect. I would draw out what Vörös strongly implies, namely, that such indefinite toleration by the Constitutional Court of unconstitutional conditions that endanger (by the Court's own definition) both fundamental liberties and the democratic workings of institutions is itself unconstitutional.[23]

4. The decisions concerning the role of the president in appointments and dismissals, were much better formulated in the legal sense. Here, my objections will be on a more theoretical level. But before I turn to critique formulated on the level of political theory, there is at least one more narrowly legal issue to take up here as well. Miklós Haraszti has pointed out one remarkable feature of Prime Minister Antall's strategy, with respect to his attempt to get a Constitutional Court ruling on president Göncz's refusal to sign his recommended appointments and dismissals under the Appointments Law.

Instead of asking the Court directly about the president's obligations under this law (the enactment of which required a 2/3 majority and received an over 90% majority), the Prime Minister requested a ruling on the meaning of "appoints" and "dismisses" under the Constitution. Thus, he deflected, Haraszti implied, not only from the historical context which produced the consensus of the leading parties, but also from the justification appended to the Appointments Law in 1990, according to which "the right of appointment must be taken from the Government and given to the president in order to actualize non-partisanship and the freedom of press in the public media".[24] Evidently, the legal advisors of the Prime Minister sought to move the consideration of the issue to a context where, in the majority of cases, the appointed powers of the president were indeed only formal. But, and this is my question, did the Court also have a good reason to leave out of its consideration the meaning of the actual law which regulated the president's right in a specific contested case?

Evidently the Court was not, and could not be asked to decide the concrete specific case. But when it reviewed all the various meanings of the presidential role what is the justification for not considering the specific meaning of this role in the relevant law? The President, in his statement to the Court, sought no general share in executive power, nor a right to substantively and independently practice his power

---

[23]   Case No. 431/B/1992/5, supra note 4, at 2.

[24]   Telehir, August, 1992 at 40-41.

of appointment in all cases where he formally possessed such power.[25] Rather, he only wanted to exercise this authority in the specific instances he mentioned, when the appointment (of the official) was not to an organ of public administration. Specifically, President Göncz referred to the appointment of the presidents and vice-presidents of the media pursuant to the Appointments Law. Indeed, Parliament's Cultural Committee, who asked for the initial constitutional review, also specifically referred to the Appointments Law.[26]

Did the Court have the right to leave this law's meaning out of consideration, as the law is linked to the appointment power set forth in Article 61(4) of the Constitution? Article 61(4), by requiring a 2/3 majority for the enactment of an Appointments Law, (and thereby requiring consensus), was obviously consistent with the claim that the law passed must incorporate such a consensus. The Court, without considering either the relevant law or the relevant constitutional article sought to derive the meaning of and constraints on, the range or scope of the President's ability to make independent political decisions,[27] from instances of such actions actually described in the Constitution as the extraordinary calling or dismissal of Parliament.[28] But while its taxonomy was convincing to a point, it was not at all evident that it must exclude *independent political decision* by the President, in specifically stated instances of lesser gravity than those mentioned by the Court. This would presumably refer to situations when the President could

---

[25] Thus, it was unnecessarily polemical and set up a strawman when the Court majority repeatedly argued that "one cannot derive a construct form the constitution according to which the government and the president would be at the head of executive power, who, mutually controlling and balancing one another, arrive at decisions by consensus". Magyar Közlöny, No. 103, at 2118. Does the constitution exclude such consensus in all specific domains? Hardly.

[26] Id. at 2113; see also Case No. 765/G/1992/3, supra note 3, at 1-2. The confusion may stem from the fact that though the Cultural Committee mentioned the Appointments Law, it referred it only to Article 30(A) of the Constitution, which deals with the rights of the president in general, and not to Article 61(4) on which the relevant law of appointment was primarily based.

[27] Under which heading they group negative decisions concerning appointments and dismissals that logically cannot require counter-signing by a minister. Magyar Közlöny, No. 103, at 2119.

[28] It sounds nevertheless absurd to say that the weight of reasons for the denial of an appointment or dismissal must be similar to those relevant to these two instances: the extraordinary calling or dismissal of the parliament. Case No. 765/G/1992/3, supra note 3, at 21-20.

exercise his authority by insisting on a shared role in making an appointment, (i.e., in a decision by consensus).

If, on the other hand, the Court believed that the exclusion of this option was warranted by several paragraphs of Article 30 of the Constitution, as well as other considerations derived from the non-existence of a political responsibility in the case of the president (he can be impeached only in a legal proceeding) as well as the inviolability of his person, etc., then the constitutional status of the Appointments Law should have been considered, because of the strong presumption that it incorporated a striving for consensus in the case of appointing the leaders of the Hungarian media.[29]

There are good reasons for this presumption. First, it was evidently the aim of the Constitution makers, the politicians who constructed the pact between the MDF and the SzDSz and who devised the wording of both Article 61(4) of the Constitution, which required 2/3 majorities for enactment of the law on the media[30] and the Appointments Law itself. The overwhelming majority vote for the latter law proved that Parliament assumed that the requirement of consensus was a definite implication. Whatever one thinks of interpreting laws through "original intent", it remains a question whether it was wise and legitimate to totally disregard, only two years after the enactment of the Appointments Law, the intent of legislators who were still engaged in constructing the rest of the laws regulating the media.

Of course, one could argue that the majority and minority parties agreed to the law and voted for it only because they gave it a different interpretation all along. A sloppy wording, now conceded by the SzDSz, certainly allowed for such a possibility.[31]

---

[29]   The Court minority repeatedly pointed out the arbitrariness of this derivation. In their view, the letter of the Constitution established a divided sphere of responsibility wherever sharing the power of appointment between the one who recommends, the one who appoints (i.e. the president), and the one who countersigns. Id. at 21-22. President Göncz himself did not claim such broad powers, which, however, still do not mean a "division of executive power".

[30]   Or, in the later MDF interpretation, laws on the media, that include the law of appointments.

[31]   See the various remarks of Haraszti on this question at Hankiss's hearing and after in Telehir, November, 1992 and in Beszélö, December 1992. Whatever their original intentions, they did not insist on a law that would, similarly to appointing the judges of the Constitutional Court, have incorporated Parliamentary consensus in the new law. Evidently, they hoped to actualize controls on the executive in the role of the president who was to be a member of their own party. But, given the

Nevertheless, given the fact that the president is supposed to be above and independent of political parties and to represent the unity of the nation, his inclusion in the appointments process did incorporate the notion of some kind of important limit on the executive. In other words, the Prime Minister would need to achieve consensus, if not with other parties, than with a fully independent public official, the head of state. If one denies such an intention, one would have to maintain that the Opposition in parliament gave away important prerogatives to the ruling parties and especially to the Government for absolutely no concessions at all. Moreover, one would have to deny the existence of the justification appended to the law which includes the phrase "the right of appointment must be taken from the government and given to the president".

Even if the Court wished to deny the role of original intent, was it right to disregard the "justification" appended to the law which even the majority did not object to at that time? Finally, while it is possible to derive the requirement of consensus among parties from Article 61(4) of the Constitution only in terms of specifying voting on the law of appointments (a matter of 2/3 majority), one cannot derive such a consensus requirement being the necessary content of the law. Nevertheless, one can derive the legitimacy of an incentive to the minority being incorporated in the law itself.

At a minimum, such incentive is the full *participation* of the president in appointing and dismissing, and it is this incentive that is incorporated in the justification whose stated principle is the freedom of the press. The Court may be right in arguing that no such political solution or incentive can by itself realize the principle in question. But it is wrong to dismiss the possible contribution that consensus can make in defending the freedom of the press. The inclusion of a 2/3 majority requirement in passing a media law (Paragraph 4) in the Constitutional article on the freedom of expression and press (Article 61) indicates the opposite perspective.

To conclude this argument, had the Court actually considered the constitutional-based Appointments Law, it ought to have come to the conclusion that since the law incorporates consensus, either its own definition of the appointment role of the president ought to be expanded to incorporate the option indicated by the law, or the law ought to be declared unconstitutional in terms of Article 30 of the

---

form of election of the president actually provided for, such an outcome would be an exceptional one!

Constitution. If, in other words, the Court had come to the inescapable conclusion that for example because of the absence of political responsibility the president cannot play a substantive role in making appointments, it might have been better to declare the law that provided for such a role unconstitutional instead of rewriting it in such a way that the intention behind it, its stated justification, and the constitutional principle behind it were all subverted.[32]

Of course, this option was the least desirable of all to the initiators of judicial review. And one cannot, of course, exclude the possibility that the Court could have come up with some other alternative than either accepting the President's claims or declaring the law unconstitutional even after considering the status of the Appointments Law. But not considering the relevant law at all, given its constitutionally based status, simply short circuited the process of constitutional review.

---

[32]   A point argued over and over again with much force by the court majority, but disputed by Justice Kilényi who asked why the legal responsibility of the president as defined under Article 31(A) of the Constitution and his delayed political responsibility (if he can still stand for reelection) should not be considered an equally strong form of responsibility given the fact that the members of government and the prime minister do not themselves have legal responsibility of the same form of that of the president.

Case No. 765/G/1992/3, supra note 3, at 13-14. Formally Kilényi's argument is strong, but he forgot that in reality if 50% + 1 of the deputies have another candidate for prime minister, the prime minister is removed and continues to have normal legal responsibility in the courts for his acts. The president on the other hand can be removed only through the vote of 2/3 of the deputies plus the majority of the Constitutional Court, before his ordinary legal responsibility may be assessed or reviewed. Thus, there is a weaker set of constraints on him, justified as long as he is much weaker in power. It is another matter, however, whether one can derive from this state of affairs the inability of the president to fully share the power of appointments in specific instances. Here, I agree with the thrust of Kilényi's argument.

CHAPTER IV

THE MEDIA AND THE POLITICAL ARENA

THE HUNGARIAN MEDIA WAR OF INDEPENDENCE

by Elemér Hankiss

I.   Introduction

It is better to have a war of words and political strategies centered around the media than to have a war fought with tanks and guns in the fields. And it is better to have public television fighting for its independence than to have one which has accepted, and resigned itself to dependence. In this light, the Media War in Hungary, which has been fiercely fought for two years, may be considered as a sign of relative peace and maturity. At the same time, it is the exception that does not make the rule. One has to be careful, though, with the use of the word "normal" in the East-Central European context. This region has such a long history of absurdities and abnormalities that one is frequently at a loss to know what the words normal and abnormal really mean. If one wants to understand, for instance, contemporary developments in East-Central Europe one has to take into account a bewilderingly wide gamut of facts. History, and the last four decades, may, at least partly, explain also what has happened in the field of the media in the last two years.

The gentle revolution brought to East-Central Europe the long expected freedom of the press. At the same time, however, in most of these countries it has not liberated the electronic media, public television and radio, from the control of those in political power. There has been, of course, a substantial change in the character and intensity of control, but the fact remains that in most of these countries public television is government television or presidential television, according to the political system in the countries in question. Changes in government have been routinely followed by changes in the leadership of public television. In most cases, one of the first steps of new prime ministers and presidents has been to replace the old television leaderships and new staffs by new ones with loyalties to the new government. This seems to be the norm in present day East-Central Europe.

A. Sajó (ed.), Rights of Access to the Media, 243-257.
© 1996 Kluwer Law International. Printed in the Netherlands.

Hungary was, in many ways, a happy and unhappy exception for more than two years. It entered the process of transformation with a different and better legacy than most of its neighbors. A couple of other East-Central European countries, too, began to experiment with economic and political reforms already in the late 1950's or 1960's. But these processes were halted, and even reversed, in Czechoslovakia in August 1968 and were interrupted in Poland in 1981, while in Hungary, the changes continued, with temporary setbacks, throughout the 1970's and 1980's. Czechoslovakia was frozen in its sclerotic communist regime until the moment of revolution in November 1989. In Poland, a major confrontation developed between the communists party and Solidarity in the late 1980's and this political confrontation absorbed most of the energies of the country until mid-1989.

In Hungary, important economic reforms had been implemented already in the early 1980's, (opening the field, for instance, for small scale enterprises). In the late 1980's, well before the revolution, some basic institutions of the market economy were established by the communist Parliament. In addition, the disintegration and inner pluralization of the communist party went farther in Hungary than in any other East-Central European Country. It was there that the younger and more dynamic generations of the communist oligarchy discovered, earlier than anybody else in the region, the possibility and need to "convert" their political power into economic assets to prepare themselves for their new roles in the emerging market economy. Having discovered this escape-route, they were able to open the country politically and, by engaging in a dialogue with the opposition groups, managed the smoothest transition to a democratic polity in the region.

Hungary, with her deeply divided communist party, and well articulated opposition forces had a better chance in 1989 and 1990 to establish a pluralistic, multi-party parliamentary system. It was further luck that at the general elections in March and April 1990, none of the parties got a decisive majority. Even the governing coalition won only a slight majority in Parliament. All these factors together contributed to the establishment of multi-party parliamentary machinery in Hungary. This situation and, on the other hand, the slower than expected pluralization of the Hungarian polity and society in general, led to what has been called in Hungary, the Media War.

In those countries in which, after the collapse of the communist regime, a dominant party, or a dominant personality, came to power, public television and radio could not escape government or presidential control. This was, or has been the case in Czechoslovakia, Poland, Romania, Bulgaria, Serbia, Croatia, and Slovenia.

There were good and bad reasons for exercising control over the media. Among the good, let me mention that the extremely difficult process of transition to democracy and market economy calls for common goals, national unity, and broad national support of government plans and policies. For the success of a strategy of national unity, television and radio are indispensable. In several, if not in most of the cases people appointed to top jobs in the television and radio companies sincerely believed, and some of them still believe, that their duty is to serve, or at least to help, the government. In Hungary this was not the case.

II. The Background

The first free elections since 1947 were held in Hungary in March and April 1990. After the elections, the MDF (Hungarian Democratic Forum), the main governing party, having only a slight majority, had to make a pact with the strongest opposition party, the SzDSz (Association of the Free Democrats). One of the first points in this pact was that they would pick two independent persons to be the presidents of Hungarian Television and Hungarian Radio. This was not an easy task since in the buoyant years of 1988-1989, and in the heat of the 1990 electoral campaign, few people could resist the temptation to jump headlong into party politics. Rising to the position of a leading politician became almost overnight the most glamorous and attractive social role. This could bring one not only power but also fame, prestige, and a new identity after so many years spent in anonymity if not in anomia.

It was in this situation that in June 1990, after the elections, the prime minister and the leader of the main opposition party came to us (both my friend, Mr. Csaba Gombár and I were political scientists teaching at the University of Budapest) and offered us these jobs. They told us that we had been proposed as two independent candidates. We were supposed to be able to keep a middle course between the governing parties and the opposition and ensure the impartiality of the two media institutions. At that time, in the post revolutionary euphoria, all the parties seriously believed in the sanctity of the freedom of the press. They did not know yet how annoying the practice of this freedom would soon become for many of them.

For several weeks we said no. Finally, we gave in and told them that we would accept the nomination under the condition that the law regulating the appointment of the public media presidents would change. During the communist regime, the Council of Ministers had the right to appoint the presidents of the Radio and Television (under the almost overt and imperative control of the Party Politburo). We made it clear that we would not accept the appointment from the hands of the Prime Minister because we did not want to be dependent in any way on him or on the Government. Our point was accepted and the law changed overnight. According to this new law, only the Prime Minister had the right to nominate his candidates, who, after hearings in a Parliamentary Committee, were, or were not, appointed by the President of the Republic of Hungary.

Even with this amendment, we accepted these positions only for six months, or more precisely until a new media law would be passed. This was in July 1990. More than two years passed from this date and there was still no media in Hungary. Instead, we had a Media War.

After our appointment in August 1990, the honeymoon (if there was any) with the governing parties came to a quick and early end. They realized very quickly that they had picked the wrong persons. The Government's biggest mistake was that they forgot or ignored the fact that we, too, suffered from a disease which was widespread among East-European intellectuals in the four decades of communism. It was an uncomfortable giddiness, a feeling of lightness, of weightlessness, a feeling of uncertainty about ourselves. We also faced the fear that one day we could be called to account for the seriousness of our ideas.

We were suddenly asked to prove that we had opposed communism in our writings, discussions, and books, for almost four decades. We were also called upon to demonstrate that the idea of justice and democracy, civic courage and tolerance, truth and freedom, were more than mere words and intellectual frivolities. That, instead of speaking only about them, we could live up to this ideas. In 1989, the moment of truth finally came. This was a happy and slightly alarming surprise. We had to prove the integrity and consistency of our ideas and actions.

On the one hand, this was an easy task since we were convinced that the freedom of the press and the independence of the public media from any political or governmental influence was one of the main imperatives of a democratic polity. Therefore, we acted accordingly. On the other hand, the situation may have prompted us to embark on a potentially quixotic experience.

For two and a half years, Hungarian Television and Radio were the most independent public media not only in East-Central Europe but also in Europe as a whole. And this was not a pure blessing. Due to the new law regulating the election and appointment of the public media presidents and also to the absence of a new

Media law, which would have created a good balance between the independence of these situations and their social control, the two newly elected presidents had virtually absolute control over their institutions. Anecdotally, one might almost say that if we had decided to transform our institutions into, say, shoe factories, it would have been quite difficult to legally stop us from doing so.

Actually, we set out in a less (or more) absurd direction. We made an attempt to transform these formerly party controlled institutions into European public television and radio companies, with a high level of public responsibility, impartial news and current affairs programs, and a wide range of educational, cultural and entertaining programs. We did and did not succeed. We did succeed, because by 1992, our programming could already stand its ground against most European public televisions in spite of a much weaker financial background. But, on the other hand, we failed because after more than two years of successful resistance, we have finally been defeated by party politics.

This was not a big surprise since almost all the power was on the other side throughout the Media War. The governing parties and the Government used all their legislative and executive means. Though we, too, had some protection and some important partners. We could, first of all, rely on the letter and spirit of the law. Second, in the course of the Media War, we were more and more supported by the greater and, in my opinion, better part of the written press and by the parties in the opposition. And, last but not least, we had the power of being independent. Our adversaries knew our positions. We did not want to accumulate power for ourselves. We could not be blackmailed or intimidated into any bad compromise or conformity.

III. The Facts

Let me begin with a *caveat*. I have been one of the actors of this conflict and so my report is necessarily and inevitably biased. I am going to list the main steps and developments of the conflict. However, I am sure that even these facts would be seen, or at least interpreted, in a different light and a different way by those people who have stood on the other side of this conflict, namely the Government and the governing parties, and mainly the populist-nationalist right wings of these parties.

People at the other side would certainly emphasize that they have been for the freedom of the press at least as much as we have been and that the Government was forced, by various factors - among them our misbehavior - to curb the autonomy of Hungarian Television and Radio. I have no reason to question the sincerity of the Government, or at least that of the Prime Minister, Mr. Antall, when he spoke of his dedication to freedom of the press. For forty years, freedom of the press was a Holy Grail to be attained for all of us who were in the opposition of the communist regime. And it is beyond doubt than in the euphoric months around the first free elections, in early 1990, most of the new politicians, as a matter of course, supported freedom of the press, including freedom for the electronic media. It would have been an anathema and an unacceptable absurdity on the part of any of the parties in the electoral campaign to propose control of the media by the future government.

The question of who is responsible for starting the Media War is still a controversial issue. According to the Government the main responsibility lies with the written press, which, sympathizing with the opposition, launched a wholesale attack against it and against anything the Government did or failed to do in the first days of its being in office. In this situation they were forced to find a solution. First, they tried to establish a pro-Government press, or at least some newspapers and weeklies sympathetic to the Government. After the failure of this attempt, they turned toward the two great electronic media and began to lobby for an increase from them. Since these media were, according to the Government, controlled by former socialists turned liberals, it was justified, even in the name of freedom of the press, to extend a kind of government control over them, to force them to achieve a better balance in their reporting.

According to the opposition parties, all this was unfounded accusation and empty rhetoric to conceal the efforts of the Government and of the governing parties to concentrate all power in their hands and to extend a direct political control over the electronic media. And to do so in order to be able build up an authoritarian type of democracy and, by winning the next elections, establish themselves as a permanent coalition of dominant parties.

I believe that, on the one hand, the liberal press was, biased against the Government in the first months of the new regime and throughout 1990. Since mid-1991, however, the best organs of the press had become more and more neutral and impartial. By 1992, they had reached a relatively high professional quality. As far as Hungarian Television and Radio were concerned, I think that they were less biased against the Government than the written press. Their programs had been well balanced between various political forces since early 1991 (in spite of the survival of some pro-government and pro-opposition programs). It was the fault of the

Government and the governing coalition that they could not profit from the openness of these two institutions. It was simply a cynical strategy when they justified their attack against these two institutions by the alleged pro-opposition bias of these institutions.[1]

The fact, however, that in the last months of the conflict, the Government lost its patience and invaded the realm of public television and radio before a court could have ruled whether it had the right to do so, was not the most serious offense it committed. It did real harm by destroying the autonomy of two important public institutions in a country, and in a region, which were kept in a semi-colonial and backward state by centuries of authoritarian rule, bureaucracy and centralization. By reinforcing this destructive East-European tradition, instead of helping development of a pluralistic democracy of interactive autonomous institutions, the Government has, in my opinion, dangerously slowed down the post-1989 process of democratic transformation in Hungary.

I may be mistaken, but, nevertheless, I shall interpret and assess the facts and developments of the Media War in the light of this conviction.

IV.   The Events

July 1990. The two media presidential candidates were proposed by the Prime Minister and after being unanimously approved by the Cultural Committee of the Parliament, they were appointed by the President of the Republic.

December 1990. Conflicts with the governing parties and the Government began. Government politicians did not see any "guarantees" in the persons I had appointed to lead positions in Hungarian Television. They cut our budget subsidy by half.

From January 1991 on. We began the radical reorganization of our institution with the aim of transforming it from a rigid bureaucratic state institution into a modern

---

[1]   The Hungarian government is not the only government in Europe, including the western part of the continent, which has made successful or unsuccessful attempts at extending its control over the public media. And I have to admit that in the first two years of the conflict - in which the Hungarian government observed the legal regulations of the country and tried to win the Media War by the help of the legal means - used by some of its western counterparts.

250

and flexible television company, which operated like a commercial television station in its organization and management, but kept its public values and duties intact. Right wing groups and the governing parties began to attack us on various counts. For instance, we were criticized for:

a) "Commercializing" national television.

> **The fact:** We quickly developed our commercial activities, founded a joint company with one of the world's greatest media agencies and doubled our income from publicity in a year (so we could survive in spite of the budget cuts, to the dismay of our Governmental adversaries).

b) "Americanizing" national television.

> **The fact:** We began to screen the episodes of "Dallas" and other American television series. But the proportion of Hungarian and European made productions has remained much higher in our programming than in most European public televisions.

c) Allowing our journalists and programs to be overly critical of the Government.

> **The fact:** In the first month after the elections in 1990, this was at least partly true. In the first half of 1991, however, our programming was already well balanced, with some pro-government and pro-opposition programs still remaining.

d) Reorganizing the institution and thus ruining the old production workshops.[2]

> **The fact:** We dismantled the big departments of the old institution and replaced them with a number of small production units which

---

[2]   As a result, we allegedly jeopardized the dominance of Hungarian national cultural values in the programs.

had to compete for the production orders of the two channels. This outcry came from those who lost their departments and the power which they had under the communists and who were now sailing under nationalist and pro-government flags.

From April 1991 on. The Prime Minister, supposedly under the pressure of the right wing of his party, began to propose various persons for vice-presidents for Hungarian Television and Radio (with the less and less veiled intention to have somebody there through whom the Government *could exert* its influence over these institutions).

From May 1991 on. Government experts excavated an old decree of 1974 (Directive No. 1047/1974) of the communist Council of Ministers. This directive gave the Council the right to "supervise" Hungarian Television. The Prime Minister used this anachronistic decree as one of his main instruments or weapons in the ensuing Media War.

November 1991. I started a new evening news program to counterbalance the increasingly right-wing tendencies of the existing news programs. In the budget debate in December, the Government punished us by practically cutting all our budget subsidy.

March 1, 1992. The Prime Minister finally succeed in forcing new vice-presidents on the two public media institutions.

March 3, 1992. I suspended my vice-president from his position in Hungarian Television. This led to a long and passionate legal controversy between the Prime Minister and myself.

May and June 1992. Not being able to win the legal controversy, the Prime Minister proposed to the President of the Republic, to dismiss me and my colleague at Hungarian Radio, Mr. Gombár, from our positions. After hearings in a parliamentary committee, the President rejected the proposal.

August 1992. Mr. Csurka, vice-president of the MDF (Hungarian Democratic Forum), published his ill-famed pamphlet in which he drew the outlines of a vaguely populist and nationalist ideology and program, with xenophobic and anti-modernist overtones. This made the nationalist versus European, and conservatives versus liberals controversy even more passionate and absurd. In Mr. Csurka's mythology there was a Judeo-Bolshevik-liberal-cosmopolitan conspiracy against the Hungarian nation. Mr. Gombár and myself, were unmasked by him or some of his followers as chief agents of this conspiracy.

September 1992. Hunger-strikes were staged by nationalists against me and my colleague at Hungarian Radio. Right-wing groups also organized demonstrations against the President of the Republic, my colleague Mr. Gombár and myself in the streets of Budapest. A crowd of about 15,000 men requested my resignation in my favorite square in front of the Hungarian Television building. A week after, a counter-demonstration of about 60,000 people protested against these attacks and supported human rights and basic democratic values.

September and October 1992. I dismissed the editor in chief of the main news program (a former party secretary who became the mouthpiece of nationalist and populist forces) and the editor in chief of our main foreign news magazine (a former member of the communist party presidium in Hungarian Television, who, after 1989, became the untouchable hero of the nationalist forces in Hungary). Mr. Gombár took similar steps at the Hungarian Radio a few weeks earlier.

November and December 1992. Retaliating, the Prime Minister started a disciplinary procedure against me and later, suspended me from my post. I protested immediately and questioned his right to initiate such a procedure and to suspend me since, in my reading, he was and could not be my employer. (Such a dependency would be against the law and would jeopardize the freedom of the press.) I then brought a suit against the Office of the Prime Minister for this, according to me, illegal action. The first trial was held and postponed in February 1993.

December 1992. In the debate over the 1993 budget, the parliamentary majority voted a paragraph into the Law according to which the budgets of Hungarian Television and Radio were incorporated into the budget of the Prime Minister's Office as of January 1, 1993.

December 27, 1992. The media bill collapsed in Parliament.

January 6, 1993. Together with Mr. Gombár, we submitted a letter to the President of the Republic asking him to relieve us of our office. He did not accept our request.

March 6, 1993. According to the Prime Minister, with our "resignation", we ceased to be the presidents of these two institutions. According to the President of the Republic we did not resign, or if we did, he had not yet accepted our resignation. We were placed in the absurd and slightly comic situation of being and not being the presidents of these two institutions.

As I have just mentioned, on the 6th of January 1993, Mr. Gombár and I wrote a letter to the President of the Republic asking him to relieve us of our duties as presidents of these two public media institutions. We gave the following reasons: first, after the failure of the media bill in Parliament in December 1992, and with no conceivable hope of the enactment of a new bill until the general election in 1994, we felt ourselves exempt from our promise to stay until a media law was passed; second, when our institutions lost their financial independence with the new Budget Law, they lost their hard-won autonomy. Instead, the public media institutions once again become an East-European, government-controlled state media. Third, we did not want to assist in the destruction of two of the most important autonomous institutions in our new democracy.

The Prime Minister eagerly jumped on the opportunity. In his letter of January 20 he wrote us that he accepted our "resignation" and entrusted the two vice presidents with running the two institutions. Next day, on the 21st of January, the President of the Republic issued a statement according to which: (i) we did not resign, (ii) it was the President's *exclusive right* to accept or not to accept our request to be dismissed, (iii) if the Prime Minister proposed our dismissal, and that was his sole right, then (iv) the President would consider the proposal and would make his decision in due time.

It was absurd that Mr. Gombár and I were forced to decide whether the President of the Republic or the Prime Minister was right. And it would have been nonsensical and cruel if each of our several thousand colleagues, managers, producers, cameramen, editors, security guards, cleaning women and others had been forced to decide day by day whom to obey: us, or the new men delegated by the Government.

We did not want to involve our innocent colleagues into this ordeal and we did not want to get entangled in a hopelessly vicious and degrading squabble with the Government's men. Having pondered all the pros and cons, we published an open letter on the 20th of January, in which we explained our dilemma. We stated that we considered ourselves the lawful presidents of these institutions but would not exercise our rights until the President of the Republic and the Prime Minister, or the Parliament, or the Constitutional Court had resolved our status.

V.   The Rules of the Game

There were several episodes in the Media War which may be of some interest for those who study the situation and the role of the media in the process of democratization in East-Central Europe. One among them were the parliamentary hearings of the two presidents in mid-1992.

As it has been mentioned already, the Prime Minister, when he saw that legally he could not prove and win his case, looked for direct political ways and means to bring me and my colleagues at the Hungarian Radio to our knees. In May 1992, he asked the Cultural Committee of the Parliament to investigate our "ability" to run these two institutions. Having a Government majority in this Committee, he did not take too of a much risk.

Mr. Gombár and I chose different strategies. Gombár went to his hearing and read a short statement saying that he did not accept the authority of the Committee because it was not a neutral body, - and walked out. *Scandal.* The next week, I walked in with five experts and thousands of documents and announced that I was happy to be there and to be able to discuss important matters with distinguished politicians. *Hilarity.* But, I added, "I shall force you to take these hearings seriously, since parliamentary hearings in a decent democracy should be taken seriously. I shall make your lives miserable in the coming days. I shall do my best to make it very difficult for you to pass judgment without considering the facts, figures and proofs which I shall submit to you." And the hearings lasted for thirty hours in three long days.

During the hearings, deputies from the governing parties first argued that I had not observed some rules and laws in the course of the transformation and management of Hungarian Television. When we proved that they were wrong, they tried to convince the public, and themselves, that Hungarian Television did not serve enough the interests of the Hungarian nation, that it had become too international, Americanized, commercialized, "anti-magyar". When we proved with figures, statistics, analyses that the contrary was true, they finally lost their temper, swept all the documents, figures, proofs, pieces of evidence off the table and retreated to the *ultima ratio* of party politicians: "We, the governing parties, have lost confidence in you and this is a sufficient reason to propose your dismissal even without any further facts, proofs, or arguments."

It was an interesting exercise in learning about democracy. It was almost moving to see how governing party deputies, or at least some of them, struggled with their conscience. To see how they tried to squeeze their party interests (and their antipathies for this meddlesome president) into the forms and strait jacket of legal rules. By that time, almost the whole country was watching.

Those who watched may have understood, for the first time in their lives, that democracy was not an abstract construct of a couple of sublime ideas but simply and very prosaically a well defined set of rules of the game. They realized that a democratic polity needs well-defined rules agreed upon by all the interested parties and the willingness of its citizens to observe these rules even if their momentary interests would be better served by breaking these rules. Hundreds of people have admitted, and hundreds of thousands would certainly agree, that these hearings were an elevating and traumatic experience for them.

Half a year later, in January 1993, the same ceremony was repeated but, by this time, without the respectable personal drama of some of the participants. By that time, after having been more than two years in office, government politicians seemed to have lost their former timidity and chastity. They seemed to have realized more and more that they were *in power*. With the national congress of the MDF approaching, they went out of their way to prove their unrelenting patriotism to the forces of the right. In the disciplinary procedure started against me, the Prime Minister appointed the Minister of Justice as commissioner and three other ministers as members of the disciplinary committee. After making, with lordly nonchalance, one legal and formal mistake after the other, they played the cynical comedy of a formal trial to the end.

A real scandal resounded in the country. The minutes of the trial were published (in a form and under circumstances reminiscent of the good old days of samizdats) and they became a best seller overnight; in one of the theaters of Budapest actors read passages of it with the audience roaring with laughter and indignation; the Media War turned into a kind of tragi-comedy.

Some of the journalists went so far as to label the procedure the "first show trial" since the free elections in Hungary in 1990. This was, of course, a metaphor which stretched similarities far too far. It is true that the whole process was motivated by the political will to get rid of the presidents of the Television and Radio. It is true that the whole case was prefabricated and the judgment had been passed before the trial. It is true that the disciplinary committee passed judgment without considering the hundreds of facts and pieces of evidence that proved the innocence of the defendant, etc. But everything else was different. All this took place in a democracy, in 1993, and not in a dictatorship in 1953. The stakes were much lower. Instead of the hangman, cheering crowds and sympathizing journalists greeted the condemned who appealed the verdict and stated that they would go to Strasbourg, to the European Court of Human Rights, if they did not find a truly independent court of appeal in Hungary.

VI.   Lessons Learnt

It is too early to judge the social impact of the Media War but it may have been quite substantial since this conflict became a major political confrontation already in the second half of 1991 and remained one of the most publicized political issues throughout 1992 and early 1993. In their stubborn fight for autonomy, Hungarian Television and Radio became the major actors of a society protesting against the centralizing and authoritarian efforts of the Government. The country was watching, with fears and hopes, the ups and downs of this conflict between the Davids of television and radio and the governmental Goliath. It was, I think, an exciting show, full of important lessons for those who watched and who wanted to understand.

After 1989 it came as an uneasy surprise how difficult it is to be a democrat... in democracy. This was a real surprise since it had been comparatively easy to be a would-be democrat in a dictatorship. After 1989 we have had to learn that democracy cannot be imported, it cannot be bought off the peg. And that it is not brought about and established overnight by a first and single free election. It may be generated only in the course of a long and tedious learning process in which everybody has to take part and has to take up his or her responsibilities. The fact that we have a government responsible to Parliament does not mean that everybody else is relieved of all responsibilities. That we can go on living in the Heaven and Hell of childish irresponsibilities which we enjoyed, and suffered from, in the four decades of communism. When it was easy and legitimate to blame the communists for everything miserable in our lives. The Media War may have shown to many that there is no democracy without citizens acting with responsibility and, if necessary, civil courage.

I have tried to show that, in spite of all the negative effects, Hungarian society has also profited from the Media War. Let me add that the very existence of a Media War proves the relative strength of the emerging democratic polity in this country. The fact that two fragile public institutions, which could rely only on the letter and spirit of the law, were able to protect their newly won autonomy against extremely strong pressures and attacks coming from the side of the Government and the governing parties, proves that all the main political actors observed, at least until the last act, the rule of law and have accepted the basic rules of the democratic game. Including one of the most important rules or principles: that in a democracy interests can be achieved only within the framework of laws and rules that have been accepted by the community.

A "war" that proves the strength of democracy: this is another example of those absurdities which characterize the region called East-Central Europe. It is one of those absurdities from which, I assume, people living in less absurd societies may also learn a few lessons.

THE DEVELOPMENT OF RIGHTS OF ACCESS TO THE MEDIA: THE ROLE OF MEDIA IN LUSTRATION

by Jan Kavan

I.

It is a truism that the collapse of the communist governments in 1989 did not automatically lead to the emergence of democracy. Equally, the abolition of censorship did not automatically lead to a free and independent press capable of balanced and objective reporting.

An American research team noted a year after the departure of the censors that "the press is mainly an advocacy press, still connected to governments and political parties or factions, rather than being truly independent".[1] In their chapter on the former Czechoslovakia the authors asserted that "press freedom is widely enjoyed". In their evaluation of the quality of the press they stressed "a tendency among journalists to favor commentary over reportage" and acknowledged that "the line between reporting and editorializing, fairly well defined in American journalism, is not so clear for the Czechs".

It seems to me that these observations are still true today. The legal guarantees of the freedom of press have been anchored in the Bill of Human Rights and Freedoms, passed by the Czechoslovak Federal Assembly in January 1991. These legal guarantees as well as an absence of institutions of censorship are crucial preconditions for a genuinely free and independent press, but they do not secure it. I shall try to illustrate some of the problems which still have to be tackled concerning the lustration debate.

The American authors of the above mentioned report thought that one of the problems associated with the emergence of a free press stemmed from the difficult "transition from opinionated, polemical samizdat writing to objective news reporting". It is easy to see why they thought so in early 1990. At that time, books previously published only in "samizdat" were either reprinted or imported from Czech émigré publishers in the West and flooded the market. Former dissident

---

[1] See generally Everette E. Dennis & John Vanden Heuvel, *Emerging Voices: East European Media in Transition*, (Media Center, Columbia University, eds., Oct. 1990).

A. Sajó (ed.), *Rights of Access to the Media*, 259-279.

journalists recounted their experiences in a variety of leading publications. These journalists expressed their opinions on a multitude of conceivable subjects. Today many of these books cannot be sold even at rock-bottom remainder prices. Some of the former dissident journalists are dissidents again. The strong opinions presented as facts in leading dailies and in Television news coverage are frequently expressed by people who under communism cautiously kept their opinions to themselves. Some of them probably did not have the courage to even read the samizdat press.

W.L.Webb, former assistant editor of the English newspaper, *The Guardian* also agreed that the ex-samizdat journalists come from a tradition in which opinions, because heretical, were news-worthy. Webb was also able to point to another tradition which emerged just last year - the tradition of journalists willing to place their pens in the service of those in power. Webb noted that the word "enemy" "plays once again a frequent role in politics". This time it is used against "people linked to communism and the broadly understood left" but also against the social democrats or even the centrist liberals "with their suspicious, "European" talk of pluralism and civil rights".[2]

Former communists, for example from the 1968 Prague Spring, or people with sympathies for the social democrats or other parties left-of-center, (these parties are also comprised of former dissidents) can become targets of a kind of a double resentment. The anti-dissident resentment was described by President Havel in an interview with Adam Michnik, published in *Gazeta Wyborcza* in Poland.[3] However, Havel did not express similar views in his own country Czechoslovakia. Václav Havel drew attention to the:

> "[s]ort of hidden, rather psychological conflict between the so-called dissidents who were in the opposition and put up resistance to the regime, and the new, fresh, juniors who were not in evidence before, and who did not cooperate either with the communists or the opposition... [T]hey consider the opposition fought the communists for so long that they got their own hands dirty during the fight, and their role is now played out. In addition they hold it against the opposition that some of them were previously members of the communist party, in the 50's or 60's, and they hold that all communists are the same, whether from the 60's or the 80's. Meanwhile, public opinion tends to identify with the non-dissident politicians for the simple reason that the majority of people were neither dissidents nor

---

[2]   W.L. Webb, *Press and Politics in East Central Europe: The Fourth Guardian Lecture at Nuffield College*, 12 (Oxford University, 1992).

[3]   Gazeta Wyborcza, Warsaw, December 1, 1991.

members of the [communist] establishment. Such politicians are... closer to them mentally."[4]

Adam Michnik, in his response to Havel's remarks, summarized the conflict unambiguously when he stated that "dissidents are in a way pangs of conscience for people who were conformists and now practice the rhetoric of de-communization".[5]

Today, Michnik's *Gazeta Wyborcza* is in the forefront of the struggle against the new threats to democracy posed by people whom Michnik aptly describes as "anticommunists with Bolshevik mentality".[6] The stubborn intolerance of "the right-wing Bolsheviks" (a term used by Jiří Dienstbier, former Czechoslovak Foreign Minister), a sad, but inevitable legacy of the ancién totalitarian regime presents, in my opinion, a much greater obstacle to the establishment of a genuine free press than the amateurishness of some of the former dissidents, which I do not wish to underestimate.

The high degree of politicization of and the corresponding political polarization of issues, combined with the absence of any experience with a free press for more than half a century helps to solidify a set of approaches and perceptions which are not conducive to bipartisan reporting. A Prague-based American journalist researched the attitudes of her Czech colleagues, who talked to her about "issues they will not cover, politicians they will not antagonize and a latent timorousness toward the government that so far has kept the press from fulfilling its role as the eyes and ears of the people".[7]

Many journalists candidly admitted to her that they view themselves primarily as "citizen-journalists", i.e. as reporters who put their civic duty and the

---

[4]   Id.

[5]   Id.

[6]   One could possibly contend that *Gazeta* leads this struggle not just in Poland but in the whole of Central and Eastern Europe. It may be a source of optimism that *Gazeta* boasts today the largest circulation of all Central and Eastern European newspapers. I find it less optimistic that the runner-up is a daily paper *Blesk*, a Western-financed tabloid paper in the Czech Republic, a country whose population is less than a third that of Poland.

[7]   Michele Kayal, *The Unfinished Revolution: The Czech Republic's Press in Transition*, in "Creating a Free Press in Eastern Europe", The James M. Cox, Jr., Center for International Mass Communications, Training and Research, Henry W. Grady College of Journalism and Mass Communications, The University of Georgia, Athens, Georgia, 1993. p.261.

health of the republic, as they perceive it, before their journalistic freedom and duty to inform. The editor of one of the main dailies acknowledged that reporters "are so personally involved in politics, in what they are living as citizens, that they can't look at the government in [an aggressive] way".[8] In their daily reporting, journalists often tailor their coverage to support a party or goal that they believe works for the "good of democracy".

For example, an economics reporter, Petr Husák, said that he considered it part of his role as a journalist to motivate support for those government's economic reforms which he feels would benefit the country. Thus, if he reported corruption scandals of the privatization process, people might lose interest in the process. Such lack of interest has to be discouraged because privatization is the only good solution for the Czech economy. "Not as a newspaper man, but as a citizen of this country, I want privatization to be successful", stated Husák.[9]

In this context, an assertion by the leader of the Czech Social Democratic Party serves as a further illustration. Mr. Miloš Zeman, elected Social Democratic Party leader in February 1993, told me that at a press conference he made available to the media a list of privatization corruption scandals which his party researched. Not a single example was published.

More ominously, many journalists argue that during this critical transition time, it is necessary to suppress voices that may be hostile to the existing fragile democracy. This reflects what many government politicians believe in but it seems a paradox that journalists would try to ensure democracy - and its most basic element, a free press - by squelching that press.

II.

Such defence of democracy by undemocratic means is further illustrated by many of the arguments employed during the bitter controversy provoked by the "lustration" law, passed by the Czechoslovak parliament in October 1991. The term "lustration" comes from Latin, meaning to "cleanse", "to illuminate". The principal purpose of the law was legitimate and the original motivation for it was clear: to

---

[8]   Id. p.268.

[9]   Id.

find a mechanism which would ensure that those who carried out the repression in the former totalitarian regime, and those who secretly helped them to do so, would not infiltrate the new democratic institutions and sabotage the transition in order to facilitate a reversal of the post-1989 achievements. The lustration law concerned the need to come to terms with the past and the need to understand and know the truth and face one's responsibilities. Furthermore, it purported to do so without resorting to revolutionary tribunals or other forms of revenge.

The lustration law denies certain categories of Czech citizens the right to hold specified public and private positions because of their prior affiliation with certain politically-related organizations. Other citizens could be denied positions because their names were found in the Secret Service archives, allegedly registered there as various kinds of collaborators or because they studied at specific schools in Moscow, etc.

The legalized discrimination would affect only persons in top and influential positions and only for a limited period of five years. Such measures were justified by the need to protect the new and fragile democracy. But such restrictions must be narrowly tailored to further such legitimate objectives and restrict individual rights only to the extent necessary to achieve that objective.

As reported in a detailed submission produced by Helsinki Watch, the International Helsinki Federation for Human Rights and the Center for Human Rights and Humanitarian Law at the Washington College of Law at American University, the lustration law failed to meet these criteria. These organizations argued that the denial of certain public and private positions could not be justified by a need for safeguarding the Czech transition to democracy, for retribution or in order to deny wrongdoers the fruits of ill-gotten gains.

Many people affected by the law were not involved in any activities which represented any threat to democracy. Also, many people guilty of a clear violation of basic human rights and who represented a tangible threat to democracy have not been covered by this law. Furthermore, the law itself violated many Czechoslovak human rights obligations as expressed in the International Covenant on Civil and Political Rights, the International Labor Organization's Discrimination Covenant No.111/1958, the European Convention for the Protection of Human Rights and Fundamental Freedoms and the Treaty of the CSCE as elaborated by the CSCE Vienna and Copenhagen Concluding Documents. The law relied on the prior status of a person and not on the individual's past actions or behavior.

Most importantly, the lustration law legalized collective guilt and the presumption of guilt. It did not allow individual evaluation of a person's guilt and responsibility. It violated the principle that people should not be subject to retroactive justice. The evidence against the subjects is based on incomplete, inaccurate and otherwise unreliable State Secret Police ("StB") files.

In the above mentioned interview with Adam Michnik, President Václav Havel accused the lustration law of being harsh and unjust, of failing to define where justice ends and revenge begins. Havel argued eloquently against such witch-hunts, persecutions, fanaticism and generally against the creation of atmosphere of fear. His words were not published in Czechoslovakia, but Havel expressed his negative attitude to the law, though in more restrained terms, on several public occasions in the country. This led some journalists to suggest that Havel might wish to protect former collaborators. Other journalists reminded people that the problem was created by Havel's original velvet, soft approach to communists immediately after November 1989.

Mr. Jaroslav Bašta, chairman of the former Independent Commission of the Ministry of the Interior empowered to examine the most controversial category of so called "conscious collaborators", drew attention to the fact that the lustration issue was raised:

> "[e]xactly at the moment when Parliament began discussing the responsibility of the communist nomenclature for the state of the country... this was a classic political manoeuver, whereby people's attention was diverted from the main issue to a less important question, which is, however, more attractive and more easily tackled..."[10]

Martin Palouš, the former Deputy Foreign Minister of Czechoslovakia (1990-1992), argued even more explicitly that the lustration law was designed as an instrument of the political struggle not against:

> "[t]he shadows of the past" but against current political opponents. . . . The purpose was to polarize the society, publicly label some people as enemies, enable people to learn who is who, who is against us and who is with us, whose policies are hesitant, unreadable or full of compromises and, on the other hand, who

---

[10]   Drahuše Proboštová's interview with Jaroslav Bašta, in *Práce*, October 29, 1992.

possesses all the rights and all the preconditions (moral and objective) to be entrusted with political power in this society."[11]

Mr. Palouš made these comments during a Prague conference on lustration organized by the Helsinki Citizens' Assembly in the Czech Republic and attended by more than 100 people. The audience listened to presentations by lawyers, human rights activists, journalists and politicians from Czechoslovakia, Poland and Hungary. None of the papers presented at the conference were published in the Czech press or even mentioned in a positive manner.[12] The tendency to perceive problems as conflicts in which there is a recognizable enemy against whom it is justifiable to fight even by unlawful or unethical means, was once again prevalent.

I believe that this adversarial mind set is part of the legacy of totalitarianism. Many of the journalists I spoke to could not imagine that today innocent people could be actively discriminated upon. If, however, they were innocent of things they were accused of, but guilty of disagreeing with the government's chosen method of transition to democracy, then any outrage at a possible injustice became quickly very muted. An opponent is perceived as an enemy. And an enemy has to be treated as an enemy. This approach applies generally, not just to lustration cases.

The 1992 arrest of Mr. Zdeněk Porybný, the editor-in-chief of *Rudé Právo*, on nebulous fraud charges, his short term detention, the search of the newsroom and other politically motivated illegal actions did not raise too many eyebrows. As a former editor of *Lidové Noviny* optimistically asserted "it can't become a habit and it won't once democracy is firmly established".[13]

---

[11] Martin Palouš, *Bez Paměti a svědomí [Without Memory and conscience] in Co Se S Námi Stalo? [What Has Happened to Us?]*, (Helsinki Citizens's Assembly, eds. 1993). This volume is a dossier of contributions to a seminar on lustration organized by the Helsinki Citizen's Assembly in Prague on November 21, 1992. The English version of the brochure was published by the Helsinki Citizens' Assembly in November 1994.

[12] The one exception was a bi-monthly LISTY, transferred to Prague from Rome when it was published since 1971 by Jiří Pelikán, a Czech born member of the European Parliament for the Italian Socialist Party. The current editor is Petr Uhl, who courageously spoke up against the lustration (and defended me) in the Federal Assembly (Parliament).

[13] Kayal, supra note 7.

Incidentally, the terminology used almost daily in the media, for example, in connection with the politicians of the current Communist Party, an established parliamentary party, is designed to leave no doubt in readers" mind as to who is the enemy. It is not really surprising that Martin Weiss of the right-wing *Český Deník* (which means "Czech Daily") uses the term "Bolshevik whores". However, it is disquieting that newscasters on the main television news programs, when, for example, describing formal communist MPs' proposals automatically add adjectives such as "absurd", "pathetic" or "dangerous".

From my own experience, I am familiar with the argument that the truth is unacceptable if it undermines our fragile democracy. I have been accused of being a former collaborator of the Czechoslovak Secret police, the StB. This accusation was levied against me while I was a Member of Parliament in March 1991. This occurred seven months before the lustration law was passed. There were no rules of any kind in existence concerning lustration. I was asked to resign quietly and promised that if I did so my name would not be published and my alleged collaboration [with the former communist regime] would not be exposed.

I refused to resign, quietly or otherwise, and I began to defend myself. As Martin Palouš reminded his listeners in the above mentioned speech, I was primarily reproached for not showing sufficient magnanimity and not accepting that society has to defend itself against the consequences of the past and that there simply was no better, applicable solution. By defending myself I proved to be "selfish" because I, allegedly, placed my "individual interests" above those of the state.

The argument used by my opponents was not that I was wrong or that my arguments were false, but that my defence could discredit government's policies. Thus, I would provide a helping hand to those who would like to reverse the reforms and reintroduce a form of pre-November 1989 communism. I would thus be helping the very people against whom I fought for more than two decades. Surely, I was told, I did not want to do that simply out of a selfish desire to save my own reputation. A similar version of this argument was presented to the public by Mr. Petr Toman, the press spokesperson of the former Parliamentary Commission of November 17. He argued that even if some of the accused members of parliament were innocent they "should resign quietly because to contest the accusation would create doubts about the whole screening process which would help the real agents".[14] This reminded me of the argument used in the 1950's against

---

[14]   Interview with Toman quoted by Andrew Nagorski, *Newsweek*, October 14, 1991.

my father and some other communists accused of being "imperialist agents" by the Stalinists in the leadership of the communist party. The innocent defenders were told to confess in order to help the party punish the *real* enemies. Most of them did so and were then executed for their loyalty.

It was therefore, understandable that I rejected this logic and contested the accusation. I did so not because I think that the transition to democracy is secure and that democracy is no longer fragile. I fought the accusation precisely because I thought that it was still fragile and that it could not afford to be undermined by undemocratic methods, by measures lifted directly from the arsenal of the Stalinists. Unfortunately, however, the Czech media was virtually closed to me. The only journalists prepared to ask me about my side of the story (with the possible exception of *Rudé Právo*, the former communist party daily, now an independent left-wing paper) and to publish my answers were foreign ones, most of them from the West but also from Poland, Bulgaria and elsewhere.

My story received considerable publicity in the West. The Czechoslovak Press Agency ("CTK") under its first post-November Director General Mr. Petr Uhl fairly regularly reported this publicity when it appeared in major newspapers, such as *The New York Times*, *The New Yorker*, the *Times of London*, etc. Czech subscribers invariably ignored these dispatches unless the articles were critical of me.

One of the arguments used against Petr Uhl after he was sacked last year was the fact that CTK mentioned me in about 70 dispatches while an allegedly comparable case of a fellow MP similarly accused was mentioned in only 40 news items. Petr Uhl earned himself a label of the "defender of StB agents".

The author of the attack stressed that Petr Uhl had worked closely with me for years in the dissident times and had defended me in the Parliament. The author declined to mention that the "comparable case" of the other MP was not really comparable. The case concerns a former dissident who did not challenge his accusation in the courts, did not conduct his own public defense and was virtually unknown abroad.

The fact that I was prepared to defend myself abroad when faced with hostile Czech media was also been turned into a strong argument against me. Lawrence Weschler, a leading reporter of the prestigious U.S. magazine, *The New Yorker*, wrote a long article on my case and interviewed for it, among others, Jan

268

Ruml, the current Czech Minister of Interior. Ruml knew me from our dissident days.[15]

Ruml explicitly acknowledged that there was no justification for the media accusations levied against me concerning three alleged incidents which took place between 1981 and 1989. He checked the allegations carefully and rejected each of them. He explained that my case both stands and falls on my conversations with a Czech educational attache in London in 1969-1970. He also admitted that the information I provided this diplomat had zero value.

Nevertheless, Ruml came to the conclusion that I was guilty on two grounds. First, given my intelligence, I must have known, 23 years ago, who the diplomat really was. Second, I was lustrated correctly because by defending myself abroad, I had damaged the interests of the Czechoslovak Republic abroad.[16]

The Czech media found me guilty on the first day that my name was read in the Parliament among ten MP's who had allegedly been registered under various categories as being Secret Service collaborators. This presumption of guilt was, of course, facilitated by the Parliamentary screening commission. This commission did not explain clearly and publicly that being registered as a collaborator did not necessarily mean being a collaborator. The commission was not equipped or empowered to establish the guilt or innocence of individuals. They simply reported names which were registered in the StB's papers. The media, of course, interpreted the commission's findings as a verdict of guilty.

My case proved to be the most controversial and became almost symbolic for the disputes provoked by the lustration process. On the other hand, it soon transpired that the Parliamentary screening commission could not collectively make up its mind on my case. Finally, following a major quarrel on the eve of its public report the commission decided by 6 to 5 vote, to include my name among the denounced MP's. Six months later it transpired that I have been registered under a very controversial category as a "secret service collaborator-confidential contact".

---

[15] Lawrence Wechsler, *The Velvet Purge: The Trials of Jan K*, The New Yorker, October 19, 1992; and Lawrence Wechsler, *From Kafka to Dreyfus*, The New Yorker, November, 1992.

[16] This phrase corresponds to an article in the communist Penal Code under which I was previously accused both before Prague Spring under Novotny's rule as well as under Husak's normalization regime in 70's and 80's.

This meant that I need not have known about my registration and even if I had known, the category meant that I had strong reasons for not collaborating with the Secret Service and was only prepared to be in contact with other official authorities. Furthermore, the category of "secret service collaborator-confidential contact" in which I was the only registered person in the country, did not even exist at the time I was allegedly included in it.

These facts were published only by *Rudé Právo*. Much later, at the end of 1992, the Constitutional Court of Czechoslovakia removed this category from the lustration law as "unconstitutional". It made no difference to the media campaign.

In February 1992, these facts and arguments led the Ministry of Interior to issue me "a negative" lustration certificate. I was cleared, and had a piece of paper signed by the then Federal Minister of Interior Mr. Ján Langoš, in my possession. However, the resulting uproar forced Mr. Langoš to change his mind. He announced reversal a few days later on television thereby violating the lustration law itself. The law explicitly forbids any public revelation of a "positive" finding, especially in a category which was still subject to further evaluation and confirmation by a special commission and even before I was informed personally. His story was disseminated widely, although he gave one explanation for his positive finding in Prague and the very opposite one in Slovakia.[17] My response was not published anywhere.

The gap between the publicity which portrayed me as a dangerous and important agent and the conversations of a 22-year-old student which took place 23 years ago in London began to appear too broad. It had to be filled in. The media obliged.

I have been in contact with the leaders of the Czechoslovak opposition for 20 years. I regularly organized journeys of smuggling foreign literature for them and smuggled their materials to the West. In the 1980's, I even met most of them on three occasions during my clandestine trips to Prague, when I used my British passport and an assumed name. I facilitated contacts between the Czech opposition and many opposition groups in the other East-European countries, especially in Poland, Hungary and the former East Germany. I also facilitated contacts between Charter 77 and the anti-Soviet section of the West European peace movement between 1983 and 1989. I was a member of the Labor Party and my views critical

---

[17] Compare the statement by Ján Langoš published by ČSTK on February 27, 1992 and an interview conducted by Luboš Homolka with Ján Langoš and published in the Slovak newspaper *SMER, Banská Bystrica*, on April 7, 1992.

of Thatcherism and shock therapy were quite well known. If my alleged collaboration with the StB extended beyond my 1969-70 conversations with the Embassy's education officer into two subsequent decades, or at least if it could have been presented as such by the media to the public, then it would have been possible to use my case to discredit the majority of leading Czech dissidents especially those with left of center views.

The official accusation lodged against me could not include any such allegations. Even the courts in their difficult and traumatic phase would have dismissed them and exposed the pathetic motivations behind such accusations. The official accusation thus remained restricted solely to the above mentioned conversations on student affairs with the Czech education officer.

However, some right-wing journalists began to speculate about my situation and to present their speculations as facts. Soon they were assisted by the leak of my StB file, still highly confidential, to some of my political opponents and to their journalist friends. Extracts taken out of context and some even wilfully distorted were published. Further absurd speculation was encouraged. Despite the fact that the law was grossly violated, the source of the leak was never discovered and the publication and distortion of confidential information was not even criticized, let alone prevented. My demands for a right of reply were ignored.

The most outrageous and libelous accusations were published in the weekly *RESPEKT* which, in 1991, received the U.S. World Press Review international award for promotion of freedom of press and for defense of human rights and for professional journalist work. In its desperate attempt to argue that I must have been collaborating even during the 1980's, *RESPEKT* even suggested that there were "suspicious circumstances" surrounding the seizure of one of my smuggling vans, (the only one of my vans ever caught) in April 1981. The magazine made this criticism despite the fact that the name of the person who betrayed the van had been established and I had been cleared of any suggestion of negligence, let alone any wrongdoing.

Furthermore, the journal quoted an alleged extract from my StB file which suggested that I was in contact with the StB in 1978. The extract was willfully distorted to convey the very opposite meaning then that of its original form. In its original form, the document proved that I was under surveillance in London as "an enemy person" and specially targeted by a StB agent. The then chief editor of the journal, Mr. Ivan Lamper, however, refused to publish my detailed and documented response as well as responses written by other former dissidents who were outraged by the publication of such lies.

This example is only the very top of the pyramid of similar experiences which I had with other media, especially with television. And television is undoubtedly the most popular and influential media. Unlike in the West, in this region, roundtable political debates enjoy consistently high viewer rating figures. In the most popular of such programs, "What the week served" (in Czech, "Co týden dal"), Mr. Petr Toman, the former spokesperson of the parliamentary lustration commission, was encouraged by the moderator, Mr. Otakar Černý, to talk about me as if I was already a convicted StB collaborator. Toman also quoted with impunity from confidential StB files as if their contents were authenticated evidence. My requests for a correction or for the right of reply were ignored.

On another occasion, while I was still a Member of Parliament, the television news team recorded an interview with me but then they transmitted just a fraction of it (the rigors of editing and time constraints are known equally well in the West). In the process, the news reporters slandered and denigrated my words. Furthermore, they added several comments from prominent politicians who simply stated that I had lied without bothering to mention any evidence for such assertions. The recorded statement by one of my supporters, Dr. Jaroslav Šabata, then a Minister in the Czech government, was pared down to few toothless words.

The tradition that TV is controlled by the state and influenced by the "leading political party" is established firmly in the minds of both politicians and the majority of television viewers. It will be very difficult to tackle. The ray of the hope that a commercial channel would be able to provide a freer alternative has yet shone very persuasively.[18] Only *Rudé Právo* and on one occasion the trade union daily

---

[18]   There is, for example, speculation about the criteria used for the selection of an American company which was allocated a nationwide franchise for the only commercial television channel which commenced transmission in 1994. (A special commission for broadcasting elected by the Parliament and chaired by a member of the Civic Democratic Alliance ("ODA"), one of the ruling coalition parties, awarded this lucrative franchise to a US-financed company, CET 21.)
Among the new television station's Czech bosses are people known for their sympathies to ODA. ODA received in 1993 alone, gifts and donations of up to 60 million Czech crowns, most of them from abroad. ODA refused to identify the donors, although the law demands such disclosure.
A report in *Rudé Právo* suggested that among the ODA's donors one might find the U.S.-based Central European Development Corp ("CEDC"). CEDC is a consortium of US financiers who invest in Central European countries. They have, for example, invested in five Hungarian newspapers, a major Hungarian bank and trade firm Novotrade, and Estonian cement works. In the Czech Republic it controls

Práce, were prepared to publish interviews with me. Other papers did not dare publish my own words. Some, at least showed restraint, and did not publish the unverified slander which appeared in the newspapers known for their staunch support for the lustration law.

I have spoken with a number of Czech journalists. Some did not want to antagonize their chief editors, as happened to some of those who argued in my defense. Some former dissidents did not want to be labelled as "friends/defenders of StB agents". Non-dissident journalists did not wish some modern-day jacobins to rummage in the cupboards of their past.

Some members of the Parliamentary Screening Commission were dismayed by the good publicity my case received in the West. Therefore, in December 1991, they broke the law and showed my StB file to a U.S. broadcast journalist. The Commission even played a videocassette which had nothing to do with the accusations levelled against me. The videotape had been secretly filmed in November 1989 when the StB interrogated me in their villa shortly after my return to Prague (and following my 12-hour interrogation at the airport). A few seconds from the videocassette were later aired on Czech TV and described it as a "friendly meeting" between me and StB officers. (Since then, of course, still illegally, my entire StB file was smuggled to the West and sold to a British TV journalist).

In December 1991, a World Monitor television correspondent disclosed to more than 25 Prague reporters at a press conference that he videotaped members of the Parliamentary Commission displaying for him my confidential StB documentation. Only one - a journalist - accepted this offer and went to see the video and then wrote about it. He soon stopped because - as he later explained to Michele Kayal - "I didn't want to put a gun into the hand of the ones who say that *Rudé Právo* is attacking the government . . . [and our reporters are] plotters who were preparing to discredit the commission."[19]

No other newspaper picked it up, but when returned to the story a month later, when journalist Jan Urban obtained the documentary evidence, commission

---

majority shares in CET 21. (Rudé Právo, November 19 and 20, 1993.)

[19]   Kayal, supra note 7.

members and other politicians reacted fiercely.[20] Urban explained that his editors made it clear they wanted the issue dropped and so he dropped it.

There was one article published in the West in *The Observer*, an English newspaper, that was critical of me.[21] It has been quoted extensively in the Czech media. My reply which *The Observer* published the following week was, of course, ignored. The Czech media did not mention articles which argued in my favor, including the unprecedented major coverage in *The New Yorker*. At the same time, a CTK correspondent in New York filed a brief story which the media did not pick up.

I regarded the CTK dispatch as fairly objective, being used to some of the really vicious and slanderous coverage in Prague newspapers. The American author, Lawrence Weschler, disagreed and complained to Radio Free Europe ("RFE") that:

> [T]he report concentrated on my [Wechsler's] interview with Jan Ruml and create[d] the impression that I regard him as an authority and that I agree with his opinions. That is not the case. Furthermore it conveyed the impression that I have washed my hands and am doubtful about Kavan's case. But I published many other testimonies and evidence which prove that it is justifiable to doubt Ruml's conclusions. And I stressed that according to all criteria of normal due process Kavan is innocent because his guilt cannot be proven beyond reasonable doubt. And that is omitted from the CTK report.[22]

Weschler went on to attack the Czech media coverage of my story and pointed out that although he does not believe that a journalist can be absolutely objective, he must be transparent and fair. "If you have your prejudices", he said, "then it is necessary to place them on the table and not to present them as objective findings. Let people judge for themselves. This approach is absent in the Czech media...".[23] Weschler aptly reminded RFE listeners of the relevant Karl Kraus" observation:

---

[20]   Urban is no longer on the staff of the newspaper.

[21]   The article was written by John Sweeneg, who received his "information" from *RESPEKT* editors and agreed to coordinate simultaneous publication with this Czech journal. *RESPEKT* also violated the law by obtaining my confidential StB file, quoting extracts from it and making it available to other journalists, both Czech and foreign.

[22]   Transcript of studio recording of interview with Lawrence Wechsler conducted by Karel Jezdinský, October 22, 1992.

[23]   Id.

"Politicians tell lies to journalists and then believe what they've read in the newspapers".[24]

III.

The media treatment of the lustration issue raises many more serious questions than the injustice experienced by myself. During the 1990 Prague conference on the media, Václav Havel and his then press spokesperson Michal Žantovský made clear to the U.S. journalists present, their determination not to allow - under the threat of severe punishment - the publication of a list of 150,000 alleged StB collaborators. Havel and Žantovský talked about a respect for law and about journalists" responsibility. The Czech Parliament later reiterated the same sentiments.

Nevertheless, the list was published. It was an unverified list of names compiled by the former secret police. The list almost certainly included names of corrupt collaborators who denounced fellow countrymen for money or for promotion. But the list also contained the names of people who promised to inform and never did, the names of people who had been broken down by being subjected to violence or long-term imprisonment as well as the names of people who never knew that they were registered as informers.

These latter names were complied by the secret police possibly to help some agent to fulfill his quota and get a reward. The list included the names of people who have been dead for a long time and could not defend themselves and finally, many names of the list were there simply in error. Some of the "errors" were later admitted but not explained.

Those who lived to find their names on the list became second-class citizens, ostracized by some, unemployable by many others. Some foreigners from Third World countries, who were recruited by Czechoslovak intelligence at the time of their studies, and who informed, for example, about Middle East terrorists, were said to have been shot in their home countries. The list included real collaborators as well as victims, victims from the 1950's as well as 1970's and 80's, and entirely innocent people who had proved their civic courage in a number of dangerous situations. Missing from the list were the conformists whose passive loyalty to the communist regime did not earn them any interest by the StB. Today they use their

---

[24]   Id.

absence from these lists as evidence of their anticommunist past and legitimation of their power ambitions.

Jeri Laber of the U.S. Helsinki Watch pointed out the irony that in order to accept the authenticity of these lists, in order to be able to implement the lustration law and have an essential test of suitability for responsible work in a democratic society, the supporters of the lustration process had "put their faith in the Secret police, who were known to have lied consistently and to have misled and abused the population".[25]

In April 1992, another list was published. This time, as a first step in the pre-election campaign, a list of journalists, who were StB agents, according to the StB files, was published. The list was published in the daily press less than 24 hours after Members of Parliament were assured that it would not be leaked. Havel responded to the list critically: "I myself personally have found out under what contentious and highly disputable circumstances one can find oneself in this category".[26] In the current atmosphere for which the media bear their responsibility, the lists also compelled some employers to sack those whose names appeared on the lists.

The lustration issue has subsided by now as it has fulfilled its role. The lustration law, however, did not fulfill the purpose for which many of us supported the search for an adequate lustration mechanism in the first place. My adverse experience with the media, however, continued.

In November 1993, the publishing house LIBRI published an encyclopedia of espionage. To my horrified surprise under "Affair Kavan", I read that according to "newspaper reports", I was jointly responsible for the seizure of my van in 1981 and the subsequent detention of my friends, that I accused a British journalist of causing this disaster, and that I had a working meeting with the StB in November 1989.[27]

A few days later people close to this publishing house organized a press conference in Prague where a New York-based Czech cameraman Jiří Gajda claimed

---

[25]   Jeri Laber, *Witch Hunt in Prague*, The New York Review of Books, April 23, 1992.

[26]   Václav Havel on Czech Radio, May 3, 1992.

[27]   This was a purely absurd contention as the Ukrainian Slovak Mr. Pavel Muraško, who betrayed the arrival of my smuggling van had previously confessed to this in early 1990.

that dissident films filmed in Czechoslovakia in 1970's and 80's by dissidents working for my agency, Palach Press, were in fact filmed under the supervision of the StB. These films were regularly smuggled to the West by my couriers and Palach Press then offered them to various television companies, mainly in the United Kingdom but also in the United States. Gajda astonishingly argued that I selected for Western TV stations only those dissidents whom I and the StB wanted to acquire "a good image" in the West before they emerged in top positions after the collapse of the communist government.

The implication of Gajda's remarks is clear. According to his theory, the November "Velvet Revolution" was only a conspiracy between the StB (and Soviet KGB) and some power-hungry dissidents controlled by an StB agent, Jan Kavan. Václav Havel is not a courageous human rights activist but an StB puppet. The evidence for this absurd construction is equally simple: First, Jan Kavan is "a proven" StB agent. Second, it was impossible to film Havel and others without being caught by the StB. Finally, it was equally impossible to smuggle this filmed material to the West. Or rather, Mr. Gajda and his journalist friends could not imagine how it could have been done. They assumed that nobody was courageous and nobody could have ever outsmarted the StB.

IV.

Restrictions on the press in the Czech Republic are more subtle than in some other countries and therefore, more difficult to identify and combat. In many cases they come from editors and reporters themselves reflecting their desire to support a particular political party and a policy expressing their convictions as "citizen-journalists". The fact that they can present such an approach as normal and desirable without encountering a strong and viable opposition reflects the problems the country is encountering on its cumbersome way to democratic behavior, respect for basic ethical standards, including journalist ethics, and to the rule of law.

At the same time these transformation problems accelerate the development of civil society and provoke the emergence of a number of NGO's willing to tackle some of the most pressing problems and work for the involvement of larger number of people who come from all walks of life outside the political class. I am personally involved, for example in the Helsinki Citizens' Assembly in the Czech Republic which has its roots in the pre-1989 dissident struggle for the respect of human and civil rights and for the integration of democratic Europe as well as in the most recently founded Policy Center for the Promotion of Democracy: for research, education and training ("PCPD").

PCPD attempts to link people from the political world with social scientists and NGO activists and to address both the social and political consequences of the economic transformation. The organization also focuses on the problem of coming to terms with our past and learning to think and act democratically and live in a legal state based on plurality, tolerance and solidarity. The success of these and similar endeavors would, of course, also solve the problems mentioned in this paper. It will necessarily take a long time but we have to eventually succeed because it does not concern the fate of just one small nation in Central Europe.

Since 1993, as before, Václav Havel have spoken up against lustration witch-hunts that lead to "human tragedies". The use of this term brought Havel to court as a defendant in December 1993, for the first time since 1989. He repeated it again in court and in one of his most emotional and eloquent speeches explained that only a minority of people registered in the StB files were active informers and "a large percentage is represented by people, who were persecuted in a way, which cannot be even imagined by the majority of those, who managed to slip through the previous regime without the StB finding them worthy of any notice".[28] He went on to assert that "...only someone really cynical or fanatical will fail to understand what does it mean for a person, who was persecuted throughout his life by the communist regime, and spent even a number of years in prison, to find his or her name on a list of collaborators - without ever committing anything. Everyone around him ceases to talk to him. The world collapses for such a person".[29] Havel confirmed that innocent people lost their jobs and careers, families divorced, people were ostracised, some even committed suicide, including several children of accused fathers. He then angrily and correctly described the unofficial publication of the

---

[28]   Quoted from President Václav Havel's speech delivered in court in response against charges of libel submitted by Petr Cibulka, chief editor of *Necenzurované Noviny*. The full text was published as "Trvám na tom, že zveřejnění seznamů údejných spolupracovníků StB způsobilo četné tragédie" (I maintain that the publication of the list of alleged StB collaborators caused numerous tragedies), *Rudé Právo*, December 15, 1993.

[29]   Id.

StB's list of alleged collaborators[30] as "one of the greatest successes of the StB, which has managed for many years to poison the atmosphere of a democratic state, to mobilize all the rabble whose greatest joy is to harm others and to cynically offer it the flag of radical anticommunism as a protection suitable for these times. It managed to throw in doubt those basic values which are the foundations of a legal and democratic state".[31]

The ardent lustrators, who brought Havel to court because he dared to criticize their vitriolic publication, Havel tellingly depicted as "the successors of the communist ideology of hate, revenge and totalitarian contempt for the law".[32] It seems to me that it is precisely this contempt for the law, the habit of the powers-to-be that may jeopardize not only attempts to come to terms with the past but also the transition to genuine democracy.

My belief, that this transition will not be too long and painful, was fleetingly strengthened in September 1994 when the court has finally cleared me of the slanderous accusation and declared unambiguously that I have never been a secret police collaborator. But the official justification of the verdict did not seem to reflect that my case was under review by the court for three and half years. On the contrary, it gave the impression of being written quite hastily, with scant regard to the content of the StB file and other available evidence. The verdict received a cursory attention from the media, uncomparable with the attention paid by the journalists to the accusations. The Ministry of Interior appealed against the verdict and eight months later I am still awaiting to hear anything from the appeal court.

---

[30]   The list of over 100.000 names was published by *Necenzurované Noviny* (Uncensored Newspaper) in three volumes. Later the editors offered the list for sale also on computer diskettes. No one was ever prosecuted for this violation of the law. Jaroslav Bašta revealed that the published version is identical with the database compiled by the Parliamentary Commission of 17th November. He concluded that on the basis of his investigation he can identify the person responsible for the leak and described as someone, who: "1) Had access to the database and was a member of the commission... 2) For ideological reasons supported the publication of the confidential list of agents. 3) Suffered from 'agents-mania' (preoccupation with agents). 4) Displayed in the past his willingness not to respect the law for the protection of confidential facts and was able to have access to strictly confidential file on the Kavan's case, for example, to American television company..." (Only Stanislav Devátý, current provisional director of the FBIS, fits these criteria).

[31]   Havel's speech, see note 28.

[32]   Id.

In the meantime, reflecting probably the rise in popularity of the opposition's Social Democratic Party and my own position within it, the media attacks against me were resurrected. Despite the court's verdict I was again labeled as "the agent of the communist intelligence service".[33] The same newspaper also published one of the most vicious and absurd concoctions of lies and speculations I ever had the misfortune to read.[34] In it I was accused of being a former agent of the British Intelligence Service, which I, allegedly, betrayed to the Czechs by sending them an anonymous letter. The Czech espionage apparently planned to work with me since I was a toddler in London. After the alleged discovery of my "treachery", the British, according to the article, made me an outcast. And the fact that, despite being a "traitor", I was seen lunching with British diplomats in Prague, the author explained away as "new intelligence games". He went on to assert that I never worked for the opposition, never organized any literature smuggling trips and never sent any couriers with documents to and from the opposition.

An article of this kind would never have been published in any democratic country which respects the rule of law. I decided to test the rule of law in my country and sued the publisher and the author for libel. Among witnesses, who have agreed to testify on my behalf are not only many former top dissidents, who are now again in the opposition but also Mr. Jan Ruml, the current Minister of Interior, who had been personally receiving books, documents, letters and so on from me for many years during our dissident collaboration. The outcome of this case, as well as the outcome of the appeal court, will be for me a litmus test on how far we are on the road towards a democratic state based on the rule of law.

---

[33]   Dušan Šrámek, *Devátý odmítá nařčení z manipulace se svazkem exploslance Jana Kavana*, Denní Telegraf, Praha, February 22, 1995.

[34]   Václav Eminger, *Konec lustračního případu Jana Kavana*, Denní Telegraf, Praha, March 11, 1995.

POLITICAL SPEECH AND POLITICAL MONEY

by Zsolt Krokovay

Liberalism is a boring philosophy insofar as it supposedly provides, as a theory of social cooperation, ready answers, at least in a rough way, to the practical problems of constitutional democracy. The standard activity of a liberal philosopher consists simply of the illustration and the appropriate application of the principles which determine what is right and wrong. This occurs in a social structure where free, equal and reasonably rational citizens consider the facts of pluralism, primarily, their different conceptions of the good, as a permanent condition.

Our electoral and other basic political rights certainly derive from such a principle, the constitutional principle of political liberty. It also seems evident that a similar general principle lies behind our basic right to freedom of speech. And it is a well-known fact that these two clusters of basic rights can be in conflict with each other in particular cases. If one does not wish to have these conflicts resolved by an ad hoc balancing by courts or, what is worse, by civil servants, and if we do not want thereby to consent to the prevailing judgement of the political majority, we need to adjust the constitutional principles themselves. We need to determine, to the extent possible the scope of basic rights which derive from these principles, on the grounds that they have a central role in a fair social cooperation.[1]

This essay deals with some questions raised by such a theoretical venture. First, I wish to explain the concept of political speech and the term "political money". Second, I shall refer to the idea that there is an underlying notion of justice. In other words, there are background conditions which must be satisfied for the effective practice of equal political liberty. Third, I shall deal with the circumstances that endanger the "one man, one vote" principle. I shall isolate three problems. Accordingly, the fourth section in my paper touches upon the problem of governmental speech and more specifically, the requirement of the neutrality of the state in the electoral context. My fifth section will discuss on the workings of the

---

[1]   It is no secret for those familiar with the questions of modern political philosophy that this is based on John Rawls' ideas. See especially his essay, *Basic Liberties and Their Priority* which, in sections VII and XII, deals entirely with the problem. The essay was delivered as The Tanner Lecture on Human Values at The University of Michigan, April 10, 1981, *reprinted in Liberty Philosophy and the Law: Tanner Lectures on Moral Philosophy* (S.M. McMurrin ed. 1987).

A. Sajó (ed.), Rights of Access to the Media, 281-292.
© *1996 Kluwer Law International. Printed in the Netherlands.*

modern media and the sixth will explore the circumstances of corruption and incompatibility. Finally, I will mention two points about certain kinds of regulations which appear to be suitable for handling these problems.

I.

Whatever the role of freedom of speech is in the process of self-realization, self-expression and the development and exercise of a rational conception of good, or as a great philosopher of the 19th century said, in the continuous daily exercise of "moral and intellectual muscles",[2] our most important special interest in this basic liberty is the protection of the free discussion of public affairs, or as we say more solemnly, the pursuit of full development and expression of our sense of justice.[3] First of all, it should be evident that there are no free elections without freedom of political speech. This principle permits a candidate to state his or her conception of the public good, and the voter to cast her vote in a rational and well informed way. Once a constitutional regime guarantees the full possession of equal political liberties, no one can reasonably deny that citizens must adhere to those rights which derive from a free speech principle.[4]

In this context, we may use the term "political money" to refer to those sums that are spent either independently or as a contribution to promote certain political programs, and above all to support election campaigns. It is evident that the effective expression of opinion in public affairs in modern constitutional democracies necessitates such monetary expenditures. In other words, these sums serve for all intents and purposes as an entry point for the effective exercise of the right of political speech. Generally, the most important expense is incurred for access to political broadcasting, especially the different campaign events which attract

---

[2]   J.S. Mill, *On Liberty*, Ch. 3, 6 (1989).

[3]   The pioneer of this reasoning was Alexander Meiklejohn in his seminal essay *Free Speech and Its Relation to Self-Government*. Some of the most important followers of his consideration include Harry Kalven, Thomas Scanlon, Vincent Blasi and, of course, John Rawls. For a general survey, see Eric Barendt, *Freedom of Speech* (1985).

[4]   See T.M.Scanlon, *Contractualism and Utilitarianism in Utilitarianism and Beyond* 110 (A. Sen and B. Williams eds. 1982).

television cameras. Only after this come the expenses for newspaper advertisements, transportation, direct mailing, personal phone calls, and distribution of materials and bulletins, posters and flyers during the election campaign.[5]

The competition between candidates shall always be limited, as long as the facilities required for considerable publicity and for reaching the broadest public are not freely available. Whomever is not capable of paying the entrance-fee for access to publicity, is not able to effectively introduce his or her views to the voter. Even though a more peripheral, less expensive or free public forum is available to all, the truly effective means of communication via the mass media are dominated by those candidates who have the greatest budget. And if the competition between the candidates turns out to be a competition of money, the voter will not be able to gather information about the different alternatives. Hence, the principle of "one man, one vote" and the fairness of the election, no longer prevails. This is the dilemma.

Let me make an important caveat. I am only going to discuss campaign funds and the financing of election campaigns. I shall completely disregard other questions which are concerned with the cost of freedom of political speech generally. The reason is quite simple: the assurance of an acceptable political equality plays a very special role in the context of free elections.

II.

An old popular criticism of liberal philosophy states that such a philosophy merely provides formal advantages without the realization of certain background conditions, or in effect, only a small powerful elite is capable of exercising basic freedoms. This is seen primarily as a consequence of the great social and economic inequalities present in society. "Freedom of the press is guaranteed only to those who own one", is one comment that appeared in a study on newspapers in the United States. "The millionaire as well as the beggar is free to sleep under the bridge and they are both forbidden to steal bread", states the writer. "What may the Egyptian peasant do with

---

[5]   See generally, *Campaign Financing of National Elections in Foreign Countries* (Law Library of Congress ed. 1991).

his freedom of speech if he has no bread to eat?" asks the philosopher.[6] It is equally in vain to carefully create the adjusted family of equal basic liberties, where a great majority of the citizens do not have a true prospect of fully exercising and enjoying their liberties as they do not have the resources to purchase the necessary mediums of communication.

One does not imply that human rights necessarily be accepted in the nations where the fulfillment of the required conditions has to be provided in a state of emergency. One supposes instead that constitutional democracy can only develop to an acceptable degree under the favorable conditions of material civilization and political culture.

When these favorable conditions are satisfied, the problem, as it is usually stated, is the difference between liberty and the worth of liberty.[7] Often not much material wealth is required for a person to enjoy and exercise freedom of religion. However, the expression of certain viewpoints and the goal of reaching a broad general audience renders specific requirements, and instruments, such as money, indispensable. Moreover, what is especially important is the guarantee of appropriate political equality.

For many people their entire constitutional rights will remain solely on paper if the fair value of electoral and, in general, political equality cannot be assured. The United States Supreme Court has previously addressed this very point in two landmark cases. In *Wesberry v. Sanders*, the Court stated that "[o]ther rights, even the most basic, are illusory, if the right to vote is undermined".[8] In a second case, *Reynolds v. Sims*, the Court concluded: "Full and effective participation by all citizens in state government requires . . . that each citizen has an equally effective voice in the election of members of the state legislature".[9]

---

[6]   A.J. Liebling, *The Press* 30-31(New York, Pantheon Books, 1981); see the citation included in the inaugural lecture of Professor Eric Barendt, *Press and Broadcasting Freedom: Does Anyone Have any Rights to Free Speech?* (London, 1991). The writer is Anatole France, the philosopher is Sir Isaiah Berlin.

[7]   John Rawls, *A Theory of Justice* 32 ff. (1972). For a criticism, see N. Daniels, *Equal Liberty and Unequal Worth of Liberty in Reading Rawls* (N. Daniels ed. 1985). For a clear interpretation of this distinction in the analysis of the concept of liberty, see Joel Feinberg *Social Philosophy*, Chs. 2 and 3 (1973).

[8]   376 U.S. 1, 17 (1964)

[9]   377 U.S. 533, 565 (1964).

According to a well-known liberal precept, the solution to the problem of political inequality lies in a thought-experiment, in a multi-stage procedure involving a hypothetical original position in order to create a basic and just structure for a society.[10] In this procedure, one develops an appropriate system or rather a well-adjusted set of "equal basic liberties" subject to the adoption of certain necessary moral constraints. This is followed by the provision of equality of opportunity for all citizens in the distribution of society's economic goods and social positions. Then one selects the level of social and economic inequalities which are the *most beneficial* for the least fortunate members of society.

The two principles of justice, as the result of this hypothetical social contract, are not composed merely of these three principles (i.e., a well adjusted set of equal basic liberties, equal opportunity of access and necessary beneficial inequalities). Rather, one may consider the guarantee of the fair value of basic liberties as the fourth principle, and the special requirement of sufficient political equality as the fifth principle. In order to avoid circularity, following the stipulation of just inequalities, and the acceptance of difference, one must return to the first principle of equal basic liberties. This principle serves as the basis for providing the indispensable means for all citizens to effectively exercise and fully enjoy their basic liberties. While we may consider the previous conditions as well as the necessity of the particular requirement of political equality in advance, the justice of social and economic distribution requires the stipulation of a subject matter.

Inherently, this highly abstract discussion does not even touch on the question of how the specified requirements for political and social liberty can successfully be fulfilled. However, they are not superficial. If we are not able to define the objective, we needlessly debate on the method.

III.

A number of scholarly commentators in the area of free speech theory infer that the state does not exercise censorship when it restricts the use of political money. They base their argument on the grounds that the writing of a check is not an expression,

---

[10]   Rawls, *A Theory of Justice*, supra note 7.

but an action.[11] This argument is suspiciously circular. On the one hand, it is conceivable that in many cases where an act clearly carries a message for the general public, even if it is not expressed verbally, it nonetheless constitutes "speech", namely "symbolic speech". On the other hand, it seems to many observers that whenever we do not wish to allow certain expressions because they cause clearly unacceptable harm, we call them speech acts, performatives or fighting words.

We characterize these harmful acts as speech acts in the sense that these are not "speech" or "expression" in the proper constitutional sense but "more than speech" or "speech plus something else". This completely elastic classification is not only attractive because in certain cases it appears rather intuitively convincing, but also because such a classification contains the necessary distinction between speech restrictions that trample on civil rights and the more appropriate regulations of time, place, and manner in the exercising of these civil rights.[12]

Consequently, one should regulate the writing of a check during an election campaign not only because it is the words that these funds help to publicize which deserve constitutional protection rather than the act of check writing itself. Surely we could not speak of freedom of painting in a country where certain colors, canvas and brushes are confiscated by authority. One has to take the expression "money talks" literally. Whomever sacrifices money for a noble or ignoble cause in the course of an election campaign, is able to give expression to his or her political views in an effective way.

But it does not follow that the restriction of campaign expenditure is always unacceptable. It is not simply a question of legal definition and whether freedom of speech has its boundary where the rights deriving from it infringe upon the rights of others. If it can be shown that without restrictions on campaign expenditure, the fairness of the elections would come into jeopardy, then such regulation would not be unconstitutional.

The first danger is the use of public power to influence the political contest. One cannot speak of free elections in a country where candidates of the governing party are given an advantage over their challengers. The requirement that the state

---

[11]   See T. Emerson, *The System of Freedom of Expression,* 8 (New York, Random House, 1971).

[12]   Laurence Tribe, *American Constitutional Law,* 12-20 (1988),

should stay away from electoral debates is so self-evident, that its crude infringement is quite rare in developed constitutional democracies. However, in places where the structure of self-governing public institutions has not developed, where state officials in leading posts regard themselves as dependent on the current government, these crude infringements could occur during the legal gaps of the political transition and because of a lack of a long experience with political culture. In the countries which emerged from behind the iron curtain, the greatest problem, I believe, is the political strategy of the dominant governing party to stabilize its governmental power while having to face the enormous task of stabilizing rule of law in a new democracy.

The second danger is most prevalent in Western democracies. This danger involves permitting the dominance of certain social groups and of powerful financial circles in public debates. If one can imagine the debate over public affairs as a town meeting of free, equal and suitably rational citizens in the former New England, then it is apparent that we need to limit the lengths and the number of contributions to the discussion. Without such a limitation, some persons would be overshadowed or would miss completely the opportunity to speak.

If there are especially important and less valuable fora, then primary fairness dictates that the most significant of these should only be used in accordance with certain ground rules. In modern societies, the most important fora are those which aim at the widest public. These fora play a primary role in the orientation of the population and in public life. As everybody knows, these are the prime time political programs of radio stations, and of national television networks.

The first two dangers accommodate the third, which is corruption. Naturally, a democracy has never openly espoused political corruption. Nevertheless, it is the disillusionment and the cynical pragmatism of citizens that leads to the corruption of the future legislator. This is a direct consequence of the failure to solve the first two problems.

IV.

In the West and in modern societies that are based on notions of private property and on a competitive market economy, there is a tendency to repeatedly make a breach in the wall raised in defence of the tyranny of the majority. Such a defence, is, for example, manifest with a two-fold strength in Hungary and in the whole post-communist world. Here, the government is not only the largest contractor, but it is also the greatest direct economical force in every respect.

The Soviet regimes left behind enormous state-owned sectors. Their reduction, the so-called privatization, also creates the potential for direct state guidance. Old and new governing bureaucracies pour out official information and allocate enormous funding to propagate certain patronized ideas in the press and in publicly funded "nationally spirited" foundations.

In the process of both confidential data management and development of a superpower empire of information the old and new "etatisms" meet under the interpretation of a "mission" in the form of an extremely simplified majority rule. The government, which was only elected for four years, hopes to validate its policy of force through the press, the culture and in the distribution of public funds in the name of a patriotic and often nationalistic communitarianism. The regime uses every effort to establish a loyal press. Moreover, the governing regime will also create a "national" media that is not overly critical toward the government.

The independent institutional press is by far the most effective instrument of freedom of speech in modern societies, the most basic forum, the guarantor of constitutionally protected control of public power, displacement, and electoral and political freedom. In societies that are in the process of modernization, as is Hungary, it is equally the open and the concealed instruments of the state press that pose the greatest danger for civil rights and for future free elections.

It is self-evident what it means when ministers, cabinet members and public servants actively join in the election campaign of their party. Such government officials not only deploy governmental power but also public funds through various transfers in support of their campaigns. They may create funds close to the government which they fill with donations by state enterprises. Thereby, the national objectives of a country's progress become one with the objectives of the government. The latter becomes synonymous with the electoral interests of the largest governing party. Furthermore, all those measures with which the government must actively secure the effectiveness of the "one man, one vote" principle in developed countries, only create further possibilities for infringements in post-communist societies.

V.

The opinion of political scientists today differs greatly concerning the actual effectiveness of campaign funds. Many commentators believe that traditional estimates are overstated.[13] According to this view, the great political influence that is supposedly exerted with available campaign funds, is not justified in practice. It cannot be shown that political funds thrown in for a re-election or for a successful challenge significantly increase the odds of a candidate's victory.

I touch upon this subject in order to demonstrate that its outcome does by no means conflict with the specific requirement of political equality, which states that all candidates must have sufficient opportunity to present their program, irrespective of the advantage a given candidate gains by the performance. And likewise, the voter's right to gather information demands an unrestricted discussion, irrespective of the evidence concerning the effect of the realization of these requirements on his or her vote.

The stipulation of unrestricted discussion means that we legally differentiate, at least during the narrower span of the campaign, between the more and less important fora of the electoral campaign. It is not enough to guarantee that somewhere and by some means even the poorest candidate can find himself or herself an audience. It is essential that all views worthy of consideration be delivered at the most important fora. Consequently, the right to appear means two things: based on the practical criteria of importance and significance, we have to develop the requirements of primary fairness and proportionality.

As I have previously suggested, the most important fora in modern constitutional democratic electoral contest are television advertisements and editorial broadcasts. When radio and television are brought under a public service regulation, and, as in European countries, also serve as some kind of a national or public service forum, the requirements of balance and minimal fairness must be most strictly observed. This stands in contrast with American constitutional principles which clearly require that "we limit the contribution of some in order to strengthen the voice of others in our society".[14]

---

[13]   D. Lowenstein, *A Patternless Mosaic: Campaign Finance and the First Amendment After Austin*, (21) Cap. Univ. L. Rev. 381, 391 (1992).

[14]   *Buckley v. Valeo*, 424 U.S. 1, 48-49 (1976).

VI.

Electoral laws have made an effort to forestall the corruption of politicians and public servants ever since the first days of democracy. In the case of a public official we can easily define what counts as a bribery and as a gratuity. According to a United States federal bribery statute, writes one commentator, a public servant commits bribery if "he corruptly asks, demands, ... or agrees to receive anything of value for himself or for any other person or entity, in return for ... being influenced in his performance of any official act".[15] In essence, all donations given to and accepted by a politician with the purpose of practicing influence on his or her official activity constitutes bribery. When the expectation of a service in return for the political donation is not present, the same anti-bribery statute defines the "gratuity" offense. This offense is defined as a situation where a federal official, without "proof of corrupt intent or proof that the value was given specifically in return for performance by the official", receives "otherwise than as provided by law for the proper discharge of official duty ... anything of value for himself for or because of any official act performed or to be performed by him".[16]

But how can we apply the notion of bribery or gratuity for a member of parliament, to a prospective member and above all to those contributions and independent expenditures which play a major role in an election campaign? The difficulties with such definitions are of vagueness and overbreadth. It is the moral responsibility of a legislator to do his or her work conscientiously. However, if he or she is thought to be lazy, works badly or is unsuitable for some other reason, the voters we still have to wait for such an MP's dismissal until the next election, unless he or she breaks a law. The only punishment which may be used against him or her is a symbolic "death penalty" of being voted out of office.

Nevertheless, it is evident that an MP is elected in the hope of seeing him or her act in the desired way. A person's vote is cast based on the performance of the member or the party during the latter part of the previous parliamentary period. Therefore, there is nothing to object to, at least at first sight, the financial support

---

[15]   Note, *Campaign Contributions and Federal Bribery Law*, (92) Harv. L.Rev. 451, (1978).

[16]   Id.

of a party or a candidate as some sort of return service for their efforts. Surely, one only wishes to ensure an MP's success for no other reason but that one is satisfied with his or her performance. When the candidate discloses the plans for his or her future legislative activity, such disclosure is evidently done explicitly in order to gain new supporters. Moreover, the essence of an election campaign is the debate of rival candidates. As a result of the communicational feed-back between voter and candidate an agreement is made, which formally is no different from bribery.

We must still ask in what instances the use of spending of political money qualifies as "corruption". In other words, when does the danger and appearance of bribery come about in the process of an election campaign? The most obvious example is the direct selling of votes and internal or confidential information. Both activities are most likely to benefit the majority, but an influential member of the opposition might also have valuable goods to offer.

Lobbying within legal boundaries consists of an interest group attempting to convince the undecided members of parliament of the importance of its views. If the group's efforts are successful, the legislator collects the group's votes. But in a stable political system not all types of lobbying are legal, as not every motive for voting is permissible. If the reason for a "yes" is demonstrably or even presumably some soft material reward, then the politician's vote for an article or his or her motion for an amendment is based on "sinful" interest, in return for some other pecuniary or political gain. Perhaps it is done against the party's or MP's personal political conscience.

The sale or trading of inside political information, which may have an exceedingly great value for those concerned, must, after all, be leaked from government offices. If the mismanagement of secret information gets out of hand, we are back to the problem of state corruption. In Hungary and in other post-communist countries, the state is not only the greatest economic actor but could also be the greatest potential corrupter. In a stable political structure there are constitutional restrictions on the purchase of MP's by the state. These restrictions prevent the current majority from collecting loyal votes by offering lucrative positions, making arbitrary decisions in competitions and distributing other privileges.

VII.

The constitutional principle of freedom of speech and the press, along the lines of the First Amendment of the United States' Constitution, calls for a strong legal immunity[17] from interference from all three branches of government. At the same time, even the most crucial political free speech has to be compatible with and adjusted by other basic rights.

Naturally, in this short paper, I was not able to discuss - even as a boring liberal philosopher - the practical questions of regulation. All I can do is to mention two very general points which could play a role in the considerations of Hungarian electoral regulation.

First of all, openness and strict disclosure rules are the most important requirements of fairness in a free election, against the abuse of power, either public, or private. It might be required at a minimum that the parliamentary parties keep accounts of all contributions from private individuals and organizations, as well as of expenditures made to promote their candidates. Greater transparency, with a clear-cut law against conflicts of interest, also diminishes the chances of the abuse of governmental power.

On the other hand, if parties are to receive public funds and other benefits - either in a direct or indirect form - in proportion to their support, then it is possible to fix limits on private contributions, independent expenditures and a number of categories of expenses. Nevertheless, the acceptance of such "house-rules" type of regulation is possible only if it is neutral and rational. On one hand, such regulation should not impose any undue burdens on the various political groups or any single candidate. On the other, the regulation should not extend beyond what appears to be required by fairness.[18] In the course of this regulation, as a part of the electoral law, the order of the distribution of public service campaign programs and campaign advertisements on the radio and television may also be decided in the same manner.

---

[17]   For a discussion of the classical analysis of this absolutist concept see W.N. Hohfeld, *Fundamental Legal Conceptions*, 35-64 (1919).

[18]   See Rawls, *Basic Liberties*, supra note 1, at 73.

CONCLUSION

by Monroe E. Price

The essays in this book come from an extraordinary moment in time: an awakening to the complexities of transition, not only in the political system itself, but in the communications infrastructure so basic to democratic values. The moment was not only a change in Central and Eastern Europe, or, in an isolated way, in efforts to design new laws or engraft new ownership patterns for television and radio. The very concept of access was itself changing as geopolitical approaches to television and popular culture shifted.

In this conclusion, we want to focus on three points not so strongly emphasized by the contributors to this volume, all related to the impact of technology (and its adoption) on access in the future. The first involves determining what globalism really implies, how it should be defined, and how it affects the idea of a civil society related to the state. The second point, the distorted mirror of the first, is the implications for national identity, namely the positive steps the state takes to ensure democratic values and a local sense of loyalty in the face of centrifugal pressures. Finally, we note ways in which changes in the communications technology, within the state itself, may affect ideas of access in the future.

The future of access, in the face of globalism, is important because of the role of concepts of access in the very acceptability of societal constraints. Access is a lubricating doctrine. Access works at the edges to render the harsh realities of power and the distribution of wealth more acceptable. Access provides the notion that particular cultures and individual states can endure. Within access doctrines are buried concerns about how individuals receive the information that shapes them, their attitudes toward themselves, their fellow citizens and the state.

Given the importance of access, the impact of globalism is important to consider and monitor. The developing countries sought to deal with globalism, alone, during the period of the ill-fated New World Information Order debate of the 1970's which had too ideological and too regional focus. Now, the question of dealing with information flows is a general one. Global access has to be refigured so that it is not a denial for individual states - particularly smaller states, of their particular identities. Language, the marker of distinction, is especially at risk. Cumulatively, the changes in the patterns of communication take their toll on traditional approaches to access.

A. Sajó (ed.), Rights of Access to the Media, 293-303.
© 1996 *Kluwer Law International. Printed in the Netherlands.*

All these changes, springing from a combination of technology, politics and the flow of capital, make it more difficult for traditional notions of access and communications in society to hold sway. The German ideas of communicative freedom, thoughtfully delineated by Ulrich Preuss, could be in jeopardy because they relate to the internal strength of systems of discourse. Technology may mean that, in the distinctions drawn by Eric Barendt between various approaches to pluralism - access approaches as compared to competition and mergers policies - greater emphasis will be placed on the latter. The essays in this book deal, primarily, with the state, in its regulation, looking inward, mediating among competing producers of information and visions of society. As the world becomes one of multiple satellite-delivered channels, the challenge for the nation-state will be looking outward, scrambling for ways to protect its identity, rather than to use the media as a mechanism of control. Here are some conclusions that we draw, looking forward from the essays presented in this volume:

1. Traditional national approaches to regulating television imagery will adjust to those transformations that Ithiel de Sola Pool presciently called "technologies of freedom".[1] Rather than thinking of broadcasting entities as primarily "public" or "private," our mental categories will have a new divide: global broadcasting enterprises, regional (supranational) broadcasting enterprises, and then, a residual category of broadcasting entities that work primarily within traditional borders, often more locally than before.

It has already become almost impossible, consistent with maintaining democratic values and following international norms, to determine means of "protecting" domestic audiences, or dividing markets through government supervised restraints. In most of the essays in this collection, the assumption is that the state is capable of continuing to be a significant factor, an element of force, in determining who has access and for what purpose. On the other hand, the debate may be shifting to means of screening out technology, if possible, and the programming that traverses it, rather than determining the nuances of domestic discourse.

In the new environment, it will be particularly difficult to engage in the kind of recuperation of the public sphere that is at the heart of Jean Cohen's discussion of the concepts of Jurgen Habermas. If a healthy public sphere is to exist, then television may play less and less of a role. Perhaps the lesson of global

---

[1]   Ithiel de Sola Pool, *Technologies of Freedom*, (Harvard, MA: Belknap, 1984).

technology is a turn toward enriching robust public debate - in Owen Fiss' memorable term - through the printed press, or possibly through radio.

Another possibility is that a new kind of public sphere is emerging, one that, itself, transgresses national borders and one that attaches itself to the decision-making of global bodies or builds a transnational civic society. The growth of the BBC World Service or CNN are initial steps in that direction. Then, the question of what constitutes "news" and the narrative of information will change; and with that the question of who has access to the process of depicting what is important in the world and to the viewer.

Karol Jakubowicz has outlined the approach national statutes take to quotas for domestic production or foreign ownership. These are the elements of law that will be under the greatest strain in a new communications era. There are, however, related problems of access such as whether cable systems will be required to carry the national or government service channels. At a time when BBC and Radio Free Europe are granted radio frequencies, as in the Czech Republic, it is relevant whether a preference or mandate for national programming services ought to exist.

Global broadcasting generally implies the search for a transnational - perhaps even intercontinental - virtually universal audience. Inherent in the muscular challenge of the global is a television largely unmediated by any state, or any government entity including a public broadcasting authority.[2] Obviously, the new generation of producers and reconstructed broadcasters - the great multinationals - have the goal of reaching audiences regardless of locality and without negotiating with governments to reach their audiences.

Globalism, in this definition, depends not just on the reach of the producer but on the power of the state. Only if the state has little control over the capacity of the signal to be received or exercises no such control is a scheme of spreading narratives considered global.

Signals can become global because they are selected by "the market" rather than by a public broadcasting service. A clearer way of defining unmediated global television is to confine it to that set of signals beyond the control of the receiving state. To say that the programming is global does not mean that it comes from nowhere, or has no cultural impact. Deciphering its impact is already a small

---

[2]   A more standard meaning of global relates primarily to content. See Marjorie Ferguson, "The Mythology about Globalization," *European Journal of Communications*, 7 (1992): 69.

industry. It is becoming important to determine how the global menu of programming gets developed; what constitutes the relationship between the global menu and the national; what means are or ought to be available to improve the global menu, make it more responsive to audiences, more efficient in terms of choices available and means of expressing intensity of interest on the part of the consumer.

The counterpart to "global" imagery is broadcasting that must pass through the skein of governmental authority. "National" radio and television involves some combination of the furtherance of state power and of a state-defined national identity. The proliferation of new nation-states, or newly assertive nation-states, underscores a need to reexamine what is meant by national television, and how national television functions in an era of greater globalism and pressures toward regionalism as well. National television, in this definition, implies a television (and broadcasting structure) that has some implicit or explicit obligation to reinforce the community that constitutes the state, whether it is one or more "nationalities", and is seen as an instrument of the state to shape the image it holds within the populace. Public service television becomes a vital cultural institution, as Jean Cohen has put it, to form part of civil society, to be in between government and the economic structures. Perhaps concepts of access, including ideas that the public gets prescribed opportunities to receive important information, become all the more important in a period of growing global communication.

These are hardly neat categories. The point, rather, is that emerging broadcasting patterns are not congruent with the borders of existing countries and have the potential to undermine them and build new loyalties. The new patterns can be accidentally or purposefully redefining. Broadcasting to the Basques in Spain and France, straddling borders, or to Palestinians in Jordan, Israel and contested territories are examples. But broadcasting policies are also arranged to help support the integrity of a group of states or substantial portions of states. Concepts of access have as much to do with self-determination as they do with the fulfillment of notions of the marketpalce. Europe is a region in that sense, and its Broadcasting Directive is an effort to use television and radio to undergird a European culture and identity. Without hyperbole, it could be said that the history of American broadcasting involved the creation of a more homogeneous United States out of its culturally dissimilar and previously antagonistic parts. Access doctrines may help to pave ways of asserting the self-determination of groups and the relationship of groups to geographical space. They may, on the other hand, become means of imposed cultural homogenization.

2. In such a world, the confounding question is determining what constitutes access and the public interest and how that public interest implicates the state. If the broadcasting structures of the past have been so closely tied to national identity, the question will arise what kind of identity is associated with a transnational communications period. Additionally, the shift will be to considering what supranational structures, if any, can be constituted as a match for the transnational program providers.

Trying to determine the correct conceptual way of thinking about radio and television structures in this moment of change is far from an idle task. Changes in political thought and political boundaries, artifacts of the post-Soviet era, make the invention of new broadcasting structures a matter of great political and economic importance. Both in the West and in the transition societies, fundamental problems exist that bring planning for change to a stalemate. New parliaments seek to determine which combination of models to adopt, both among the public service and private, wholly market-based, structures. To the extent "state" television is considered an option, there are difficulties in defining what the state should be for these purposes, how to finance cultural and political dreams, and the relationship that should exist between the state and the furtherance of particular national or cultural goals.

Since the operative categories are shifting, there is the classic problem of policy makers engaging in meaningless conflict over outmoded outcomes and failing to take advantage of the opportunities clearly enough to think through the broadcasting structures that will inevitably evolve. In other words, policy makers may be working primarily with the vocabulary of the old axis (state/private) while the context in which they are operating requires decisions that recognize the new (global/national/regional).

Canada's history of mediation between a national whole and decentralized diversity is similarly reflected in creating the reality of a region through the media.[3] What is important is whether, as technology alters the space for the delivery of

---

[3] The former Soviet Union, or part of it, may turn into a "region" with the devolution of control over television accompanied by some pan-Republic television signal or cooperative policy.

television signals, regional governing mechanisms emerge or are adapted to supplement or displace the now less-significant state.

In the transnational arena, concepts of human rights and free speech are the forward guard of the narratives of the West. The questions of openness and competing narrative are being fought around the world on the ground of principle - the principle, variably stated, of freedom of speech and the right to receive and impart information. Hard, cruel, difficult struggles have to do with the pain of political speech: whether to allow Nazis to march in Skokie or anti-semitic pamphlets to be published in Budapest or Kiev. The rhetoric built on these impossible cases is used, however, to argue, insistently, for privatization, for broadcast stations with no obligation to carry news or information on for cable systems to compete against the carriers of national identity without including them in the signals offered to subscribers.

The significant debate over principle surrounds the question of who and what is protected by limitations on state intervention in the field of speech. For example, is there some area of human communication - not classified as indecency, or obscenity or violence - that relates to the overall culture of a community and which the community can protect? And is there a way to distinguish between the great corporations, in terms of their capacity to envelope the culture, and the area of political discourse? Is there a difference between the promulgation of the stuff of immediate political discourse, news, information, debate, and the stuff of popular culture, entertainment, advertising and commercial speech?

Is there a difference between establishing the architecture of communications: concerns about monopoly and competition, rate regulation, access and controlling speech itself? Put differently, for the purpose of determining the level of immunity from government regulation, who constitutes a speaker?

The sanity of a community may rest on its capacity to make meaningful, principled, honorable distinctions among these categories. As we have seen, these distinctions are eroding and enhanced discourse and freedom are not the only result. In the United States, cable television corporations and telephone companies, successfully arguing that they are "speakers", rather than instruments for other speakers and listeners to use, have depleted the power of the Congress (or of the states) to impose regulatory standards. Denying the legislature authority to separate maintenance and operation of the highways of speech from their traditional uses is an important departure of the last decade. Whether it is convergence of technologies, disappearance of editorial categories or a more libertarian attitude of hostility to the state, the expansion of the principle of immunity from government intervention in American jurisprudence would undermine many approaches of Western democracies and efforts to construct a public sphere.

The First Amendment, and similar doctrines of free speech throughout the world, can become not an instrument for the realization of democratic values, but a severe and significant block to vision. Those who benefit from the expansion of the American rule, find it much more comfortable and efficient to couch the question of state power in terms of principle than in terms of a vision of society, a narrative of the desirable course of history. Two prevailing metaphors, used *ad nauseam* during recent decades of broadcast regulation, demonstrate the new mentality. The first is government as "traffic cop", or as little more than facilitator of movement among competing private interests. The second, which implies a remedial activism, ascribes to government the task of "leveling the playing field", with the leveling function usually limited to overcoming advantages earlier conferred on competitors. These are both metaphors of orchestrated neutrality; both are *formulae* to deny a positive role to the decision-maker. Of course, the mother of all metaphors is "the market", the market economy, the free market, the marketplace of ideas. The market is, by definition, a place of no intrinsic loyalties except to the market itself.

But what appears to be a form of nonintervention may be merely the reconfiguring of the collection of American and other myths. A new sense of concern must emerge, new structures of thinking, if there is to be hope of cultural, educational and civic redemption. At the least, alternate conceptions of the role of government and society are needed so that we, collectively, are not powerless to adjust to shifting circumstances in the circulation of images. Cass Sunstein, the noted University of Chicago legal scholar, has called for a new understanding of freedom of expression that would draw a sharp distinction between a "marketplace of ideas" and a "system of democratic deliberation".[4] Sunstein breaks through the problem of language and conception by arguing that the "marketplace of ideas" (the reigning metaphor) is not a thing found in nature. "Markets generally promote both liberty and prosperity. But when the legal criterion of a market has harmful consequences for free expression - and it sometimes does - then it must be reevaluated ... If our

---

[4]   Cass R. Sunstein: *Democracy and the Problem of Free Speech.* (The Free Press. New York, 1993.) p.xviii.

Madisonian goal is to produce attention to public issues, and exposure to diverse views, a market system may well be inadequate."[5]

3. There is yet another concern that affects the understanding of access in the future. The impetus for access, as a mode of democratic enhancement, is based almost entirely on a model of communications technology in which the public sphere exists in a forum largely open to the common gaze. The questions for the future are not only whether the services of the media will be universal or ubiquitous, but who will control the narrative and how participatory the forum will be.

Openness of the speech terrain is not alone sufficient for a properly operating public sphere. There must be modes of reflection, of private communication, of discourse that is within enclosed terrain, the electronic equivalent of a right of association.

For the essays in this book, given the structure of the mass media, the undergirding of public policy, the preoccupation is with the open terrain of speech: ensuring that it exists and providing access to it. The great communications institutions, such as the television networks shape national identity, define attitudes and character, and mold political attitude. The fact that they are such a public theater of presentation invites concern about access to the stage.

But openness is declining as a paradigm. The new technologies, redolent with addressability (the capacity of producers to reach individual households rather than the mass) and complex interactivity (the capacity for senders and receivers to communicate) are distinguished by their capacity to be closed. The power to establish closed channels efficiently, and to collect money from individuals based on the intensity of their response to a particular set of offerings, is a hallmark of these new systems. Newspapers are filled with diagrams attempting to describe the frontiers of the information world of the future. In the forest of arrows and metaphors, something important is obfuscated: contrary to what might be anticipated, the very abundance of channels may mean more, not fewer calls for government intervention to ensure that something remains of the public space. Access becomes a different question in the world of the information infrastructure.

The dynamic that is occurring, insufficiently noticed, must affect strategies to generate an effective public sphere since it encompasses a shift in the way information is transmitted and distributed within society. Consider a world of

---

[5]   Sunstein, op. cit. p. 50.

channels of communication that are transparent, commonly received, pervasive and everywhere available. Think of these as a kind of "open terrain", like the spaces that have been used for public speech in the television in its first half-century (or, like the streets, from time immemorial). In opposition, consider channels of communication that are reserved and private, encrypted and privileged, channels in which important discourse takes place, but which are not open to the public view.

In each society there is a balance between these two modes, a balance which influences the nature of control and the sense of access. The shift in the balance in the United States has occurred as a consequence of deregulation, but also as the new technology develops. In a number of sectors (television is only one) there is a privatizing of speech (not in the sense of being offered by commercial interests, but in the sense of being offered *privately*), a contraction of the public realm, and, with that, a change in patterns of discourse.

The move toward closure in the electronic media are especially important because they are part of a larger trend, a systematic transformation in the distribution and presentation of speech. Its full expression has not been realized, but the tendency is definitely away from the broadcast to the narrowcast channels, away from channels underwritten by advertising or government - and therefore seemingly free and open to offerings in which information is metered, the distribution is limited, and individuals pay for what they receive. There are benefits to this new approach, and it would be wrong to be Luddite in the face of technological enrichment. The pace that market forces are creating such new relationships between producers and consumers of information suggests that old assumptions about the structure of discourse and democracy are becoming obsolete.

Consider the transformation of newspapers as they are absorbed into the electronic era. Rather than the fixed text publicly available, the newspaper of the future will be highly customized, created for the individual, the group, the neighborhood. The charge for information will alter how information is used, how it is shaped, what is placed on the data base, what in fact is covered. The historic relationship to a space, defined by geography and political subdivision, will be further reduced. The shift to payment for individual programs on television will alter the structure of networks, change the mode of financing for new projects, alter the relationship among modes of distribution (such as broadcasting, video and theatrical exhibition of films). The main effect, however, regarding the common and open terrain of traditional broadcasting, is that it will tend to disappear. Increasingly, quality programming will migrate to the channels where viewer choice will be expressed through individual paid experience.

Great sports events, critically acclaimed films, and the highest quality news may all be delivered along the channels of the closed and privatized terrain. Consumer and other interest groups will find increasingly sophisticated techniques to control or affect the narratives of the open terrain, and the contraction of the open forum means these contestations will become even more bitter. In the United States, already, there have been political battles over access by the public to what were once thought to be commonly available goods, an aspect of citizenship entitlement.

There is another aspect of access: the scarcer the open terrain, the higher its value for the shaping of public views. If the ratio of openness to the closed alters, access to the open terrain may become even more complex. And the more difficult it is to reach consensus on what should be on the open channels - the more subject to negotiation and regulation that may be - the more rapid the inclination will be to the unregulated alternatives. A society that is fractured cannot easily tolerate a public space. These elements feed on themselves: technology and its industrial organization reduce the common narrative and reduced common narrative makes the remaining public space more contentious. The vanishing of public space is more acceptable precisely because there can no longer be adequate consensus on what its content should be.

Traditionally, the cry has been that the answer to offensive speech is not censorship but "more speech". But in the world of the closed terrain, more speech does not necessarily mean more public communication or the enriching of the public sphere. It may mean more stratification, more division and patterns of increased separation within the community. The attempt to define a proper role for government in relation to the architecture of the media has been clumsy enough in the era of broadcasting.

The idea that government should not intervene was based on the very notion that so much of speech would take place in the public setting of the mass media, or that the very function of the mass media was to expose and air, commonly, the issues of the day. The role of government alters direction as the transition to a technical system of particularity and narrowcasting, of interactivity and the information superhighway takes place. The very metaphor of twentieth century First Amendment analysis has been the "marketplace of ideas", a teaming forum for public discussion; and, given that marketplace, the issue for government has been the very limited one of intervening to correct extreme cases of market failure. But if the purported marketplace as a locus of public discussion is diminishing, a government role in reconstructing a public sphere becomes essential, setting rules so as to include an ideal of equality of access among potential speakers.

Technology, global politics and national claims all, then, have their impact on concepts of access, and concepts of access are used to affect national and transnational trends. Claims to access, as we have seen, are central to consideration of democratic values, in terms of the development of a public sphere and, in the very mechanics of the political process. Access claims transcend, however, concern with the "robust public debate". They are also aspects of defining meaning and representation within the state. They involve problems of self-determination, language survival, the protection and nourishment of diversity within a strengthened whole. Communicative freedoms - the right to receive and impart information are in need of cherishing in the emerging world as well as the restrictive world from which the transition takes place. Thinking about access, as we have explored in this volume, is a key way for those communicative freedoms to be defined.